The Multifaced Aspects of Atrial Flutter Interpreted by Precision Electrocardiology

Editors

GIUSEPPE BAGLIANI
FABIO M. LEONELLI
ROBERTO DE PONTI

CARDIAC ELECTROPHYSIOLOGY CLINICS

www.cardiacEP.theclinics.com

Consulting Editors
JORDAN M. PRUTKIN
EMILY P. ZEITLER

September 2022 • Volume 14 • Number 3

ELSEVIER

1600 John F. Kennedy Boulevard • Suite 1800 • Philadelphia, Pennsylvania, 19103-2899

http://www.theclinics.com

CARDIAC ELECTROPHYSIOLOGY CLINICS Volume 14, Number 3
September 2022 ISSN 1877-9182, ISBN-13: 978-0-323-91981-4

Editor: Joanna Collett
Developmental Editor: Hannah Almira Lopez

Cardiac Electrophysiology Clinics (ISSN 1877-9182) is published quarterly by Elsevier Inc., 360 Park Avenue South, New York, NY 10010-1710. Months of issue are March, June, September, and December. Subscription prices are $247.00 per year for US individuals, $525.00 per year for US institutions, $259.00 per year for Canadian individuals, $549.00 per year for Canadian institutions, $315.00 per year for international individuals, $549.00 per year for international institutions and $100.00 per year for US, Canadian and international students/residents. To receive student/resident rate, orders must be accompanied by name of affilliated institution, date of term, and the signature of program/residency coordinator on institution letterhead. Orders will be billed at individual rate until proof of status is received. Foreign air speed delivery is included in all Clinics subscription prices. All prices are subject to change without notice. **POST-MASTER:** Send address changes to Cardiac Electrophysiology Clinics, Elsevier Health Sciences Division, Subscription Customer Service, 3251 Riverport Lane, Maryland Heights, MO 63043. **Customer Service: 1-800-654-2452 (US and Canada). From outside of the US and Canada, call 314-477-8871. Fax: 314-447-8029. E-mail: JournalsCustomer-Service-usa@elsevier.com (for print support); JournalsOnlineSupport-usa@elsevier.com (for online support).**

Reprints. For copies of 100 or more of articles in this publication, please contact the Commercial Reprints Department, Elsevier Inc., 360 Park Avenue South, New York, NY 10010-1710. Tel.: 212-633-3874; Fax: 212-633-3820; E-mail: reprints@elsevier.com.

Cardiac Electrophysiology Clinics is covered in *MEDLINE/PubMed (Index Medicus)*.

Contributors

CONSULTING EDITORS

JORDAN M. PRUTKIN
Assistant Professor of Medicine, Division of Cardiology/Electrophysiology, UW Medical Center, Seattle, Washington, USA

EMILY P. ZEITLER
Cardiac Electrophysiology Assistant Professor of Medicine, Geisel School of Medicine, Assistant Professor of Health Care Policy, The Dartmouth Institute Dartmouth-Hitchcock Medical Center

EDITORS

GIUSEPPE BAGLIANI, MD, FAIAC
Cardiology and Arrhythmology Clinic, University Hospital "Ospedali Riuniti," Department of Biomedical Sciences and Public Health, Marche Polytechnic University, Via Conca, Ancona, Italy

FABIO M. LEONELLI, MD
Cardiology Department, James A. Haley Veterans' Hospital, University of South Florida

Morsani College of Medicine, Division of Cardiovascular Diseases, Tampa, Florida, USA

ROBERTO DE PONTI, MD, FHRS
Department of Heart and Vessels, Ospedale di Circolo - Department of Medicine and Surgery, University of Insubria, Viale Borri, Varese, Italy

AUTHORS

MARTINA AMADORI, MD
Department of Experimental, Diagnostic and Specialty Medicine, Institute of Cardiology, University of Bologna, IRCCS Policlinico S.Orsola-Malpighi, Bologna, Italy

FABIO ANGELI, MD
Department of Medicine and Surgery, University of Insubria, Department of Medicine and Cardiopulmonary Rehabilitation, Maugeri Care and Research Institutes, IRCCS, Tradate, Varese, Italy

GIUSEPPE BAGLIANI, MD, FAIAC
Cardiology and Arrhythmology Clinic, University Hospital "Ospedali Riuniti," Department of Biomedical Sciences and Public Health, Marche Polytechnic University, Via Conca, Ancona, Italy

FEDERICO BLASI, MD
Department of Heart and Vessels, Ospedale di Circolo, Department of Medicine and Surgery, University of Insubria, Varese, Italy

ALESSANDRO CAPESTRO, MD
Departments of Paediatric and Congenital Cardiac Surgery and Cardiology, University Hospital "Ospedali Riuniti," Ancona, Italy

MICHELA CASELLA, MD, PhD, FAIAC
Cardiology and Arrhythmology Clinic, University Hospital "Ospedali Riuniti," Department of Clinical, Special and Dental Sciences, Marche Polytechnic University, Ancona, Italy

CLAUDIO CAVALLINI, MD
Cardiovascular Disease Department - Arrhytmology, University of Perugia, Perugia, Italy

GIUSEPPE CILIBERTI, MD
Cardiology and Arrhythmology Clinic, University Hospital "Ospedali Riuniti," Department of Biomedical Sciences and Public Health, Marche Polytechnic University, Ancona, Italy

LAURA CIPOLLETTA, MD, PhD
Cardiology and Arrhythmology Clinic,
University Hospital "Ospedali Riuniti," Ancona,
Italy

PAOLO COMPAGNUCCI, MD
Cardiology and Arrhythmology Clinic,
University Hospital "Ospedali Riuniti,"
Department of Biomedical Sciences and Public
Health, Marche Polytechnic University,
Ancona, Italy

ROBERTO DE PONTI, MD, FHRS
Department of Heart and Vessels, Ospedale di
Circolo - Department of Medicine and Surgery,
University of Insubria, Viale Borri, Varese,
Italy

ANTONIO DELLO RUSSO, MD, PhD
Cardiology and Arrhythmology Clinic,
University Hospital "Ospedali Riuniti,"
Department of Biomedical Sciences and Public
Health, Marche Polytechnic University,
Ancona, Italy

IGOR DIEMBERGER, MD, PhD
Department of Experimental, Diagnostic and
Specialty Medicine, Institute of Cardiology,
University of Bologna, IRCCS Policlinico
S.Orsola-Malpighi, Bologna, Italy;
Pharmacologic Area of AIAC (Associazione
Italiana Aritmologia e Cardiostimolazione),
Rome, Italy

LORENZO ADRIANO DONI, MD
Department of Heart and Vessels, Ospedale di
Circolo - University of Insubria, Varese, Italy

FABRIZIO DRAGO, MD, FAIAC
Paediatric Cardiology and Cardiac Arrhythmias
Complex Unit, Department of Paediatric
Cardiology and Cardiac Surgery, Bambino
Gesù Children's Hospital and Research
Institute, Palidoro-Rome, Italy

MARCO FOGANTE, MD
Cardiology and Arrhythmology Clinic,
University Hospital "Ospedali Riuniti,"
Department of Clinical, Special and Dental
Sciences, Marche Polytechnic University,
Ancona, Italy

GEMMA GAGGIOTTI, MD
Department of Biomedical Sciences and Public
Health, Marche Polytechnic University,
Ancona, Italy

FEDERICO GUERRA, MD
Cardiology and Arrhythmology Clinic,
University Hospital "Ospedali Riuniti,"
Department of Biomedical Sciences and Public
Health, Marche Polytechnic University,
Ancona, Italy

S. YEN HO, FRCPath, FESC, FHEA
Emeritus Professor of Cardiac Morphology and
Consultant Cardiac Morphologist, Royal
Brompton Hospital, Imperial College London,
London, United Kingdom

MOHAMED KHAYATA, MD
University of South Florida Morsani College of
Medicine, Division of Cardiovascular Diseases,
Tampa, Florida, USA

FABIO M. LEONELLI, MD
Cardiology Department, James A. Haley
Veterans' Hospital, University of South Florida
Morsani College of Medicine, Division of
Cardiovascular Diseases, Tampa, Florida,
USA

JACOPO MARAZZATO, MD
Department of Heart and Vessels, Ospedale di
Circolo, Department of Medicine and Surgery,
University of Insubria, Varese, Italy

RAFFAELLA MARAZZI, MD
Department of Heart and Vessels, Ospedale di
Circolo - University of Insubria, Varese,
Italy

RAFFAELLA MARZULLO, MD
Department of Pediatric Cardiology, University
of Campania "Luigi Vanvitelli," Former Second
University of Naples, "Monaldi Hospital-AORN
Ospedale dei Colli," Naples, Italy

FRANCESCA MASSARA, MD
Cardiology and Arrhythmology Clinic,
University Hospital "Ospedali Riuniti," Ancona,
Italy

AGOSTINO MISIANI, MD
Cardiology and Arrhythmology Clinic,
University Hospital "Ospedali Riuniti," Ancona,
Italy

SILVANO MOLINI, MD
Cardiology and Arrhythmology Clinic,
University Hospital "Ospedali Riuniti," Ancona,
Italy

FRANCESCO NOTARISTEFANO, MD
Cardiovascular Disease Department -
Arrhytmology, University of Perugia, Perugia,
Italy

QUINTINO PARISI, MD, PhD
Cardiology and Arrhythmology Clinic,
University Hospital "Ospedali Riuniti," Ancona,
Italy

RITESH S. PATEL, MD
University of South Florida Morsani, College of
Medicine, Division of Cardiovascular Diseases,
Tampa, Florida, USA

ANTONIO RAPACCIUOLO, MD, PhD
Department of Advanced Biomedical Science,
University of Naples Federico II, Naples, Italy;
Pharmacologic Area of AIAC (Associazione
Italiana Aritmologia e Cardiostimolazione),
Rome, Italy

ANTONIO DELLO RUSSO, MD, PhD
Cardiology and Arrhythmology Clinic,
University Hospital "Ospedali Riuniti,"
Department of Biomedical Sciences and Public
Health, Marche Polytechnic University,
Ancona, Italy

ELLI SOURA, MD
Department of Paediatric and Congenital
Cardiac Surgery and Cardiology, University
Hospital "Ospedali Riuniti," Ancona,
Italy

PIETRO PAOLO TAMBORRINO, MD
Paediatric Cardiology and Cardiac Arrhythmias
Complex Unit, Department of Paediatric
Cardiology and Cardiac Surgery, Bambino
Gesù Children's Hospital and Research
Institute, Palidoro-Rome, Italy

PAOLO TOFONI, MD
Cardiology and Arrhythmology Clinic,
University Hospital "Ospedali Riuniti," Ancona,
Italy

YARI VALERI, MD
Cardiology and Arrhythmology Clinic,
University Hospital "Ospedali Riuniti,"
Department of Biomedical Sciences and Public
Health, Marche Polytechnic University,
Ancona, Italy

MANOLA VILOTTA, EP Tech
Department of Heart and Vessels, Ospedale di
Circolo, Varese, Italy

GIOVANNI VOLPATO, MD
Cardiology and Arrhythmology Clinic,
University Hospital "Ospedali Riuniti,"
Department of Biomedical Sciences and Public
Health, Marche Polytechnic University,
Ancona, Italy

GIANLUCA ZINGARINI, MD
Cardiovascular Disease Department -
Arrhytmology, University of Perugia, Perugia,
Italy

Contents

Atrial flutter (AFL) is a regular supraventricular reentrant tachycardia generating a continuous fluttering of the baseline electrocardiography (ECG) at a rate of 250 to 300 beats per minute. AFL is classified based on the involvement of the cavo-tricuspid isthmus in the circuit. The "isthmic" (or type 1) AFL develops entirely in the right atrium; this circuit is commonly activated in a counter-clockwise direction, generating the common sawtooth ECG morphology in the inferior leads (slow descendent–fast ascendent). AFL can be nonisthmus dependent (type 2), often presenting with faster atrial rate and most commonly a left atrial location.

This article reviews the structure of the atrial chambers to consider the anatomic bases for obstacles and barriers in atrial flutter. In particular, the complex myocardial arrangement and composition of the cavotricuspid isthmus could account for a slow zone of conduction. Prominent muscle bundles within the atria and interatrial, and myoarchitecture of the walls, could contribute to preferential conduction pathways. Alterations from tissue damage as part of aging, or from surgical interventions could lead to re-entry.

Atrial flutter (AFL) is a macro-reentrant arrhythmia characterized, in a 12 lead ECG, by the continuous oscillation of the isoelectric line in at least one lead. In the typical form of AFL, the oscillation is most obvious in the inferior leads, due to a macro-reentrant circuit localized in the right atrium, with the cavo-tricuspid isthmus as a critical zone.: This circuit can be activated in a counterclockwise or clockwise direction generating in II, III, and aVF leads, respectively, a slow descending/fast ascending F wave pattern (common form of typical AFL) or a balanced ascending/descending waveform (uncommon form of typical AFL). Atypical AFLs (scar-related) do not include the CTI in the circuit and show an extremely variable circuit location and ECG morphology.

Typical Atrial Flutter Mapping and Ablation   459

Francesco Notaristefano, Gianluca Zingarini, Claudio Cavallini, Giuseppe Bagliani, Roberto De Ponti, and Fabio M. Leonelli

Isthmus-dependent flutter represents a defeated arrhythmia. Possibly one of the most outstanding successes in terms of understanding the mechanism behind it has led to an effective, relatively simple, and safe targeted therapy. Technology, fulfilling a number of the clinical electrophysiologist's dreams, has linked diagnosis and therapy in computerized systems showing real-time imagines of the right atrium, the arrhythmia circuit, and the ablation target. The entire history of clinical electrophysiology is contained in its path and atrial flutter needs to be regarded with immense respect for a large amount of knowledge that its study always engenders.

Mapping and Ablation of Atypical Atrial Flutters   471

Jacopo Marazzato, Raffaella Marazzi, Lorenzo A. Doni, Fabio Angeli, Giuseppe Bagliani, Fabio M. Leonelli, and Roberto De Ponti

Atypical atrial flutters are complex, hard-to-manage atrial arrhythmias. Catheter ablation has progressively emerged as a successful treatment option with a remarkable role played by irrigated-tip catheters and 3D electroanatomic mapping systems. However, despite the improvement of these technologies, the ablation results may be still suboptimal due to the progressive atrial substrate modification occurring in diseased hearts. Hence, a patient-tailored approach is required to improve the long-term success rate in this scenario, aiming at achieving specific procedure end points and detecting any potential arrhythmogenic substrate in each patient.

Atypical Cases of Typical Atrial Flutter? A Case Study   483

Roberto De Ponti, Jacopo Marazzato, Fabio Angeli, Manola Vilotta, Federico Blasi, Giuseppe Bagliani, Fabio M. Leonelli, and Raffaella Marazzi

Ablation of typical atrial flutter has a high safety and efficacy profile, but hidden pitfalls may be encountered. In some cases, a longer cycle length with isoelectric lines is associated with a different or more complex arrhythmogenic substrate, which may be missed if conduction block of the cavotricuspid isthmus is performed in the absence of the clinical arrhythmia. Prior surgery may have consistently modified the atrial substrate and complex or multiple arrhythmias associated with an isthmus-dependent circuit can be encountered. In these cases, electroanatomic mapping is useful to guide the procedure and plan an appropriate ablation strategy.

Atrial Flutter in Pediatric Patients   495

Fabrizio Drago and Pietro Paolo Tamborrino

Atrial flutter (AFL) in pediatric patients is a rare condition as the physical dimensions of the immature heart are inadequate to support the arrhythmia. This low incidence makes it difficult for patients in this particular setting to be studied. AFL accounts for 30% of fetal tachyarrhythmias, 11% to 18% of neonatal tachyarrhythmias, and 8% of supraventricular tachyarrhythmias in children older than 1 year of age. Transesophageal overdrive pacing can be used, instead, with lower success rate (60%–70%). The recommended drugs are digoxin which can decrease the ventricular rate until the spontaneous interruption of the AFL. Digoxin can be combined with flecainide or amiodarone in case of failure.

The macroreentrant atrial tachycardia is very frequent in the adults with congenital heart disease. The impact of the arrhythmias on this type of patients is related to several factors: the anatomy and physiopathology of the specific congenital heart disease (CHD), the sequelae of the corrective surgery or surgical palliation, the presence of residual lesions (shunt, regurgitation), and the age and the clinical status of the patient and the comorbidities. In turn, the mechanism of the MAT depends on the peculiar features of the conduction's system in the CHD and native and acquired (post-surgery) substrates.

Despite being one of the best understood cardiac arrhythmias, the clinical meaning of atrial flutter varies according to the specific context, and its optimal treatment may be limited by both the suboptimal response to rate/rhythm control drugs and by the complexity of the underlying substrate. In this article, we present a state-of-the-art overview of mechanisms, prognostic impact, and medical/interventional management options for atrial flutter in several specific patient populations, including heart failure, cardiomyopathies, muscular dystrophies, posttransplant patients, patients with respiratory disorders, athletes, and subjects with preexcitation, aiming to stimulate further research in this challenging field and facilitate appropriate patient care.

In the present article, we will focus on the pharmacologic treatment of atrial flutter aimed either at restoring/maintaining sinus rhythm or controlling the ventricular response during tachyarrhythmia. To provide a comprehensive description we will start discussing the electroanatomic substrate underlying the development of atrial flutter and the complex relationship with atrial fibrillation. We will then describe the available drugs for the treatment of atrial flutter on the bases of their electrophysiological effects and data from available clinical studies. We will conclude by discussing the general principles of rhythm and rate control treatment during atrial flutter.

CARDIAC ELECTROPHYSIOLOGY CLINICS

Preface

Atrial Flutter and Precision Electrocardiology: An Indissoluble Symbiosis

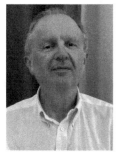

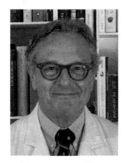

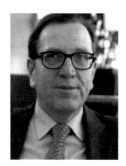

Giuseppe Bagliani, MD   Fabio M. Leonelli, MD   Roberto De Ponti, MD, FHRS

Editors

The peculiar anatomo-functional characteristics of the atria with their specificity and complexity may generate different sorts of supraventricular arrhythmias with different arrhythmogenic mechanisms. Enhanced automaticity may be responsible for both premature atrial beats and sustained focal atrial tachycardias. Focal electrical activity from the pulmonary veins combined with chaotic impulse conduction may generate atrial fibrillation with mechanisms yet to be defined in detail in specific clinical contexts. When, for different causes, a conduction delay occurs in the atria, this creates the arrhythmogenic substrate underlying a reentrant circuit.

As a consequence, macro-reentrant atrial tachycardias or flutters may become manifest, with the presence on the surface ECG of isoelectric lines between P waves or a continuously waving P-wave pattern to differentiate the former from the latter.

If, on one hand, surface ECG morphology is essential to guide the diagnosis of the typical forms of atrial flutter, usually relatively easy to ablate, then, on the other, the ECG pattern may be of limited value to clarify complex forms of atypical atrial flutter. In these atypical forms,

associated at times with complex postsurgical anatomy, accurate intracavitary mapping is needed to clarify the reentry course and identify the area critical for reentry in order to plan a rational and successful ablation strategy.

In reality, atrial flutter is a cardiac arrhythmia with a long history beginning many decades ago when served as a model to study atrial macro-reentry.

In fact, the term "atrial flutter" per se does not identify a single arrhythmia, and in clinical practice, it is commonly used to define organized atrial arrhythmias with variable atrioventricular conduction ratio. This generalization may create confusion, affecting this arrhythmia approach and treatment.

The last attempt to classify atrial flutters dates back a couple of decades ago, and the new generations of cardiologists may not be familiar with this classification, limiting their ability to distinguish different types of atrial flutters encountered in daily clinical practice.

Following our philosophy of precision electrocardiology, by reading the sequence of articles published in this issue, the readership will focus on how to discriminate the different forms of atrial flutter based on surface electrocardiogram and

Card Electrophysiol Clin 14 (2022) xiii–xiv
https://doi.org/10.1016/j.ccep.2022.07.005
1877-9182/22/© 2022 Published by Elsevier Inc.

intracavitary signals and to correctly approach these arrhythmias invasively by ablation.

Correct diagnosis and appropriate treatment in different patient populations are of the utmost importance, as this arrhythmia may have a strong impact on morbidity, especially in patients with severe structural heart disease.

Giuseppe Bagliani, MD
Cardiology and Arrhythmology Clinic
University Hospital "Ospedali Riuniti"
Ancona, Italy

Department of Biomedical Sciences and Public Health
Marche Polytechnic University
Ancona, Italy

Via Centrale Umbra 17
06038 Spello (Pg), Italy

Fabio M. Leonelli, MD
Cardiology Department
James A. Haley Veterans' Hospital
University of South Florida
13000 Bruce B Down Boulevard
Tampa, FL 33612, USA

Roberto De Ponti, MD, FHRS
Department of Heart and Vessels
Ospedale di Circolo

Department of Medicine and Surgery
Ospedale di Circolo
University of Insubria
Viale Borri, 57
21100 Varese, Italy

E-mail addresses:
giuseppe.bagliani@tim.it (G. Bagliani)
fabio.leonelli@va.gov (F.M. Leonelli)
roberto.deponti@uninsubria.it (R. De Ponti)

The History of Atrial Flutter Electrophysiology, from Entrainment to Ablation

A 100-Year Experience in the Precision Electrocardiology

Giuseppe Bagliani, MD, FAIAC[a,b],*, Roberto De Ponti, MD, FHRS[c,d],
Fabio M. Leonelli, MD[e,f], Michela Casella, MD, PhD, FAIAC[a,g],
Gemma Gaggiotti, MD[b], Giovanni Volpato, MD[a],
Paolo Compagnucci, MD[a,b], Antonio Dello Russo, MD, PhD[a,b]

KEYWORDS

- Typical atrial flutter • Atypical atrial flutter • Electroanatomic mapping • Catheter ablation
- Precision electrocardiology

KEY POINTS

- Atrial flutter (AFL) is a macro reentrant arrhythmia characterized by a continuous fluttering of the baseline of the electrocardiogram tracing. Waldo classified AFLs as isthmus (type 1) and nonisthmus (type 2) dependent.
- In the common isthmus-dependent AFL, the wavefront emerges from the cavotricuspid isthmus (CTI), travels posteriorly in a caudocranial direction ascending along the interatrial septum to the roof of the right atrium, and descends laterally toward inferior vena cava and CTI.
- The area between the inferior vena cava, tricuspid annulus, and coronary sinus is the zone of slow conduction of the macro reentrant circuit; the crista terminalis plays an essential role in creating a functional block.
- Entrainment of the flutter circuit by pacing is a fundamental maneuver able to identify the reentry as the basic mechanisms of the arrhythmia.
- Entrainment is a necessary step in the ablation procedure of type 1 AFL when the conventional approach is used to identify the CTI as the optimal site of ablation.
- Electroanatomic mapping techniques can now be used to reconstruct the reentrant path and identify ablation targets.
- After the development of AF ablation, new forms of AFL originating in the left atrium can be observed; these forms of type 2 AFL are, nowadays, among the most common arrhythmias in clinical practice.

[a] Cardiology and Arrhythmology Clinic, University Hospital "Ospedali Riuniti", Via Conca 71, Ancona 60126, Italy; [b] Department of Biomedical Sciences and Public Health, Marche Polytechnic University, Via Conca 71, Ancona 60126, Italy; [c] Department of Heart and Vessels, Ospedale di Circolo, Viale Borri, 57, Varese 21100, Italy; [d] Department of Medicine and Surgery, University of Insubria, Viale Guicciardini, 9, Varese 21100, Italy; [e] Cardiology Department, James A. Haley Veterans' Hospital, University of South Florida, 13000 Bruce B Down Boulevard, Tampa, FL 33612, USA; [f] University of South Florida, FL 4202 East Fowler Avenue, Tampa, FL 33620, USA; [g] Department of Clinical, Special and Dental Sciences, Marche Polytechnic University, Via Conca 71, Ancona 60126, Italy
* Corresponding author. via Centrale Umbra 17, 06038 SPELLO (PG), ITALY
E-mail address: giuseppe.bagliani@tim.it

Card Electrophysiol Clin 14 (2022) 357–373
https://doi.org/10.1016/j.ccep.2022.05.001

INTRODUCTION

By electrocardiographic (ECG) definition, atrial flutter (AFL) is an atrial tachycardia characterized by a continuous "fluttering" of the baseline: the isoelectric line is unidentifiable in at least a lead. The atrial activation is regular and at high frequency usually around 250 to 300 beats per minute (**Fig. 1**). AFL is caused by a reentry mechanism that, in the more common sawtooth morphology, develops entirely in the right atrium with a passive activation of the left atrium.[1]

Usually, not all the atrial depolarizations are conducted to the ventricles because of the filter effect of atrioventricular node (AVN) that prevents reaching an excessive ventricular frequency. The 2:1 atrioventricular conduction is very common in AFL, showing a rhythmic tachycardia with a frequency around 150 bpm with narrow complexes (in the absence of preexisting bundle branch block or an aberrant conduction). A flutter with an atrioventricular conduction 1:1 can be modulated by drugs increasing AV conduction to an accessory pathway.[2] A common mechanism that leads to the 1:1 flutter is the use of the 1C antiarrhythmic drug flecainide that can cause a vagolytic effect on the AVN with reduction of the refractory period.

A very common AV conduction in flutter is the 4:1. Often the 2:1 and the 4:1 can be present in the same ECG trace.

In the inferior leads, the F waves have a characteristic asymmetric "sawtooth" shape (slow descending–fast ascending) in the typical common flutter and a symmetric descending–ascending shape in the typical uncommon flutter. It is often stated that F waves are negative in the inferior leads, but, in reality, the waves are neither negative nor positive, as they represent a "continuum fluttering" in which it is not possible to identify an isoelectric line. Apart from the "sawtooth" pattern, there are also other morphology patterns

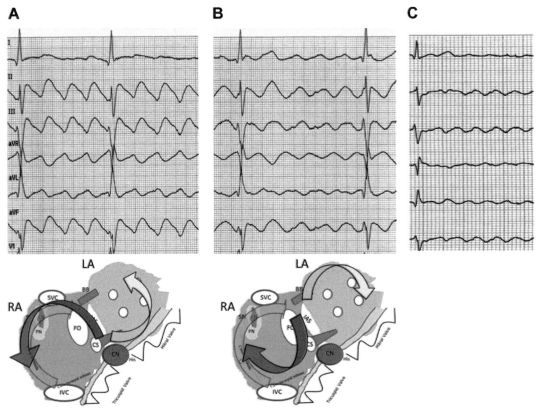

Fig. 1. Morphologic patterns of atrial flutter (AFL). (*A*) Typical AFL (isthmic) of common type: F waves with a sawtooth aspect (slow descending–fast ascending) in the inferior leads; the following cartoon highlights the electrogenetic circuit in the right atrium (*red arrow in a counterclockwise direction*). (*B*) Typical AFL (isthmic) of the uncommon type: F waves with symmetric appearance in the lower leads; the following cartoon highlights the electrogenetic circuit in the right atrium (*red arrow in a clockwise direction*). (*C*) Atypical AFL (nonisthmic): F waves with a faster rate and less delineated morphology. Several circuits not including the hollow tricuspid isthmus can give rise to the atypical form of AFL.

possible. Atrial reentry has constant atrial cycle length that correlates with the time necessary to travel the circuit instead of the cycle length variations that highly suggest automatic mechanism.[3]

When AFL is diagnosed, 4 strategies can be possible:

- Restore sinus rhythm administering an antiarrhythmic drug;
- Restore sinus rhythm by direct current (DC) cardioversion;
- Rapid atrial pacing by transesophageal or intracavitary approach (in patients with pacemaker or implantable cardioverter defibrillator); and
- Control the ventricular rate by a drug modulating the conduction in AVN.

THE HISTORY OF A FLUTTERING OF ATRIAL ACTIVITY ON THE SURFACE ELECTROCARDIOGRAM

The history of AFL begins more than a century ago, with the first mention of a rapid and regular excitation of the atria described in animal studies of McWills. Einthoven made one of the first ECG records of AFL in humans. The characteristic sawtooth waves in the inferior leads were first described in the works of Jolly and Ritchie. But it was Sir Thomas Lewis[4–6] who, in 1920, by comparing human and animal AFL, formulated an incredibly modern hypothesis regarding the electrogenesis of AFL. In his works he assumed that the right atrium was involved in a constant reentrant circuit using the vena cava and crista terminalis as a critical slow conduction zones. The hypothesis that there is a fully excitable gap between the head of the excitation wave and its tail of relative refractoriness, similar to Mines description in 1915, prevailed during the following decades. Allessie in the 70s[7] demonstrated that in the dog heart a reentry with a flutterlike activation can be obtained with rapid atrial pacing and shortening of the refractory period with acetylcholine infusion. This new observed form of atrial reentry was not dependent from a zone of slow conduction. This work showed the existence of a functional reentry circuit, in the absence of anatomic obstacles, determined exclusively by the refractory period of the atria. In this model, the wavefront travels in a circuitous route determined only by the nonuniform recovery of atrial excitability.[7,8]

The Allessie model of AFL was completely different from that described by Lewis: 2 reentry mechanisms in the atria, both able to induce a flutterlike activation of the atria and on the surface ECG.

Based on these fundamental observations the theory of reentry defines 2 types of reentries: (1) the anatomic or fixed and (2) the functional. Both types of reentry require tissue with different electrophysiologic properties favoring slow conduction and block of propagation and necessitate excitable myocardium ahead of its leading wavefront. In the anatomic form, anatomy or scar provides the milieu and determines the reentry pathway. This type of circuit shows a stability of dimensions and the presence of an excitable gap. This gap gives the capacity to an external impulse to enter the circuit, leading to the interruption of the arrhythmia or the resetting of it.

In the functional form, circuit does not have a stable anatomic location nor a constant length, as the zone of the circulating movement can vary in dimension in relation to the refractory period of the atria; no excitable Gap exists in the circuit, and for this reason this circuit cannot be interrupted or reset from an external impulse. The functional form of AFL, which can be expressed by the Allessie model can spontaneously evolve in atrial fibrillation, and in some cases, sinus rhythm can be restored following transient atrial fibrillation (**Fig. 2**).

THE WALDO CLASSIFICATION OF ATRIAL FLUTTER, A CORNERSTONE: THE CORRELATION BETWEEN ELECTROCARDIOGRAM AND ELECTROPHYSIOLOGY

In 1979 starting from the initial observations in postsurgical I AFL in which it was possible to interrupt AFL in some case but no in other, Waldo and Wells[9] made a distinction between type 1 (as previously described by Puech) and type 2 AFL.

The Waldo type 1 AFL (later named typical or isthmic) included the characteristics proposed by Lewis (anatomic determined circuit with an excitable gap); it was characterized by the following:

- An atrial frequency rate less than 340 bpm
- The susceptibility to interruption by atrial pacing

The type 1 also includes the following:

- A *common form* that shows the classic sawtooth morphology (slow descending–fast ascending) in inferior leads
- An *uncommon form* in which the descending and the ascending have a similar slope.

The Waldo type 2 AFL had similar characteristics to the experimental flutter of Allessie (a

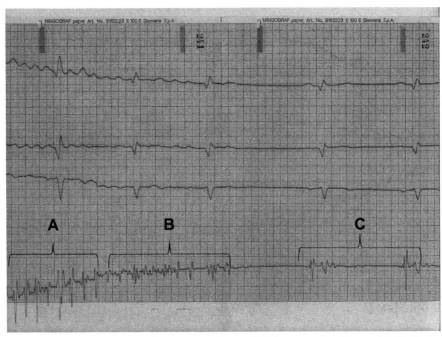

Fig. 2. Spontaneous evolution of atypical AFL. Atypical AFL (*A*) degenerating into atrial fibrillation (*B*); sinus rhythm spontaneously restores (*C*).

functional determined reentry mechanism) (see **Fig. 1**) and was characterized by the following:

- higher atrial rate (>340 bpm)
- impossibility of being stopped by atrial pacing.

Numerous subsequent clinical observations helped by improved technology changed the definition of type 2 flutter to any atrial reentrant arrythmia with a necessary isthmus different from the tricuspid valve inferior vena cava.

INTRACARDIAC RECORDINGS IN THE ELECTROPHYSIOLOGY MECHANISMS OF HUMAN ATRIAL FLUTTER

The AF analysis of the surface ECG tracings is a good method to study atrial activation at all and for the characterization of the typical flutter patterns, but it did not allow for the single analysis of each atrium or part of them: in the 70s the development of the endocavitary electrophysiologic recordings overcame the limits of the surface ECG. The conventional electrophysiologic studies included the recording and stimulation in specific points of the atria to determine the anatomic and electrophysiologic characteristics of the AFL circuit.

Intracardiac recordings (ICR) were obtained by advancing a recording catheter via femoral vein access to the right atrium, thus obtaining (**Fig. 3**)

a multipoint sequential recording. The activation sequences of the right atrium were reconstructed; the sequential activation of the left atrium was obtained by coronary sinus catheter and/or by transesophageal recording electrocatheters. By this sequential analysis of the right and left atrium, the common flutter included the following components (see **Fig. 3**):

- A circular counterclockwise activation of the right atrium
- A caudocranial activation of the left atrium proceeding from the coronary sinus

This study model also provided for the importance of the morphology of the recorded signals:

- Fragmented potentials[12] are the expression of slow conduction and are usually recorded in the isthmic zone or in the scar related zone (**Fig. 4**).
- Double potentials[10] are the expression of a reactivation of a site from 2 directions; they are found particularly along the crista terminalis that acts as a barrier between 2 wavefronts (**Fig. 5**).

By a wide use of ICR, from more than 30 years, it has become clear that the typical AFL (Waldo type 1) is due to a macro-reentry in the right atrium critically involving a zone of slow conduction in the cavo-tricuspid isthmus (CTI). In the common

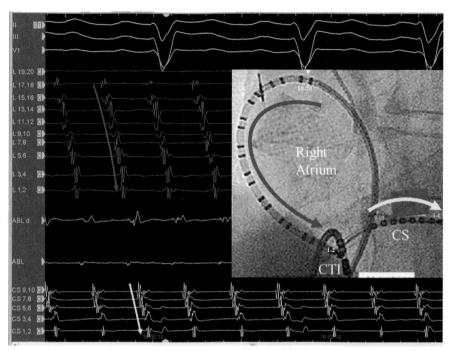

Fig. 3. Electrophysiologic study using endocavitary catheters (conventional approach) in the course of typical common AFL (isthmic, *counterclockwise*). Electrophysiologic study performed with 3 catheters: the first with 20 poles (*red arrow*) is placed from the cavotricuspid isthmus (poles 1–2) along the lateral wall and the roof [poles 19–20] of the right atrium. A second catheter is placed in the coronary sinus (*yellow arrow*). A third catheter in the lower center (scaler catheter) is placed next to the hollow tricuspid isthmus (CTI). The ECG traces from top to bottom show 3 surface leads and the recording made by the endocavitary catheters in green (D2, D3, V1). Red leads: recordings made by the catheter with 20 poles, which highlights an atrial activation (*red arrow*) from the upper part of the right atrium (poles 19–20) toward the lateral wall and then toward the hollow tricuspid isthmus (poles 1–2). White leads: obtained from ablating catheter placed in the CTI, show low voltage, fragmented atrial signals. Yellow leads: obtained from inside CS. Note how the activation front exiting the hollow tricuspid isthmus first activates the poles of the proximal coronary sinus[10,11] and then diffuses to activate the right atrium (*yellow arrow*).

form the front of the impulse wave emerges from the CTI, travels in a counterclockwise direction toward the septum and the roof, circles around the orifice of superior vena cava (SVC) and travels downward, and laterally, between the tricuspid valve and the crista terminalis, these structures tunnel back the wavefront into the CTI. The crista terminalis creates a functional transversal block, preventing an early short circuiting of the wavefront emerging from the isthmus.

In the more rare, uncommon form of typical AFL the impulse travels the same circuit but with a clockwise direction.[11]

Not always the CTI and the right atrium are included in a flutter circuit; in fact, in atypical flutters the impulse travels around an anatomic scar of a previous surgery (incisional flutter). In atypical flutter, so called nonisthmus dependent, the circular movement is confined by other anatomic structures.[13]

PACING THE ATRIA DURING ATRIAL FLUTTER: RESETTING, ENTRAINMENT, AND OVERDRIVE INTERRUPTION: A TRUE EXPERIENCE OF PRECISION ELECTROCARDIOLOGY

The observations in humans were initially made in animal models; these clinical studies were essentially based on conventional electrophysiologic maneuvers, which involved recording and stimulation in predetermined points of the atrium in order to determine the location and the electrophysiologic characteristics of the AFL circuit.

In type 1 AFL, the final demonstration of a reentry circuit with an excitable gap was obtained by overdrive atrial pacing and the so-called temporary entrainment (a temporary catching of the circuit) and interruption of AFL, as described originally by Waldo in 1977.[14]

The demonstration of the reentry mechanism is based on the ability of a premature atrial stimulus to penetrate in the circuit anticipating its basic

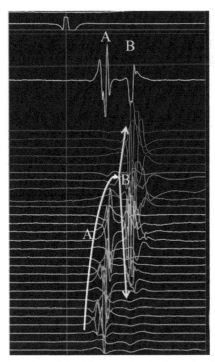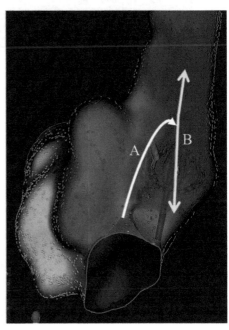

Fig. 4. Registration of double potentials in the area of the crista terminalis. Left cartoon: in the course of a typical common AFL, the electrical activity recorded along the terminal crest is highlighted; activation consists of a first series of potentials (*A*) and a second series of potentials (*B*). Right cartoon: the electroanatomical mapping of the area corresponding to the terminal crest highlights how the double series of potentials is an expression of the conductive block that occurs at the level of the terminal crest between its posterior portion (*A*) and anterior portion (*B*). The terminal crest is activated first by the activation edge A; this front then descends downward to activate the anterior region of the right atrium.

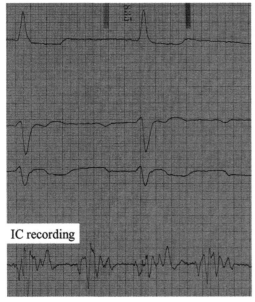

IC recording

Fig. 5. Record of fragmented electrical activity. Endocavitary recording (trace below carried out at the CTI level) highlights fragmented electrical activity consisting of long duration multiple potentials.

cycle (resetting phenomenon) (**Fig. 6**). Disertori in 1983 used this technique to localize the reentry in the right atrium.[15]

When a burst of stimuli (faster than the base cycle of AF) (n) continuously depolarize the circuit (continuous resetting), the so-called temporary entrainment is obtained. During AFL, the technique of "transient entrainment" is based on pacing the atria at a faster rate, accelerating the tachycardia at the same frequency of the pacing, causing a temporary capture of the circuit with rapid return to the previous tachycardia pattern with the interruption of the pacing (**Fig. 7**).

Fig. 8 shows that during entrainment an external stimulus (X) penetrates into the circuit propagating in 2 directions, the direction of the wavefront (orthodromic) and the opposite one (antidromic). In every paced beat (X), the orthodromic wavefront proceeds in the orthodromic direction continuing the tachycardia, whereas the antidromic front collides with the orthodromic wavefront of the previous beat (X-1), just its exit from the slow conduction zone. Waldo first defined 4 entrainment criteria, and, if at least one is verified, a reentry circuit with an excitable gap is

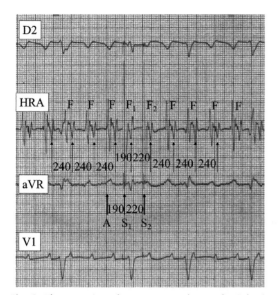

Fig. 6. The resetting phenomenon: electrophysiologic characterization of common flutter by the extra stimulus. During AFL of the common type (cycle equal to 240 ms), 2 stimuli (S1 and S2) are delivered in the upper right atrium (HRA) suitably synchronized on the spontaneous atrial depolarization of the arrhythmia (A-S1 = 190, S1-S2 = 220 ms). The 2 stimuli determine the "resetting," a global advance of the atrial flutter cycle (note how the circuit resumes with an F2-F coupling of 240 ms from the last induced atrial depolarization). The occurred "resetting" is able to establish that the arrhythmia is supported by a reentry circuit provided with an area in the excitability phase (excitable gap) through which the artificial stimulus has penetrated.

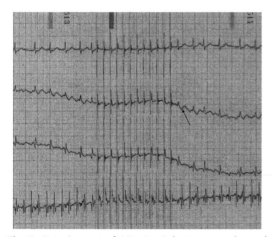

Fig. 7. Entrainment of AFL circuit by transesophageal atrial pacing during transesophageal atrial stimulation; the atrial activity is constantly induced by stimuli. When the stimulation is suspended, the arrhythmia always restarts from the last electroinduced beat that is of identical morphology to the basal flutter (*arrow*).

demonstrated.[14] The first 2 criteria are based on the variation of the morphology of the F wave during pacing, and the other 2 need a simultaneous recording in a location different from the stimulus source.

The entrainment concept starts from the idea that by pacing a zone of the circuit (usually the upper right atrium) opposite to the slow conduction, it is possible to depolarize the circuit from 2 fronts (see **Fig. 8**):

- Orthodromic front: that activates normally the slow conduction zone
- Antidromic front: opposite to the normal direction of the activation of the circuit.

In the classic entrainment, the antidromic wavefront of each impulse(x) is fused with the wavefront of the previous impulse that exits from the slow conduction zone(x-1); the final atrial activation is the result of the fusion of both wavefronts.

Waldo's criteria describe the paradigmatic electrophysiologic parameters of the classic entrainment. The first 2 criteria described by Waldo use observations derived from the surface ECG, whereas the third and fourth criteria require stimulation at a point and recording at a second point of the right atrium. Because of the complexity of the pacing/recording maneuver these last 2 criteria are seldom used in clinical practice. These are the essential content of the 4 criteria:

1. *First criterion*: a constant fusion of the atrial activation except the last impulse that is not fused (**Figs. 8** and **9**)

During the entrainment, the atrial activation seen on the ECG is the result of the fusion between the atrial activation by the paced impulse (positive in D2) and the morphology of the activation wave exiting from the slow conduction zone (negative in D2 as the basal flutter). The fusion cannot be possible for the last paced beat (x+1) that, exiting from the slow conduction zone, will not find any antidromic wavefront so it will not be fused. In see **Fig. 9** there is the demonstration of the first criterion.

2. *Second criterion*: progressive fusion (**Fig. 10**)

There is a progressive fusion that increases with the increase of the frequency of the pacing. In fact, with the increase of the frequency there is a progressive prevalence of the atrial part depolarized by the impulse (x) compared with the other one activated by the wavefront (x-1) coming out the slow conduction zone. In **Fig. 11**) there is the demonstration of the second criterion: pacing at upper right atrium, the morphology of atrial

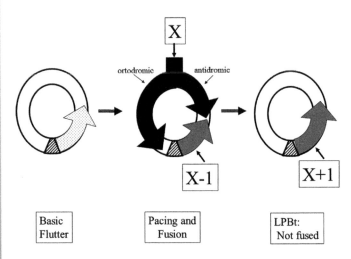

Fig. 8. Waldo's first criterion of the entrainment of the circuit of AFL: constant atrial fusion except for the last impulse (not fused). Stimulating a zone of the circuit opposite to the slow conduction zone, it is possible to depolarize the circuit from 2 fronts, the orthodromic and antidromic, in comparison to the direction of flutter activation. The front wave of each impulse (X-1) can depolarize in an orthodromic way the slow conduction being later fuse with the front wave of the following impulse (X). The last impulse (X+1) coming from the slow conduction zone will not find an antidromic impulse, and so it will not be fused having an atrial activation as the basal flutter.

complexes become more positive as the frequency of stimulation increases.

3. *Third criterion*: the demonstration that, during continuous pacing in a circuit site, the interruption of the AFL is associated, in a second site, with the block of local conduction for a beat followed by a local activation from a different direction (as evident from a change in the local recording morphology or a shorter conduction time.

4. *Fourth criterion*: for the demonstration of this criterion it is necessary, during AFL, to pace the atria in a site at 2 constant higher rates without interrupting the AFL; the demonstration of a change of activation in a second site (by the change of the atrial activation or a shorter conduction time) is the equivalent

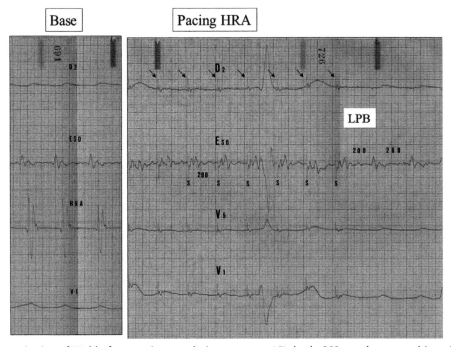

Fig. 9. First criterion of Waldo for entrainment during common AFL (cycle 260 msec): an overdrive stimulation (*arrows*) at high right atrium (HRA) level is delivered (pacing cycle length 200 msec); the transesophageal recording (Eso) shows a stable atrial capture. During the pacing, the lead D2 shows a fused atrial activity (mainly positive) except the last paced beat (LPB) that has the same cycle of stimulation (interval A-A = 200 msec) but a not fused morphology (atrial activation in D2 is the same as that of the basic flutter).

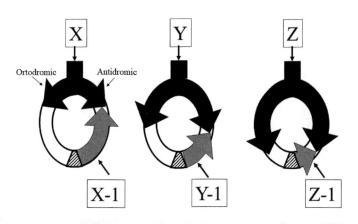

Fig. 10. Waldo's second criterion of entrainment of the flutter circuit: progressive fusion of atrial activation. Increasing the frequency of stimulation (X - > Y - > Z), there is an increase of the part of the atrial depolarization due to the induced stimulus in comparison to the one coming from the slow conduction zone (determined from the previous atrial stimulus).

of a progressive fusion into the entrained circuit.

Each one of the 4 criteria can demonstrate the entrainment of the flutter circuit; however, only the first and second criteria, derived from the analysis of the surface ECG, can be currently used. During EP Study, instead of the third and fourth criteria, the simpler analysis of postpacing interval (PPI) after entrainment can more easily identify the relationship between the circuit and the pacing site (Fig. 12). After successful entrainment, the PPI in the pacing site is the interval between the last stimulus and the next potential of the basic flutter. A PPI equal to or less than 30 msec than the basal FF interval indicates that the pacing site is within the reentrant circuit.[16,17]

Once entrainment of the circuit has been obtained, continuing pacing with minimal increments in stimulation frequency, it is possible to enter the slow conduction zone both orthodromically and antidromically: this is the condition that leads to

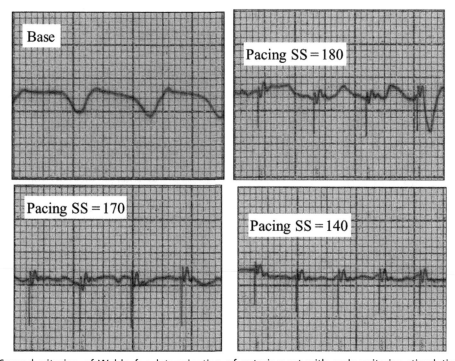

Fig. 11. Second criterion of Waldo for determination of entrainment with endocavitarian stimulation. Stimulating from the right atrium, the shortening of stimulation cycle (180 -> 170 -> 140 msec) is associated to induced atrial complexes, at the beginning (180) similar to basal flutter, then becoming more and more positive (140), as the frequency of stimulation increase.

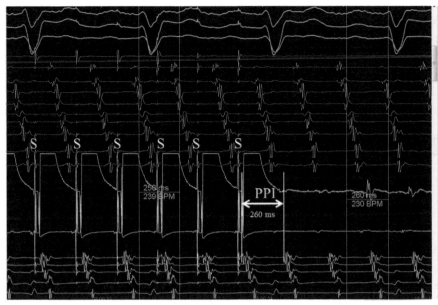

Fig. 12. Postpacing interval (PPI). During AFL with cycle 260 ms, there is a stimulation drive with cycle 250 ms in a zone near to the circuit. The PPI similar to the basal cycle of pacing demonstrates that the pacing site is within the circuit.

the interruption of the circuit (**Fig. 13**). Waldo first described the phenomenon identifying that, to interrupt AFL, should be reached a critical heart rate at which it is possible to entrain the circuit at a rate that is too fast for the flutter to reappear after end of the pacing.[15]

FURTHER INSIGHT IN THE CIRCUIT OF ATRIAL FLUTTER: THE WALDO'S CONCEPT OF CONCEALED ENTRAINMENT

Waldo noted that the second criterion of entrainment (progressive fusion) has an exception. It is

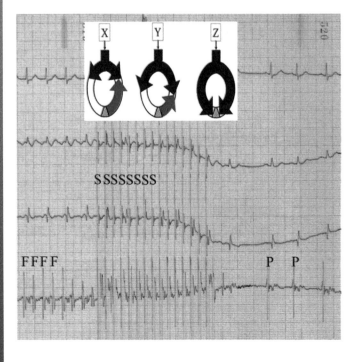

Fig. 13. Entrainment and interruption of common atrial flutter. During AFL (F), as shown from transesophageal registration, atrial stimuli are given (S) depolarizing in a stable way as the atria. Once obtaining the entrainment of the circuit it is possible to interrupt the flutter increasing the pacing frequency in order to enter in the slow conduction zone from both orthodromic and antidromic way: stopping the pacing, the flutter stops emerging a clear sinus rhythm (P wave).

possible to regularly depolarize the flutter's circuit without demonstrating a progressive degree of fusion (the atrial electrogram during pacing has the same morphology at any stimulation cycles **Fig. 14**). Waldo speculated that the so-called concealed entrainment occurs when the stimulus is delivered at a site facing the exit point of the slow conduction zone, for example, from the coronary sinus. In this case (**Fig. 15**), the slow conduction zone has a preferentially unidirectional conduction (due to functional block by the orthodromic front of the previous impulse). A functional block in the slow conduction prevents a fusion between different wavefronts, and therefore, on the ECG, the morphology of the induced atrial depolarization will remain constant at each stimulation rate (see **Fig. 15**). When the stimulation is suspended, the orthodromic wavefront of the last pulse delivered will be able to freely depolarize in an orthodromic way that slowed conduction zone perpetuating the circuit: the last electroinduced beat therefore emerges from the circuit after running through the flutter circuit in its entirety, and therefore, its PPI interval is usually longer than that of the stimulation rate and usually equal to the baseline cycle length. A concealed entrainment (no fusion in the surface ECG) was produced by pacing in the inferior CTI, suggesting that this is an area of slow conduction in which unidirectional

block of the antidromic paced wavefront probably occurs. These observations were consistent with the previous endocardial mapping studies in AFL, particularly with respect to the presence of an area of slow conduction in the low posteroseptal right atrium.[18]

CONCEALED ENTRAINMENT: THE BEGINNING OF ATRIAL FLUTTER ABLATION

The findings of concealed entrainment suggested that in type 1 AFL it is possible to identify the tricuspid isthmus as the critical area to sustain the reentry and a potential target for radiofrequency catheter ablation.[18] A delayed local activation can be detected by multiple endocardial recordings in this zone (see **Fig. 5**).

Also today, radiofrequency of Waldo type I AFL considers the CTI as the primary target for this arrythmia.[19]

For recurrent episodes of flutter, a transcatheter ablation of this critical isthmus is recommended. The technique involves electrophysiologic study of the atria during AFL to identify the location of the reentrant circuit and then to confirm that the reentrant circuit includes a critical isthmus between the inferior vena cava–Eustachian ridge–coronary sinus ostium and the tricuspid valve. When the latter is demonstrated, successful

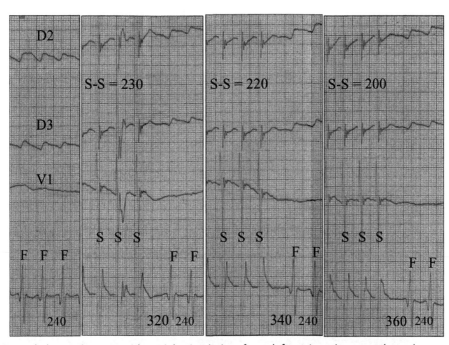

Fig. 14. Concealed entrainment with atrial stimulation from left atrium (transesophageal approach). The morphology of atrial-induced impulses given during flutter is identical to all cycle (230 -> 220 -> 200 msec). Stopping the pacing, the last electroinduced beat autoperpetrates the circuit of the flutter. See that the interval between the last induced beat and the first spontaneous depolarization is wider to the cycle of the flutter.

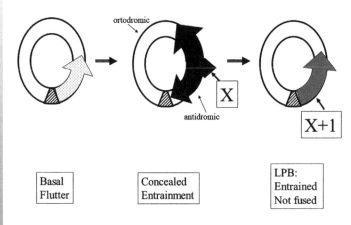

| Basal Flutter | Concealed Entrainment | LPB: Entrained Not fused |

Fig. 15. Schematic representation of concealed entrainment. It is possible to regularly depolarize the AFL circuit without demonstrating a progressive degree of fusion, that is, the electroinduced atriogram has the same morphology at all stimulation cycles. Occult entrainment occurs when, by stimulating from a site facing the slowed conduction zone, it is crossed in an antidromic direction without being able to merge with the subsequent electroinduced atrial beat. The morphology of the induced atrial depolarization will be the same at each pacing rate (see **Fig. 14**).

ablation during AFL will be followed by sinus rhythm (**Fig. 16**). The application of radiofrequency energy is able to produce a complete bidirectional conduction block in the CTI, demonstrating in the postradiofrequency ablation electrophysiology study (**Fig. 17**). The combined entrainment pacing maneuvers and mapping techniques (see next paragraph) have now evolved, allowing the reliable demonstration that the CTI is a fundamental part of the reentrant circuit.[19]

FROM WALDO TO OUR TIME—BEYOND CONVENTIONAL INTRA CAVITARY APPROACH: THE MAPPING TECHNIQUES

With the first endocavitary recordings, we began to understand the electrophysiologic mechanism of activation of the typical flutter and identify the CTI as a target for catheter ablation. The effectiveness of the ablation was identified by demonstrating the bidirectional block of the isthmus and was assessed by introducing a duodecapolar catheter along the tricuspid annulus and a decapolar catheter inside the coronary sinus.

In the last years, technology has led to the introduction of nonfluoroscopic mapping systems that helps and, in some cases, replaces the use of fluoroscopy.[20]

In the case of macro-reentrant arrhythmias such as AFL, the arrhythmia activation map has radically changed the ablation approach. The activation map represents by color code the temporality of the signals compared with reference points, which in the case of AFL, are the signals

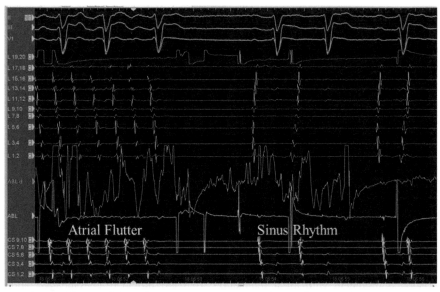

Fig. 16. Transcatheter ablation of the isthmic region: conventional recording. During AFL, energy and radiofrequency are delivered in the isthmic region: sinus rhythm restores (see **Fig. 17** for further electrophysiologic parameters).

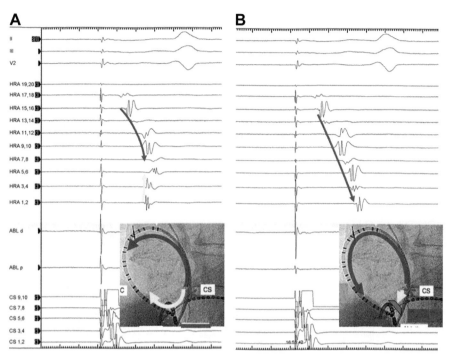

Fig. 17. Documentation of conduction at the level of the cavotricuspid isthmus (conventional approach) before and after radiofrequency delivery. In both (*A*) and (*B*) pacing (*S*) is delivered at level of coronary sinus (CS, *asterisk*). In side A, evaluation performed before ablation, the stimulus activates of the lateral wall of the right atrium from 2 fronts: an upper one (*red arrow*) coming from the terminal crest and a lower one (*yellow arrow*) coming from CTI. Figure B highlights the same situation after radiofrequency delivery in the region of the CTI: the activation of the lateral wall of the right atrium occurs exclusively from the upper and lateral region (*red arrow*); the activation from the ICT has disappeared due to the complete blockage of conduction.

recorded by a proximal dipole of the decapolar catheter inside the coronary sinus. With a detailed use of cardiac mapping, a precision correlation between ECG and the sequence of cardiac activation can be determined (**Fig. 18**).

The mapping system helps in the diagnosis of atypical flutter in which an activation pattern mimics the typical flutter and in the case of double loops around the vena cava, helps identify a mechanism that can significantly increase the degree of complexity of the ablation. Therefore, next to this additional diagnostic role, mapping systems are especially useful in the case of noninterruption of the typical flutter after radiofrequency delivery.

The lesion localization system (tag) allows the identification of the gaps in the block line (**Fig. 19**). Furthermore, velocity maps have also been created recently, showing that, during the creation of the activation map, the conduction velocities of the impulse at specific points are represented as arrows of different length and thickness (**Fig. 20**). The arrows of greater thickness and shorter length represent areas in which there is a deceleration in the conduction velocity: in these points the delivery of radiofrequency can more

likely cause the interruption of the arrhythmia and create the block line.[21]

Another fundamental aspect and important criteria for the electrophysiologist to consider is the effectiveness of the lesion performed over time. The elimination of the acute potential does not predict the durability of the lesion in the days or weeks following ablation. In recent years, therefore, catheters with contact force sensors have become widespread, which, in addition to increasing the safety of the procedure, have made it possible to create lesion indices, an "adimensional" parameter that integrates contact force, power, and delivery time into a single weighted formula. Numerous studies have demonstrated the validity of lesion indices in predicting the durability of acute lesions over time.[22]

ARE THE ELECTROPHYSIOLOGY OF ATRIAL FLUTTER CHANGING AFTER ATRIAL FLUTTER ABLATION?

In 1998 Haïssaguerre and colleagues identified ectopic foci within the pulmonary veins as a mechanism for initiating atrial fibrillation. Since then,

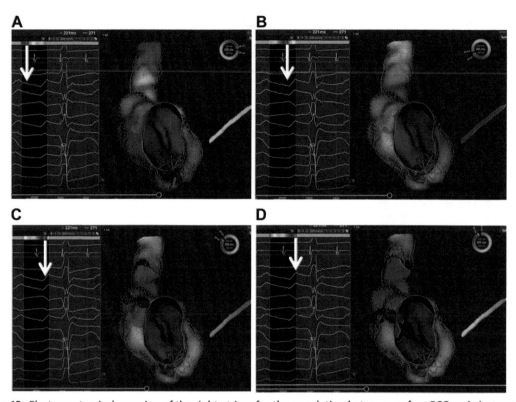

Fig. 18. Electroanatomical mapping of the right atrium for the correlation between surface ECG and electrogenesis of common isthmic AFL. The 4 panels identify and define 4 phases of the surface ECG: (*A*) the activation of the CTI: corresponding on the surface ECG (*arrow*) to the slow descending phase; (*B*) the wave front exits the isthmic area to activate the medial posterior wall of the right atrium and the left atrium through the coronary sinus: this corresponds to the rapid descending phase that follows the characteristic "notch"; (*C*) activation of the atrial roof and initiation of craniocaudal activation of the anterior wall of the right atrium: corresponds to the fast ascending component of the F wave; (*D*) activation of the lateral wall of the right atrium up to the inferior cavity: it corresponds to the positive phase of lead V1 and to the terminal positive component of D2.

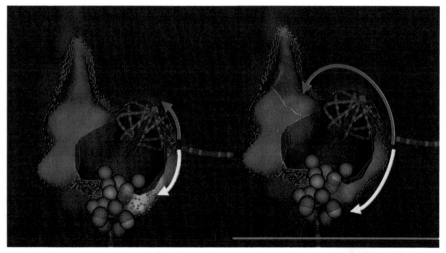

Fig. 19. Electroanatomical mapping of the isthmic conduction block after radiofrequency application. The stimulation delivered in the coronary sinus region proceeds both toward the hollow-tricuspid isthmus, stopping at this level (*yellow arrow*), and upward, proceeding regularly toward the terminal ridge.

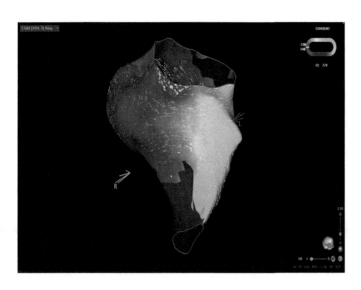

Fig. 20. Study of the local conduction velocity by means of electroanatomical mapping. At the level of the CTI, the activation front is represented by a series of micro-vectors whose length is proportional to the local conduction speed. A zone of slower conduction is clearly evident (*arrow*).

catheter ablation with electrical isolation of the pulmonary veins as a therapy for paroxysmal atrial fibrillation has become more widespread. Regarding the treatment of persistent atrial fibrillation, isolation of the pulmonary veins alone was less effective. Therefore, the ablation of other structures has become common, including the electrical isolation of the posterior wall of the left atrium; this is a structure embryologically similar to the pulmonary veins, the left atrial appendage, and the coronary sinus. The creation of ablation lines and lesions along these structures has led to the formation of physiologic macro-reentrant circuits that cause nonisthmus-dependent AFL

(**Fig. 21**). Clinically, the onset of these AFLs involves the presence of more severe symptoms than atrial fibrillation alone, often difficult to control with drug therapy. These flutters have variable cycles depending on the length of the reentry circuit and the impulse conduction velocity, which is often slowed due to areas of fibrosis.[23] The ablation of atypical AFLs is often complicated by difficulties in understanding the reentry circuit decreasing successful ablation rates.[24] These modifications of the atrial electrophysiology introduce several unquantifiable changes of the activation wave front and render the ECG interpretation of scar-related arrhythmias extremely complex.[25]

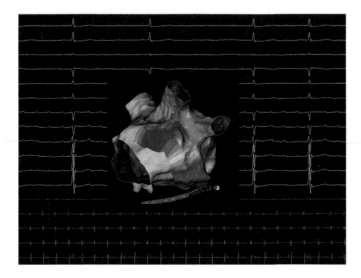

Fig. 21. Atypical atrial flutter. The surface ECG shows tachycardic atrial activities, positive in V1 (*arrows*) separated by an isoelectric line. This pattern points toward an atrial tachycardia; contrary to this, the atrial activation mapping shows an atypical AFL with a rotating reentry circuit at the level of the left upper pulmonary vein (site of previous ablation).

SUMMARY

The electrophysiologic approach proposed by Waldo (isthmus- and nonisthmus-dependent AFL) remains the best classification of AFL.

In most of the cases of isthmus-dependent flutters, the wavefront of the impulse emerges from the CTI, into a zone of slow conduction between the tricuspid annulus and coronary sinus and travels in a caudocranial direction ascending along the interatrial septum, spreading to depolarize the posterior right atrium.

This wavefront continues across the roof of the right atrium, circles around the orifice of SVC, and proceeds downward and laterally between the tricuspid valve and crista terminalis, which creates a functional block.

These structures tunnel the wavefront into the isthmus between the tricuspid annulus and inferior vena cava, then out again to the zone of slow conduction.

The crista terminalis plays a pivotal role for the development of the circuit. The myocardial cells of crista terminalis exhibit anisotropic conduction due to their transverse orientation, creating a functional transversal block. This block prevents an early activation of the anterior wall from the inferoposterior wavefront, forcing the wavefront superiorly toward the superior vena cava.

Entrainment of the flutter circuit is a time-honored, fundamental pacing maneuver proving reentry as its mechanism. It is therefore being able to differentiate among the diverse arrhythmias identifying their mechanism. Concealed entrainment, observed within the reentrant circuit, has been the starting point for ablation of AFL.

CLINICS CARE POINTS

- The circuit of Atrial Flutter can be regularly depolarized and by atrial stimuli (Entrainment).
- Pacing at critical rates can stop the atrial flutter circuit.
- In-depth knowledge of the atrial flutter circuit has allowed us to treat atrial flutter by catheter ablation.

DISCLOSURE

R.D. Ponti has received fees for lectures and scientific cooperation from Biosense Webster. A.D. Russo is a consultant for Abbott. M.C. has received fees for lectures from Biosense Webster and Abbott. All other authors declared no conflict of interest.

REFERENCES

1. Saoudi N, Cosio F, Waldo A, et al. A classification of atrial flutter and regular atrial tachycardia according to electrophysiological mechanisms and anatomical bases; a statement from a joint expert group from the working group of arrhythmias of the European society of cardiology and the north American society of pacing and electrophysiology. Eur Heart J 2001; 22:1162–82.
2. Marks J. Atrial flutter with 1:1 AV conduction. Arch Intern Med 1959;100:989–93.
3. Leonelli F, Bagliani G, Boriani G, et al. Arrhythmias originating in the atria. Card Electrophysiol Clin 2017;9(3):383–409.
4. Lewis T, Feil HS, Stroud WD. Observations upon flutter, fibrillation. Part II. The nature of auricular flutter. Part III: some effects of rhythmic stimulation of the auricle. Heart 1920;7.
5. Mines GR. On circulating excitations in heart muscle and their possible relation to tachycardia and fibrillation. Trans R Soc Can 1914;43–52.
6. Mines G. On dynamic equilibrium of the heart. J Physiol 1913;46:349–82.
7. Allessie MA, Lammers WJEP, Bonke FIM, et al. Intraatrial reentry as a mechanism for atrial flutter induced by acetylcholine and rapid pacing in the dog. Circulation 1984;70:123–35.
8. Allessie MA, Bonke FI, Schopman FJ. Circus movement in rabbit atrial muscle as a mechanism of tachycardia. III. The "leading circle" concept: a new model of circus movement in cardiac tissue without the involvement of an anatomical obstacle. Circ Res 1977;41(1):9–18.
9. Waldo AL. Mechanisms of atrial fibrillation, atrial flutter, and ectopic atrial tachycardia—a brief review. Circulation 1987;75:III37–40.
10. Feld GK, Shahandeh-Rad F. Mechanism of double potentials recorded during sustained atrial flutter in the canine right atrial crush-injury model. Circulation 1992;86:628–41.
11. Chan DP, Van Hare GF, Mackall JA, et al. Importance of atrial flutter isthmus in postoperative intra-atrial reentrant tachycardia. Circulation 2000;102:1283–9.
12. Cosio FG, Arribas F, Palacios J, et al. Fragmented electrograms and continuous electrical activity in atrial flutter. Am J Cardiol 1986;57:1309–14.
13. Wells JL, MacLean WAH, James TN, et al. Characterization of atrial flutter: studies in man after open heart surgery using fixed atrial electrodes. Circulation 1979;60:665–73.
14. Waldo AL, MacLean WA, Karp RB, et al. Entrainment and interruption of atrial flutter with atrial pacing:

studies in man following open heart surgery. Circulation 1977;56:737–45.

15. Disertori M, Inama G, Vergara G, et al. Evidence of a reentry circuit in the common type of atrial flutter in man. Circulation 1983;67:434–40.

16. Takahiko K, Shingo S, Masaomi K .Long Postpacing Interval After Entrainment of Tachycardia Including a Slow Conduction Zone Within the Circuit. J Cardiovasc Electrophysiol, Vol. pp. 1-7.

17. Kalman JM, Olgin JE, Saxon LA, et al. Activation and entrainment mapping defines the tricuspid annulus as the anterior barrier in typical atrial flutter. Circulation 1996;94:398–406.

18. Nakagawa H, Lazzara R, Khastgir T, et al. Role of the tricuspid annulus and the eustachian valve/ridge on atrial flutter. Relevance to catheter ablation of the septal isthmus and a new technique for rapid identification of ablation success. Circulation 1996;94: 407–24.

19. Calkins H, Leon AR, Deam AG, et al. Catheter ablation of atrial flutter using radiofrequency energy. Am J Cardiol 1994;73:353–6.

20. Willems S, Weiss C, Ventura R, et al. Catheter ablation of atrial flutter guided by electroanatomic mapping (CARTO): a randomized comparison to the conventional approach. J Cardiovasc Electrophysiol 2000;11:1223–30.

21. Mangat I, Tschopp DR Jr, Yang Y, et al. Optimizing the detection of bidirectional block across the flutter isthmus for patients with typical isthmus-dependent atrial flutter. Am J Cardiol 2003;91:559–64.

22. Natale A, Newby KH, Pisano E, et al. Prospective randomized comparison of antiarrhythmic therapy versus first-line radiofrequency ablation in patients with atrial flutter. J Am Coll Cardiol 2000;35: 1898–904.

23. Villacastin J, Perez-Castellano N, Moreno J, et al. Left atrial flutter after radiofrequency catheter ablation of focal atrial fibrillation. J Cardiovasc Electrophysiol 2003;14:417–21.

24. De Ponti R, Verlato R, Bertaglia E, et al. Treatment of macro-re-entrant atrial tachycardia based on electroanatomic mapping: identification and ablation of the mid-diastolic isthmus. Europace 2007;9:449–57.

25. Oral H, Knight BP, Morady F. Left atrial flutter after segmental ostial radiofrequency catheter ablation for pulmonary vein isolation. Pacing Clin Electrophysiol 2003;26:1417–9.

Normal and Abnormal Atrial Anatomy Relevant to Atrial Flutters

Areas of Physiological and Acquired Conduction Blocks and Delays Predisposing to Re-entry

S. Yen Ho, FRCPath, FESC, FHEA

KEYWORDS

- Bachmann's bundle • Cavotricuspid isthmus • Mitral isthmus • Myoarchitecture • Right atrium
- Vestibule

KEY POINTS

- Structure of the atria provides bases for obstacles and barriers to conduction.
- Tissue composition of the cavotricuspid isthmus is variable and complex.
- Myoarchitecture of the atria including interatrial connections is an integral part of atrial structure.
- Acquired aging changes and surgical interventions alter the arrangement of atrial structures.

INTRODUCTION

Atrial flutter was first described over a century ago, but it is only with developments in invasive electrophysiology that the mechanism of arrhythmia is better understood. It is recognized as a macro-reentrant tachycardia that rotates around an obstacle, nominally of several centimeters,[1,2] and it requires anatomic or functional barriers to maintain its rotation.[3]

It can occur in patients with or without previous surgery on or in the atria. Typically, it is in the right atrium involving the cavotricuspid isthmus. It can also occur in the left atrium, for example, after surgical incision or ablation for atrial fibrillation (AF). Typical right atrial flutter following left atrial ablation of AF has also been reported.[4] Clearly, atrial flutter has many clinical variants beyond the scope of a review on anatomy.[5]

This article aims to look at the anatomic structures in the normal and 'abnormal' atria focusing on the structures that could act as obstacles and barriers. To put simply, the atria are like two abutting bags joined at the septum. The bags are punctured with large holes of the tricuspid and mitral orifices and smaller holes by the insertions of the great veins that form the obstacles. The remaining walls comprising primarily of atrial myocardium account for some of the anatomic or functional barriers. Injury to the wall such as following surgery and other invasive procedures add to the normally occurring obstacles.

RIGHT ATRIUM

Generally, the right atrium is perceived as having a large appendage forming much of the anterosuperior and lateral walls. Its venous component receiving the orifices of the caval veins lies posterior to the appendage. Slightly cephalad and medial to the orifice of the inferior caval vein (ICV) is the orifice of the coronary sinus More medially is the wall that separates the right atrium from the left atrial chamber. The vestibule leads to the tricuspid orifice that is nearly vertical at an angle of about 45° to the sagittal plane.

Royal Brompton Hospital, Imperial College London, Sydney Street, London SW3 6NP, United Kingdom
E-mail address: yen.ho@imperial.ac.uk

Card Electrophysiol Clin 14 (2022) 375–384
https://doi.org/10.1016/j.ccep.2022.03.001
1877-9182/22/© 2022 Elsevier Inc. All rights reserved.

Guarding the anterior margin of the orifice of the ICV is the Eustachian valve that is usually a thin fibromuscular flap of variable height (**Fig. 1**). Extending medially from its free margin passing through the atrial wall toward the septum is the tendon of Todaro, a thin fibrous strand that is the posterior border of the triangle of Koch. This part of the atrial wall, described as the Eustachian ridge, can be more prominent in some hearts than others. The myocardium of the ridge continues into the septal musculature that forms the inferior and anterior rim of the oval fossa (see **Fig. 1**).

Cavotricuspid Isthmus

This isthmus comprising the atrial wall lies between the anterior part of the orifice of the ICV, Eustachian ridge, and the hingeline (annulus) of the tricuspid valve. Nearly quadrilateral in shape, but by no means flat, it is narrower toward the septum and broader laterally. Drawing linearly from the anteriorly situated tricuspid hingeline backward to the Eustachian valve, three isthmus lines may be described (**Fig. 2**).

The shortest and septal-most isthmus is the paraseptal isthmus (also dubbed the septal isthmus) that lies between the orifice of the coronary sinus and the tricuspid orifice. It lies at 4–5 o'clock position on the left anterior oblique (LAO) projection (see **Fig. 2**). Comprising only the vestibule, the endocardial surface here is usually smooth, and its wall is the thickest of the three isthmuses. It contains transitional cells that feed into the compact atrioventricular node and may also contain the inferior extensions of the compact node that are the targets for slow pathway ablation.

The central isthmus is sited most inferiorly, at 6 o'clock when viewed from the LAO perspective. Lying between the anterior border of the orifice of the ICV and the tricuspid valve (see **Fig. 2**; **Fig. 3**). It is recognized as a site of slow conduction.[6] Indeed, it has a complex myoarchitecture that varies considerably from heart to heart (see below).[7] This isthmus is ablated in most cases of typical flutter.

The composition of the atrial wall and its thickness varies along the length of the cavotricuspid isthmus (see **Fig. 3**; **Fig. 4**). Anteriorly, the portion nearest the tricuspid orifice is the vestibular wall. This part is smooth on its endocardial surface and is more closely related epicardially to the distal course of the right coronary artery than the paraseptal isthmus.[7] In its midportion, the wall is composed of pectinate muscle separated by variable areas of thin fibrous tissue or a mix of slender

criss-crossing muscle bundles from the terminal ramifications of the terminal crest (see **Fig. 4**; **Fig. 5**).[8] Posteriorly, toward the Eustachian valve/ridge, the isthmus wall is thinner in the most hearts, comprising slender muscle bundles sometimes separated by thin fibrous membranes especially in the posterior region. In others, this part may include the thicker muscle of the Eustachian ridge. In about 10%–47% of individuals the wall has a recess named the sub-Eustachian pouch that may cause difficulty in achieving a complete ablation line or may cause chest pain from the impact on epicardial autonomic gangli and nerves.[7,9]

To avoid the pouch, an inferolateral isthmus line may be used (see **Fig. 2**). Compared with the inferior isthmus, this isthmus is longer and has slightly thicker pectinate muscles in its middle and posterior portions. Its anterior portion remains the smooth vestibule. The distal right coronary artery passing epicardially is nearest here.

The complex architecture of the cavotricuspid isthmus lends credence to the concept of a slow zone of conduction. Waki and colleagues described a basic arrangement of the muscle bundles (trabeculae) that extend from the terminal crest. Part of the bundles extends anteriorly toward the tricuspid orifice, whereas a part passes superiorly, in parallel to the valve annulus, toward the coronary sinus orifice where they fanned out (see **Fig. 2**). In 50 heart specimens, they found 26% with a uniform trabecular pattern. In this group, there were few with almost parallel trabeculae without gaps in between. The majority lacked muscle, especially toward the ICV orifice. The nonuniform pattern (74%) was characterized by crossovers and interlacing of muscle bundles, especially in the area immediately inferior to the coronary sinus orifice.

Accordingly, this slow zone can be attributed to the nonuniform muscular content and muscular thicknesses. Considering that conduction velocity through myocytes is slower sideways than along the lengths of the myocytes,[10,11] the complex arrangement of myocardial strands interspersed with fibrous membranes supports this.

Right Atrial Myoarchitecture

Apart from a slow zone, the flutter circuit traverses over areas of the right atrium surrounding the tricuspid valve orifice. The most anterior part, immediately proximal to the orifice, is the vestibule that appears as a smooth wall with pectinate muscles inserted into it on the parietal part of the orifice. On the septal part, the vestibule blends into the myofibers at the end of the terminal crest

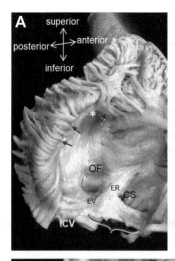
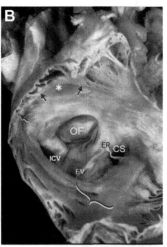
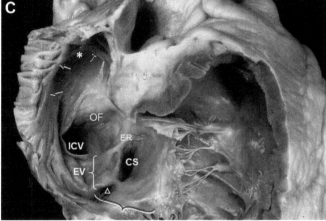

Fig. 1. Parietal wall of right atrium opened and deflected posteriorly to show the septal (medial) origin of terminal crest and its course (*blue arrows*) anterior to the orifice (*asterisk*) of the superior caval vein before descending in a postero-inferior arch toward the orifice of the inferior caval vein (ICV). Pectinate muscles extend from one side of the crest to line the membrane like wall of the appendage. The Eustachian valve (EV) and ridge (ER) vary in sizes and prominence. EV is flimsy and membrane like in panels *A* and *B* compared with *C*. The brace indicates the region of the cavotricuspid isthmus. CS, coronary sinus orifice; OF, floor of the oval fossa; triangle, pouch-like depression.

around the orifice of the coronary sinus, the Eustachian ridge and the anterior part of the muscular rim surrounding the floor of the oval fossa (see **Fig. 5**). From here, myocardial strands turn to a more inferior-superior direction toward the medial origin of the terminal crest and curve posteriorly following the rim around the fossa. The thin fossa floor comprising fibrous tissue and bilaminar crossing arrangement of myocytes[12] different from the rim could itself be an obstacle to the flutter circuit (see **Fig. 5**).

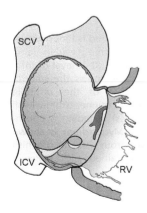
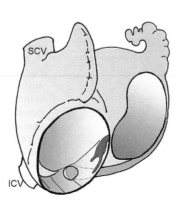

Fig. 2. Diagrams depicting the location of three isthmus (*red*) lines in the cavotricuspid isthmus as viewed from approximately right lateral perspective (*left hand panel*) and left anterior oblique perspective (*right hand panel*). The middle line is the inferior or central isthmus. ICV, inferior caval vein; RV, right ventricle; SCV, superior caval vein; blue circle, orifice of coronary sinus; red shape, atrioventricular node.

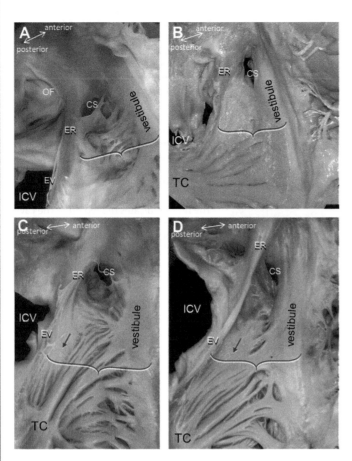

Fig. 3. Views of the endocardial surface of the inferior cavotricuspid isthmus region (brace) in four hearts (*A-D*) to show variations in terminal ramifications of the terminal crest (TC) as the muscle bundles approach the orifice of the coronary sinus (CS) to pass toward the vestibule and the Eustachian ridge (ER). Short arrows indicate areas of thin wall. EV, Eustachian valve; ICV, orifice of inferior caval vein.

On the endocardial aspect, the alignment of the myocardial strands in the vestibule seen on gross dissections tends to be circumferential or oblique relative to the plane of the tricuspid orifice.[13] Epicardially, the vestibule has a circumferential bundle that is from the right anterior crest (of Papez),[14] a rightward extension from the interatrial (Bachmann's) bundle that diverges to pass anterior to the triangular tip of the atrial appendage (**Fig. 6**).

Proximal (atrial) to the parietal vestibule is the array of pectinate muscle bundles that connects with the terminal crest (crista terminalis) posteriorly. Pectinate muscles are of varied sizes and arranged in a parallel fashion; they branch and interconnect or fan out near the vestibule or crest into further smaller bundles that connect with each other. The appendage wall between the bundles is paper thin, comprising epicardium and

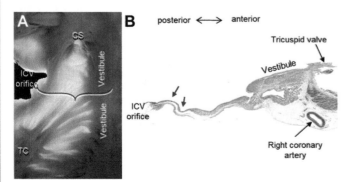

Fig. 4. The cavotricuspid isthmus transilluminated to show thin areas in panel *A*. Histologic section (*B*) at level of inferior isthmus (*brace*) shows the smooth endocardial surface of the vestibule compared with the thinner isthmus wall posteriorly (*arrows*) including a pouch-like depression. Myocardium is shown as reddish and fibrous tissue as greenish on this section stained with Masson's trichrome.

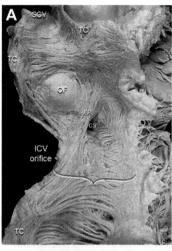

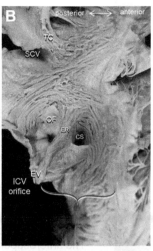

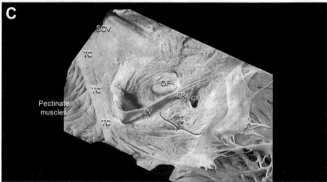

Fig. 5. Dissections of three hearts (*A-C*) of the gross myoarchitecture in the cavotricuspid area and toward the septum to the terminal crest (TC) and in the muscular rim around the oval fossa (OF). Myoarchitecture in the isthmus is complex. Note the strand-like tendon of Todaro in the Eustachian ridge on panel C. The terminal crest in this heart is rather flat, without a distinct margin at its border with the posterior (intercaval) wall. Abbreviations as in **Fig. 1**.

endocardium with scant myocardium in between (see **Fig. 1**).[15]

The terminal crest separates the pectinated lining of the appendage from the smooth wall of the venous sinus. It arises medially anterior and to the left of the orifice of the superior caval vein. It then takes a rightward course, anterior to the venous orifice before descending laterally and posteriorly to the right side of the orifice of the ICV (see **Fig. 1**). Papez termed this bundle the posterior crest that continues as the other rightward arm from the interatrial bundle.[14] The alignment of the myocardial strands is mainly longitudinal, along the length of the crest from its medial insertion until it approaches the orifice of the ICV where the muscle thins. The terminal portion branches into bundles of varying thicknesses and arrangements into the cavotricuspid isthmus. The crest itself varies in thicknesses and widths. Those that are prominent give a clear demarcation between the rough pectinates and the smooth venous component of the atrium that receives the caval veins and the coronary sinus. Others are relatively flat along their lengths, merging into the venous

component, or flatten out toward the entrance of the ICV (see **Fig. 5C**). Conceivably, the flatter or less distinct parts could be less of an obstacle for the circuit.

The intercaval bundle forms much of the epicardial surface of the posterior atrial wall between the caval orifices (see below—interatrial muscular connections). It covers the venous sinus between Waterston's (interatrial) groove and the terminal groove. From there, it becomes the external bundle of the right atrium spreading as a thin layer over the pectinate muscles.[13,14] Papez traced its origin anteriorly and medially to the left side of the superior caval vein entrance to descend obliquely, passing posteriorly.

LEFT ATRIUM
Left Atrial Appendage

Unlike in the right atrium, the left atrial appendage is small and tubular with one to several bends. A narrow ostium connects it to the atrial body. No terminal crest marks the junction. Pectinate muscles are primarily confined to within the

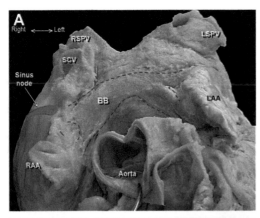

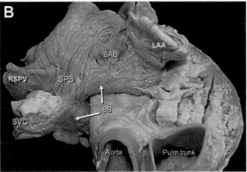

Fig. 6. Anterior views of the atria of two herts (*A, B*) following dissections of the epicardium to reveal the gross myoarchitecture of the interatrial bundle and the septopulmonary bundle (SPB) and septoatrial bundle (SAB) over the left atrium. Bachmann's bundle (BB) crosses the interatrial groove (*blue arrow*) and continues laterally on each side (*broken lines*) to branch around the right and left atrial appendages (RAA, LAA). LSPV, left superior pulmonary veins; RSPV, right superior pulmonary vein; SCV, superior caval vein.

appendage. They have been described as taking two patterns of arrangements with muscle bundles separated by thinner fibrous tissue.[16] One is like a coconut palm leaf with bundles extending in a near-parallel fashion from a 'spine' of muscle. The other is like a palmyra leaf arrangement with one short broad muscle bundle that fans out into thinner bundles.

Left Atrial Body

Distinct from the appendage, the venous component of the body receives the pulmonary veins posteriorly. Although four venous orifices are often seen, there is considerable variation in the number and arrangements. In between the superior and inferior venous orifices and between the left orifices and the orifice of the appendage are narrow parts (or isthmuses) of the wall that appear like ridges on the endocardial surface. Importantly,

the so-called ridge between the left pulmonary veins and the orifice of the appendage (**Fig. 7**) is a fold in the atrial wall that bears the remnant of the vein of Marshall and accompanying nerves and ganglia on the epicardial side. In approximately 30% of heart specimens, the artery supplying the sinus node originates from the circumflex artery of which 8% are in this fold.[17]

On the endocardial surface, the wall of the body is mainly smooth apart from a few pits and troughs. A crescent on the septal aspect marks the site of the opening for the oval fossa. The obliquely oriented septum blends into the anterior wall. Although smooth overall, the thickness of the myocardium in the atrial wall varies, usually thinner close to the orifices of the inferior pulmonary veins. The anterosuperior wall that includes Bachmann's bundle tends to be thickest, approximately 4–6 mm thick in normal hearts (see **Fig. 6**).[18] The anterior wall lying behind the transverse pericardial sinus is thinner. It continues laterally and posteriorly to the appendage. Near the orifice of the appendage, the posteroinferior wall may contain a series of small troughs with muscle in between giving the wall the appearance of pectinates.

The vestibule of the atrial body surrounds the mitral orifice. However, owing to the lack of pectinate muscles in the body, the vestibule is practically indistinguishable from the rest of the atrial wall.

Mitral Isthmus

The left atrial vestibule forms part of the inferoposterior atrial wall between the orifice of the left inferior pulmonary vein and the mitral hingeline (annulus) that is termed the mitral isthmus. Importantly, the courses of the great cardiac vein/coronary sinus and circumflex artery are along inferior and inferoposterior segment on the epicardial side (see **Fig. 7**). The venous wall that adjoins the left atrial wall has a cuff of muscle along its length usually from the coronary sinus orifice to its juncture with the vein/ligament of Marshall or slightly beyond. This juncture is also marked by a flimsy valve (of Vieussens) within the vein in the majority of hearts.[19] The thickness of the muscle cuff ranges from 0.3 to 2.5 mm in one study using histologic sections.[20] It is thicker on the side abutting the atrial wall than the outer side. Muscular connections between the coronary sinus wall and the left atrial wall are common. They vary from thin strands to broad bands that may not allow distinction between the two walls, providing the bases for interatrial connections (see below).

The muscle wall at the isthmus is not of uniform thickness (see **Fig. 7**) It is thin nearest the mitral

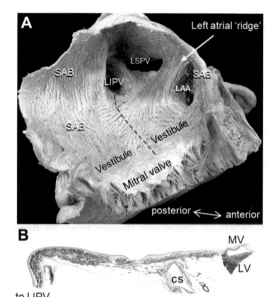

Fig. 7. View of the endocardial surface of the left atrium showing the gross myoarchitecture of the left lateral and posterior wall (*A*). The broken line marks the area of the mitral isthmus that lies between the mitral hingeline and the orifice of the left inferior pulmonary vein (LIPV). The histologic section stained in Masson's trichrome (*B*) shows the variability in myocardial thickness (*stained reddish*) along the length of this isthmus. Note the muscular connections between the coronary sinus (CS) wall and the left atrial wall. LAA, left atrial appendage; LSPV, left superior pulmonary vein; SAB, septoatrial bundle.

valve, thickens in the midportion and thins out again near the venous orifice. At its thickest, the myocardial depth measured on histologic sections in a study of 16 hearts was 3.8 ± 0.9 mm.[21] Moreover, the circumflex artery was located at the isthmus in seven hearts. It was closer than 5 mm from the endocardium in five, including three where it was closer than 2 mm and embedded within the atrial myocardium.

Left Atrial Myoarchitecture

In the majority of hearts, the most obvious bundle on the subepicardium of the left atrium is the leftward extension of Bachmann's bundle after it has crossed the interatrial groove. It bifurcates into upper and lower branches to pass to either side of the left atrial appendage (see **Fig. 6**). The upper branch continues into the lateral wall that separates the orifice of the left atrial appendage and the orifices of the left pulmonary veins. The lower branch passes inferiorly to the base of the atrium to contribute to the epicardial side of the vestibule.

Upper and lower branches merge posterior to the left atrial appendage, combining with circumferential bundles that encircle the atrial outlet around the mitral orifice to form much of the vestibule, including the inferior part that forms the mitral isthmus. The deeper septoatrial bundle comes from the anterior rim of the oval fossa together with circumferential bundles that encircle the atrial outlet around the mitral orifice to form much of the vestibule including the 'mitral isthmus' on the endocardial side (see **Figs. 6** and **7**). A detailed study using gross dissection and microscopy by Cheng and colleagues in the region of the posterior vestibule revealed a bundle parallel to the course of the coronary sinus that they termed the posteroinferior bundle.[22] In some hearts, they observed this bundle to occupy the full thickness of the vestibule. In others, they suggested the bundle might mix with extensions from Bachmann's bundle or the septoatrial bundle.

Apart from contributing to the vestibular wall, the septoatrial bundle divides into circumferential and longitudinal bundles. The latter becomes the main branch that lines the endocardial surface of the superior and posterior atrial walls, between the orifices of the right and left pulmonary veins (**Fig. 8**). Some longitudinal fibers reach into the vestibule and central fibrous body forming the inferior rim of the oval fossa.

More superficially, the septopulmonary bundle forms much of the atrial wall. It arises from the interatrial groove, passes anteriorly and superiorly behind Bachmann's bundle where it spreads out into several branches (see **Figs. 7** and **8**). The largest of these takes a circumferential course, follows Bachmann's bundle leftward, and continues into the lateral wall. The other branches fan out to the superior, posterior, and inferior walls in variable directions between the pulmonary veins. In some hearts, the branches are primarily longitudinal, whereas in others they run obliquely or laterally or are in mixed orientations.

INTERATRIAL MUSCULAR CONNECTIONS

Aside from muscular continuity at the atrial septum, the two atria are also joined by muscular bundles. Bachmann's bundle is usually the most obvious that carries conduction between the atria. Its rightward extension branches to pass to either side of the atrial appendage (see **Fig. 6**). The upper branch passes superficial to the terminal crest toward the sinus node area at the entrance of the superior caval vein. In some hearts, broad muscular bridges may be crossing the posterior or inferior regions of the interatrial groove. Although not always the case, Bachmann's bundle tends to be

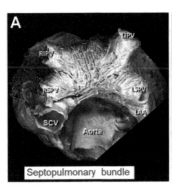

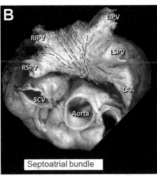

Fig. 8. Views of the dome of the left atrium following sequential dissection from subepicardium (*left-hand panel*) toward the subendocardium (*right-hand panel*). Broken lines indicate longitudinal alignment of the myocardial strands of the bundles. Dumbbell marks Bachmann's bundle. LAA, left atrial appendage; LIPV and LSPV, left inferior and superior pulmonary vein; RIPV and RSPV, right inferior and superior pulmonary vein; SCV, superior caval vein.

smaller than usual or even absent in these hearts, with implications for interatrial conduction (**Fig. 9**).[23]

Frequently, there are smaller bundles of various widths, depths, and proximity to the oval fossa that cross the interatrial groove.[24,25] Connections between the intercaval bundle and Bachmann's bundle as depicted in Keith and Flack's 1907 publication describing the sinus node, also vary in incidence and sizes.[26]

Furthermore, as mentioned earlier, muscular connections between the wall of the coronary sinus and the atrial walls are common (see **Fig. 9**). In some hearts, smaller or strand-like muscular bridges between the muscle sleeves of pulmonary veins and right atrium or between the muscle sleeve of the superior caval vein and left atrium are also encountered.

ACQUIRED CHANGES TO ATRIAL WALLS

It is well accepted that the myocardium undergoes structural and functional alterations in response to aging. At the histologic level, these include reduction in myocyte numbers, myocyte hypertrophy, apoptosis, inflammation, fibrosis, and fibro-fatty replacement. In his viewpoint article questioning how normal the human atria in patients with atrial fibrillation (AF) are, Anton Becker presented his observations comparing tissues from 20 heart specimens.[27] Ten were from patients with a known history of paroxysmal AF (aged 61–82 years) and ten were without a history of AF (aged 26–92 years). However, in the no-AF group, six had obstructive coronary artery disease with myocardial scarring. No cardiac pathology was found in two (aged 26 and 55 years). He observed that in almost all sections of the terminal crest and Bachmann's bundle, there was fibro-fatty replacement of the myocardium in both groups. In the AF group, fibro-fatty replacement was more extensive, with total replacement observed in some. The changes were so striking that he commented "this particular feature can be considered almost normal, at least in the elderly population". Further, he suggested the small patches of replacement fibrosis often seen in atrial walls are micro-scars from ischemic events and may be more common than generally believed.

Apart from pathologic changes that may or may not be associated with increases in chamber size, other changes to consider are those consequential to surgical incisions. Right atrial incisions vary in their extents and sites, especially in the scenario of congenitally malformed hearts. Trauma to arterial supply together with scars formed at suture lines then set the scene for conduction delay and lines of block.

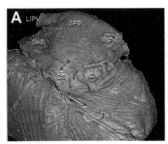

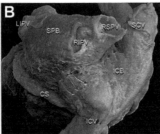

Fig. 9. Views of the subepicardial surface from the inferior(diaphragmatic) perspective following gross dissections. The muscular wall of the coronary sinus connects to both the left and right atrial walls (*double headed arrows*) in panel A. The heart in panel *B* shows a broad interatrial muscular connection inferiorly (*three arrows*) as well as superiorly where the intercaval bundle (ICV) continues anteriorly (*two arrows*) to the left atrium.

SUMMARY

There is little that anatomy can elucidate other than reviewing again the atrial structures that have been noted as electrophysiologic barriers to conduction and areas of slow conduction.

As conduction tends to follow the direction of well-aligned longitudinal strands of myocytes, myoarchitecture, ischemic, or pathologic changes to these could play a role in altering the pathways. Furthermore, it is conceivable that when pathologic changes occur in the variety of interatrial muscular connections, they may underlie some forms of atypical flutter.

Pathologic changes occur not only in aging but could begin earlier as observed in one case of 26 years old in Anton Becker's small series. Becker cited a study in the early 1960s by Maurice Lev and James B McMillan as reporting "increases in collagen and fatty replacement of the atrial myocardium from the third decade on". With his great insight, Becker concluded in his viewpoint article that "human atria of older individuals (>30 years) demonstrate a range of structural changes that should not be ignored as a substrate for initiation and maintenance of tachyarrhythmias". Indeed, observations from long-forgotten studies could well elucidate some of the facets for atypical reentry in atrial flutter.

CLINICS CARE POINTS

- The cavotricuspid isthmus occupies a quadrilateral area where three lines can be described. The most medial line, nearest to the coronary sinus orifice, is also nearest to the inferior parts of the compact atrioventricular node. The lateral-most line is the longest and is also closest to the right coronary artery. The central line traverses a pouch-like dip in some patients.

- The mitral isthmus is not of uniform thickness being thinner near the mitral valve and near the orifice of the pulmonary vein. Muscle sleeves around the coronary sinus may add to the thickness of the middle portion. The circumflex artery may be as close as 2 mm from the endocardial surface.

DISCLOSURE

None.

REFERENCES

1. Olgin JE, Kalman JM, Lesh MD. Conduction barriers in human atria flutter: correlation of electrophysiology and anatomy. J Cardiovasc Electrophysiol 1996;7:1112–6.
2. Saoudi N, Cosío F, Waldo A, et al. Classification of atrial flutter and regular atrial tachycardia accordig to electrophysiologic mechanism and anatomic bases: a statement from a Joint Expert Group from the Working Group of Arrhythmias of the European Society of Cardiology and the North American Society of Pacing and Electrophysiology. Eur Heart J 2001;22:1162–82.
3. Cosio FG, Pastor A, Núñez A, et al. Atrial flutter: an update. Rev Esp Cardiol 2006;59:816–31.
4. Chugh A, Latchamsetty R, Oral H, et al. Characteristics of cavotricuspid isthmus-dependent atrial flutter after left atrial ablation of atrial fibrillation. Circulation 2006;113:609–15.
5. Bun S-S, Latcu DG, Marchlinski F, et al. Atrial flutter: more than just one of a kind. Eur Heart J 2015;36:2356–63.
6. Olshansky B, Okumura K, Hess PG, et al. Demonstration of an area of slow conduction in human atrial flutter. J Am Coll Cardiol 1990;16:1639–48.
7. Cabrera JA, Sanchez-Quintana D, Ho SY, et al. The architecture of the atrial musculature between the orifices of the inferior caval vein and the tricuspid valve. J Cardiovasc Electrophysiol 1998;9:1186–95.
8. Waki K, Saito T, Becker AE. Right atrial flutter isthmus revisited: normal anatomy favours nonuniform anisotropic conduction. J Cardiovasc Electrophysiol 2000;11:90–4.
9. Da Costa A, Faure E, Thevenin J, et al. Effect of isthmus anatomy and ablation catheter on radiofrequency catheter ablation of the cavotricuspid isthmus. Circulation 2004;110:1030–5.
10. Spach MS, Miller WT, Dolber PC, et al. The functional role of structural complexities in the propagation of depolarisation in the atrium of the dog. Conduction disturbance due to discontinuities of effective axial resistivity. Circ Res 1982;50:173–91.
11. Spach MS, Josephson ME. Initiating reentry: the role of nonuniform anisotropy in small circuits. J Cardiovasc Electrophysiol 1994;5:182–209.
12. Marrouche NF, Natale A, Wazni OM, et al. Left septal atrial flutter: electrophysiology, anatomy, and results of ablation. Circulation 2004;109:2440–7.
13. Wang K, Ho SY, Gibson DG, et al. Architecture of atrial musculature in humans. Br Heart J 1995;73:559–65.
14. Papez JW. Heart musculature of the atria. Am J Anat 1920;27:255–77, 21.
15. Ho SY, Sánchez-Quintana D. The importance of atrial structure and fibers. Clin Anat 2009;22:52–63.

16. Victor S, Nayak VM. Aneurysm of the left atrial appendage. Tex Heart Inst J 2001;28:111–8.

17. Ho SY, Sánchez-Quintana D. Anatomy and pathology of the sinus node. J Interv Card Electrophysiol 2016;46:3–8.

18. Ho SY, Cabrera JA, Sanchez-Quintana D. Left atrial anatomy revisited. Circ Arrhythm Electrophysiol 2012;5:220–8.

19. Lüdinghausen M, Ohmachi N, Boot C. Myocardial coverage of the coronary sinus and related vens. Clin Anat 1992;5:1–15.

20. Chauvin M, Shah DC, Haïssaguerre M, et al. The anatomic basis of connections between the coronary sinus musculature and the left atrium in humans. Circulation 2000;101(6):647–52.

21. Wittkampf FH, van Oosterhout MF, Loh P, et al. Where to draw the mitral isthmus line in catheter ablation of atrial fibrillation: histological analysis. Eur Heart J 2005;26:689–95.

22. Cheng J, Yang Y, Ursell PC, et al. Protected circumferential conduction in the posterior atrioventricular vestibule of the left atrium: electrophysiologic and anatomic correlates. Pacing Clin Electrophysiol 2005;28:692–701.

23. De Ponti R, Ho SY, Salerno-Uriarte JA, et al. Electroanatomic analysis of sinus impulse propagation in normal human atria. J Cardiovasc Electrophysiol 2002;13:1–10.

24. Ho SY, Anderson RH, Sánchez-Quintana D. Atrial structure and fibres: morphologic bases of atrial conduction. Cardiovasc Res 2002;54:325–36.

25. Platonov PG, Mitrofanova L, Ivanov V, et al. Substrates for intra-atrial and interatrial conduction in the atrial septum: anatomical study on 84 human hearts. Heart Rhythm 2008;5:1189–95.

26. Keith A, Flack M. The form and nature of the muscular connections between the primary divisions of the vertebrate heart. J Anat Physiol 1907;41(Pt 3):172–89.

27. Becker AE. How structurally normal are human atria in patients with atrial fibrillation? Heart Rhythm 2004;1:627–31.

Electrocardiographic Approach to Atrial Flutter
Classifications and Differential Diagnosis

Giuseppe Bagliani, MD[a,b,*], Fabio M. Leonelli, MD[c,d],
Roberto De Ponti, MD[e,f], Michela Casella, MD[a,g], Francesca Massara, MD[a],
Paolo Tofoni, MD[a], Federico Guerra, MD[a,b], Giuseppe Ciliberti, MD[a,b],
Antonio Dello Russo, MD[a,b]

KEYWORDS

- Atrial flutter • Typical atrial flutter • Common typical atrial flutter • Uncommon typical atrial flutter
- Atypical atrial flutter • ECG recording

KEY POINTS

- Atrial flutter (AFL) is a macro-reentrant arrhythmias.
- The cavo-tricuspid-isthmus is involved in most circuits of right AFL, generating a typical AFL morphology in the inferior leads.
- Atypical (nonisthmic) AFL involves a scar in the atria, often secondary to surgery, ablation, or primary fibrosis.
- The ECG analysis is fundamental in differentiating AFL from the other forms of atrial arrhythmias and to identify the critical role of CTI in the circuit of AFL.
- The ECG identification of the critical zone of the circuit (isthmic or nonisthmic) is the primary point of every ablation procedure.

INTRODUCTION: ATRIAL FLUTTER CHARACTERISTICS AND TECHNICAL CONSIDERATIONS

Despite the enormous technological advancements in cardiac electrophysiology, the ECG remains the most useful tool in the diagnosis of atrial arrhythmias.[1] An accurate ECG interpretation (**Fig. 1**) is necessary to distinguish atrial flutter (AFL) from atrial fibrillation (AF) and from atrial tachycardia (AT)[2] and it is necessary to undertake optimal management.

From an electrophysiological point of view, AFL is a macro reentrant AT[3].[4] This definition separates micro from macro reentries based on the size of the reentrant circuit. A macro reentry is a circus movement around a large central obstacle measuring several centimeters in at least one of its diameters.[5] A wavefront of depolarization is always present within the reentrant flutter circuit giving on the 12 lead ECG, the characteristic continuous fluctuation of the baseline.[6] (see **Fig. 1**A).

[a] Cardiology And Arrhythmology Clinic, University Hospital "Ospedali Riuniti", via Conca 71, 60100 Ancona, Italy; [b] Department of Biomedical Sciences and Public Health, Marche Polytechnic University, Ancona, Italy; [c] Cardiology Department, James A. Haley Veterans' Hospital, University of South Florida, 13000 Bruce B Down Boulevard, Tampa, FL 33612, USA; [d] University of South Florida, 4202 East Fowler Avenue, Tampa, FL 33620, USA; [e] Department of Heart and Vessels, Ospedale di Circolo, Viale Borri, 57, Varese 21100, Italy; [f] Department of Medicine and Surgery, University of Insubria, Viale Guicciardini, 9, Varese 21100, Italy; [g] Department of Clinical, Special and Dental Sciences, Marche Polytechnic University, Ancona, Italy
* Corresponding author. Centro Cardiologia, Aritmie ed Ipertensione arteriosa, Via Centrale Umbra 17, 06038 Spello (PG), Italy.
E-mail address: giuseppe.bagliani@tim.it

Card Electrophysiol Clin 14 (2022) 385–399
https://doi.org/10.1016/j.ccep.2022.05.007
1877-9182/22/

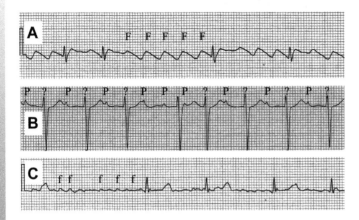

Fig. 1. Typical electrocardiographic appearance of atrial activation in the 3 most common atrial tachycardias: (*A*) atrial flutter (F), (*B*) atrial tachycardia (P), and (*C*) atrial fibrillation (f).

In AT, on the contrary, as atrial activation lasts less than the entire cycle length, there is a period of electrical inactivity which reflects on the ECG as an isoelectric line (see **Fig. 1**B): this remains the principal, although not foolproof, differentiation criterion between AFL and AT(1) .[6,7] AFL must be differentiated from AF which is characterized by a totally irregular atrial activation[2]

AFL rates usually exceed 240 beats/min but a wide range of values exist and for this reason, this parameter is of secondary value in the differential diagnosis of ATs.

Given the stability of reentry within a large circuit, the flutters' atrial rate has minimal variations. In contrast with the stable atrial rate, the ventricular rate is modulated by the AVN properties. The filter role of the AVN is manifested by the atrioventricular (AV) relationship. Most often, an AV ratio of 2:1 is observed resulting in a regular narrow QRS tachycardia. In other cases, the AV relationship can be variable and alternate between fixed ratios creating a regularly irregular SVT. In rare situations the AV ratio can randomly change from 2:1, 3:1, 4:1 giving rise to an extreme irregular ventricular rate at times mimicking AF.

The constant atrial reentrant path generates a stable, diagnostic morphology of the flutter waves.

The stereotype of AFL wave morphology, the so-called "Saw-tooth" waves (**Fig. 2**), is the classical example of correlation between the ECG and a specific substrate.[8]

The proliferation of ablative procedures to treat AF has created a large number of mixed anatomical-scar substrates sustaining a large variety of macro and micro-reentrant flutters.[9]

In these cases, widespread use of endocavitary mapping has shown the diagnostic limitations of the ECG (see Fabio M. Leonelli and colleagues', "Interpretation of Typical and Atypical Atrial Flutters by Precision Electrocardiology Based on Intracardiac Recording," in this issue).

To interpret correctly a 12 lead ECG, the substrate here the flutter occurs, and some technical aspects of ECG recordings need to be understood. Most of the literature on flutters can be generally divided into pre and postablation; the former described naturally occurring arrythmias has splendidly detailed "typical AFLs," the latter is dealing with the consequences of a profoundly altered natural substrate.

POST-RADIO FREQUENCY ABLATION TACHYCARDIAS

Nonconductive atrial boundaries usually represented by scars or prosthetic material have been described infrequently in the past.

They occurred naturally following ischemia, surgery, long-standing hypertension, among other conditions, and generate islands of nonconductive tissue among normal myocardium.

Scar-related flutters were reported infrequently in the literature until the widespread advent of surgery, cryo or radiofrequency ablation of tissue mostly in the left atrium in the treatment of AF.[10]

With the parallel development of highly sophisticated 3D mapping system, reports detailing the number and variability of mostly post-RFA have exponentially multiplied.[11]

The arrhythmias observed nowadays in clinical practice are frequently constituted by complications of these procedures appearing at variable intervals following the initial RFA.

While endocavitary mapping has detailed their variability and their relationship to previous ablation sites, the ECG has clearly lagged behind as a diagnostic tool.

This is due to a number of factors; obliteration of tissue reduces the overall voltage of the atrial recording impeding a clear ECG analysis of the arrhythmia waveform.

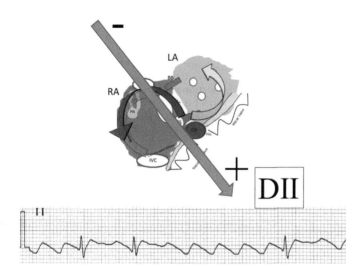

Fig. 2. Recording of the progression of isthmus-dependent circuit in lead II. The bipolar lead II by exploring atrial activation in the cranio-caudal direction is the optimal lead (as D III and aVF) to record the entire atrial reentry.

The creation of a large number of scar-related channels, bordered by electrophysiologically altered tissue, multiplies the possible paths of reentrant circuits increasing the occurrence and variations of reentrant paths.

Finally, by destroying extensive regions of the left atrium, these procedures may alter the intra and inter-atrial propagation of activation.

ECG interpretation is based on the knowledge of a certain pattern of electrical propagation. These atrial modifications, by introducing a number of unquantifiable changes in the progression of the activation wavefront, render the electrocardiographic interpretation of scar-related arrhythmias extremely problematic.

The other fundamental aspect of ECG interpretation is the understanding of this tool's more technical features.

PHYSIOLOGY AND BIOPHYSICS OF THE ELECTROCARDIOGRAM

The Importance of Unipolar and Bipolar Recording and Lead Location in Atrial Flutter

A detailed analysis of the morphology of the atrial waveform in the 12 leads is the key point in the AFL's classification.[12] The 3-dimensional analysis of the flutter wave is a complex and difficult process for the following reasons:

1. It is the result of the depolarization of 2 independent chambers
2. Some regions of the atria generate low voltages
3. Simultaneous activation of different areas of the atria can decrease or increase the resultant vector by, respectively, cancellation (the mutual elision of opposite wavefronts) or summation.

To resolve these difficulties, it is necessary for a rational choice of leads to explore the frontal and horizontal plane together with an understanding of the difference between bipolar or unipolar recording. To this end, in accordance with an approach based on precision electrocardiology, we will review some biophysical concepts of electrocardiographic recording.

Bipolar inferior limb leads

The IDFL macro reentrant circuit rotates from the inferior regions to the roof of the right atrium principally along the cardiac frontal plane. Therefore, the bipolar inferior leads (II, III, and aVF) exploring the activation of the atria in the cranio-caudal direction are optimally located to record the reentry in its entirety avoiding vector cancellation (see **Fig. 2**).

Unipolar precordial lead: the "Solid Angle Theorem"

Given this reentry main axis, the precordial leads, exploring the sagittal plane, are less informative of the global atrial electrical activation during typical AFl. Furthermore, the signal recorded by unipolar recording lead principally depends on the Solid Angle Theorem (**Fig. 3**). A solid angle delimits the imaginary space containing the electrical signal of a cardiac region with, at its apex, the recording unipolar lead.[13] The electrical signal (Φ) registered by the exploring electrode depends on:

1. The width of the angle of the cone with the recording electrode at the apex is shaped to include the explored structure; the angle is directly proportional to the radius of the structure and inversely proportional to the distance. In the case of Lead V1, the right atrium will

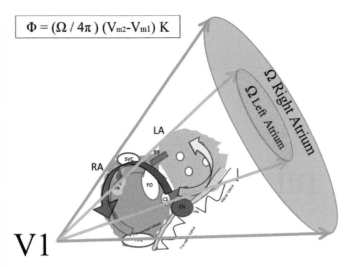

$$\Phi = (\Omega / 4\pi) (V_{m2} - V_{m1})\, K$$

Fig. 3. The "Solid Angle Theory" and the unipolar recording. The electrical signal (Φ) registered by a Unipolar Lead (V1); (1) is directly proportional to the dimension of the structure and inversely proportional to its distance from the lead; in V1 the right atrium (*green solid angle*) generates a larger signal than the more distant left atrium (*orange solid angle*), (2) depends on the strength and direction of the wavefront vector. A vector directly pointing to V1 will generate a much larger signal than a vector perpendicular to this lead.

record a larger signal than the more distant left atrium (see **Fig. 3**).
2. The strength and direction of the wavefront vector; a vector pointing to V1 will generate a much larger signal than a vector perpendicular to this lead.

The solid angle theory explains the importance of lead V1 in the analysis of AFL. The unipolar lead V6 also explores the sagittal plane, but due to its position and distance from the atria has a minor discriminating power between Left and Right atrial Vectors. The combined analysis of the peripheral leads (in particular DII and the other inferior leads) and of the precordial leads (in particular V1) is fundamental in the electrophysiological approach to AFLs (**Fig. 4**)

Isoelectric line during atrial arrhythmias
In the analysis of atrial arrythmias an isoelectric line is defined as an isopotential line of at least 80 msec^2 duration.

During a focal tachycardia, the isoelectric line corresponds to a period without any recordable electrical activity (see **Fig. 1**C). During AFI (see **Fig. 4**) whereby a continuous depolarizing wavefront exists, the isoelectric line should never be present, unless low voltage activation or cancellation phenomena occur. During IDFL the inferior leads to record a continuous activation without any isoelectric period inscribing the typical sawtooth pattern.

An isoelectric line observed during this arrhythmia could be due to different reasons depending on the recording leads:

1. In lead I, II, aVF, an initial descending phase can be so slow to mimic an isoelectric line (pseudo-isoelectric line: red arrow in **Fig. 4**)

2. In the unipolar leads, according to the solid angle theory (see **Fig. 3**), some atrial areas can be too far from the recording site to generate a potential; this is especially evident if the activation front is perpendicular to the axis of the lead. This phenomenon is noticeable in the right precordial leads (Green arrows in **Fig. 4**)
3. A cancellation phenomenon due to a spatial collision of 2 different wavefronts.

The importance of a global 12 lead ElectroCardioGram evaluation
Given these premises, it is fundamental in the electrocardiographic analysis of atrial arrhythmias to closely review not only each lead in isolation but the entire 12 lead tracings.[14]

This is necessary to be able to reconstruct, comparing the vector recorded by each lead at the same point in time the wavefront directions and the arrythmia mechanism (**Fig. 5**).

This correlation between the different leads is a necessary step in macro reentrant arrhythmias, such as the majority of AFLs, to reconstruct in great detail their entire circuit.

It will be amply shown in this book that this correlation is very robust with regard to flutters defined as "Typical" while some limitations exist for the "Atypical" (**Fig. 6**).

FUNDAMENTAL ELECTROCARDIOGRAM CLASSIFICATION: ISTHMUS OR NON–ISTHMUS-DEPENDENT ATRIAL FLUTTERS

Correlation of 12 lead ECG and intra-cavitary recordings of atrial activation has allowed us to reconstruct, fairly precisely, the path followed by the macro reentrant tachycardias and to identify the characteristic patterns associated with some reentrant paths.[14,15,16,17,18] This has generated

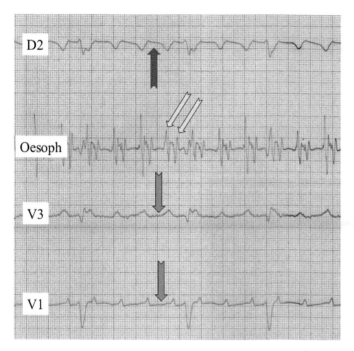

Fig. 4. Bipolar, local electrograms registered with esophageal lead, and Unipolar Recordings of common Type Atrial Flutter. The bipolar lead DII shows the typical "sawtooth" wave well highlighting the slow-descending phase (*red arrow*). The transesophageal recording shows a "local atrial activation" with the typical double potential morphology (*yellow arrows*). The precordial leads (V3-V1) show positive deflections and a pseudo-isoelectric line (*green arrows*).

an AFL classification based on well-defined ECG criteria reflecting the role played by the isthmus between the tricuspid valve and the inferior vena cava (TVIVC) in the maintenance of the macro reentry (see **Fig. 5**).

In IDFL (also referred to as typical or type I), this structure is a necessary part of the reentrant circuit which is fully contained in the RA with the LA acting as a bystander chamber.

As the wavefront rotates around the tricuspid valve, for an observer hypothetically looking at the valve from the apex of the right ventricle, 2 possible activation directions are possible: Counterclockwise (CCW) (**Fig. 7**) or clockwise (CW) (**Fig. 8**).

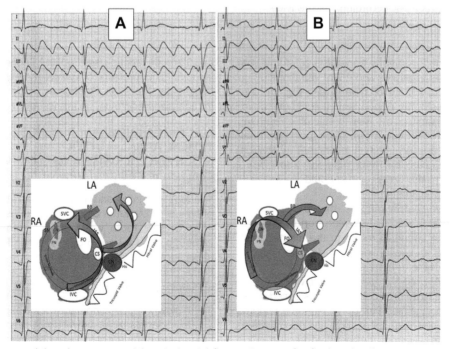

Fig. 5. Common (*A*) and uncommon (*B*) typical atrial flutter. See text for further details.

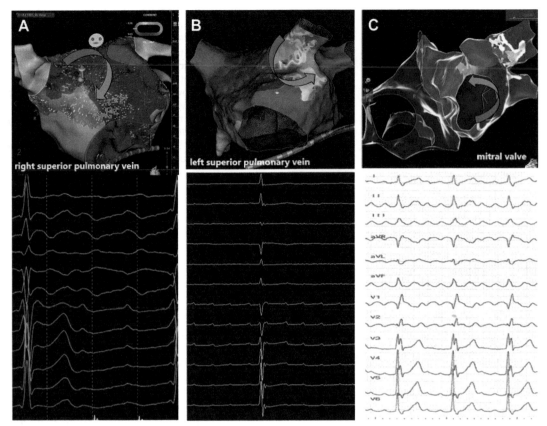

Fig. 6. Atypical atrial flutter. Three cases of atypical flutter originating from LA scars The reentry circuit is located around the right superior pulmonary vein (*A*), around the left superior pulmonary vein (*B*), and the mitral valve (*C*). Note the extremely variable of each pattern of atrial activation on the electrocardiogram. See text and Fabio M. Leonelli and colleagues', "Interpretation of Typical and Atypical Atrial Flutters by Precision Electrocardiology Based on Intracardiac Recording," in this issue.

Either of the 2 rotations generates a tracing with fairly standard features and minor variations.

In atypical flutters or type II (see **Fig. 6**), also called nonisthmus dependent, the circus movement is delimited by less predictable barriers, some anatomic but more often postincisional/ablation scars. An isthmus is present in atypical macro reentries, but it is different from TVIVC isthmus and the entire circuit could be in the R or, more often, in the LA.

In both types of isthmic AFL, the isthmus has the fundamental function of slowing conduction and allowing the circuit to rotate in the allotted path maintaining an excitable gap and preventing the extinction of the arrhythmias.

Atypical AFL has a propagation path which is often very difficult to reconstruct by analysis based solely on ECG tracings (see **Fig. 6**). While some features will suggest the chamber of origin and the overall direction of the wavefront, the complete reconstruction of this arrhythmia will require endocardial mapping and 3D reconstruction (see Fabio M. Leonelli and colleagues', "Interpretation of Typical and Atypical Atrial Flutters by Precision Electrocardiology Based on Intracardiac Recording," in this issue).

ELECTROCARDIOGRAM DIAGNOSIS OF TYPICAL ATRIAL FLUTTER (COUNTERCLOCKWISE AND CLOCKWISE)
Common or Counterclockwise

The most common and most recognizable feature of typical CCW flutter on ECG[1] [19,20,21] is the presence of saw tooth waves in the inferior leads without a clear return to baseline (see **Fig. 5**A). A close look at the components of the waves in these derivations shows a continuous tri-phasic sequence (see **Fig. 7**):

- A *slowly descending plateau* corresponding to the depolarizing wave-front reaching and crossing the cavo-tricuspid isthmus (segment 1 of **Fig. 7**),

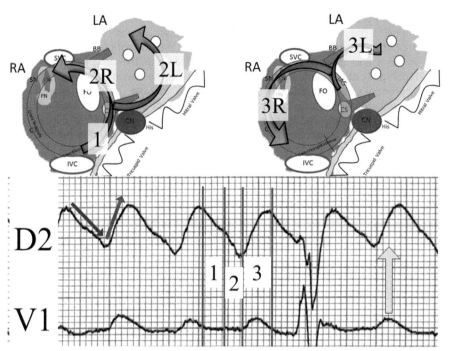

Fig. 7. Counterclockwise; isthmus-dependent atrial flutter. The sequences of the activation of the atria and the corresponding electrocardiographic "sawtooth" saw-tooth pattern (see text for further details).

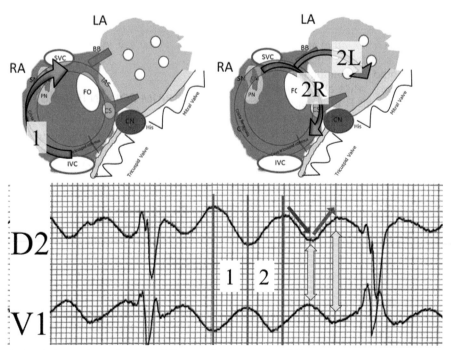

Fig. 8. Clockwise; isthmus-dependent atrial flutter. The sequences of the activation of the atria and the corresponding electrocardiographic pattern (see text for further details).

- *A rapid negative deflection, determined* by a double component: the wave-front ascends toward the roof of right atrium posteriorly between the septum and the crista terminalis (segment 2R of **Fig. 7**); at the same time, starting from the coronary sinus, left atrium is activated caudo-cranially (segment 2L of **Fig. 7**).
- *A positive deflection:* the RA propagation descends from the RA roof toward the tricuspid valve along the lateral wall (segment 3R of **Fig. 7**). From the lateral wall, the activation is forced by the Eustachian ridge into the cavo tricuspid isthmus, giving origin to the next AFL cycle. The LA contributes to the positive deflection by a depolarizing wave that from the Bachmann Bundle (BB) invades craniocaudally left atrium (segment 3L of **Fig. 7**). This second component of left atrial activation merges with the first (segment 2L) determining most of the ECG pattern of AFL (see next paragraph).

While the inferior leads will provide most of the information for the genesis of the depolarization vectors, complementary observations can be gathered by the analysis of waveforms in lead V1,[1] and to a lesser extent, in leads I, aVL, and V6.

V1 often shows only positive deflections occurring simultaneously with the positive deflections of the DII (yellow arrow of **Fig. 7**), mostly generated by the roof and lateral wall of RA. The isoelectric line between each positive deflection corresponds to the segments 1 and 2 of DII: the events of these phases (isthmus and caudo-cranial activation of R and L atria) are perpendicular to the axis of V1 and, following the solid angle theory, are represented iso-electrically. Lead I is usually noncontributory, while aVL is mostly upright due to the dominant R to L depolarization vector. A transition is observed in the precordial leads with V6 becoming positive, but this pattern is inconstant.

Uncommon or Clockwise

In this AFL the arrhythmia boundaries are the same but the propagation wavefront exits the isthmus at the free wall, therefore, engaging the other segments of the RA in the opposite direction (see **Fig. 8**). The function of the CT is again to ensure that the major anteriorly propagating wave is not short-circuited by the superiorly directed propagation with the termination of the flutter[18](22).

The following ECG waveform components are observed in inferior leads:

1. Negative deflection: The overall polarity of the flutter wave will be initially negative in the inferior leads, as the wavefront leaving the isthmus, ascends toward the SVC on the free wall until the roof of RA (segment 1 of **Fig. 8**)
2. Positive deflection: From the roof of the right atrium the wavefront proceeds simultaneously in a double direction toward the septum (segment 2R of **Fig. 8**) and through the BB toward LA (segment 2L of **Fig. 8**). Both septum and LA are activated in a cranio-caudal direction, and this generates an activation front propagating inferiorly and to the left. This front generates opposite deflections in positive in inferior leads and negative in V1 (green arrow in **Fig. 8**). This is one of the diagnostic features of CV IDFL.

A close analysis of the positive ECG wave will often show 2 components separated by a notch. The timing of the notch corresponds to the arrival of the wavefront at the lower end of the septum and to the beginning of the LA posterior wall activation along the CS. This concomitant activation of the sub-Eustachian isthmus and CS will proceed in opposite directions.

These 2 simultaneous but opposite biatrial wavefronts do not cancel each other, but create an interaction between their respective electromotive forces, and generate a distinct dipolar surface on body map distribution and a notch on 12 lead ECG.[22]

Cavo Tricuspid Isthmus (CVI) activation occurs concomitantly with Left Atrial depolarization. As a consequence, in the 12 ECG lead of CW flutter, there is no period characterized by minimal electromotive forces as in CCW flutter and no distinct plateau.

LEFT ATRIUM ROLE IN ISTHMUS-DEPENDENT FLUTTER

In typical AFL, the LA is a bystander chamber, passively activated and not necessary to maintain this arrhythmia. Nevertheless, a number of animal and human studies have shown that the activation of this chamber mostly determines the wave polarity in the 12 lead ECG.[23]

BB and CS (see **Figs. 7** and **8**). are the 2 interatrial connections determining LA activation in AFL. The former is the main atrial connection during SR. Situated in the anterior roof of the LA depolarizes the LA in a supero-inferior direction from the anterior toward the posterior LA wall. The CS, situated inferiorly and posteriorly, produces a wavefront directed in the opposite direction.

LA depolarization is a fusion between these 2 opposite wavefronts and the dominance of BB or CS is determined by the sequence of RA activation and the conduction velocity along these 2 interatrial connections.

In CCW flutter, the CS has normally activated approximately 40 msec before the BB region (see **Fig. 7**). The reverse is true in CW flutter whereby the CS follows the BB region with a delay of approximately 50 msec (see **Fig. 8**).

In CCW flutter the earliest activation proceeds unopposed caudo-cranially from the CS. This explains the inscription of prominent negative inferior flutter waves (see **Fig. 7**; **Fig. 9**A).

On the contrary, in CW flutter the BB is engaged first, generating a cranio-caudal vector and positive F waves in the same leads (see **Fig. 8**).

In both cases, the septal vector being codirectional with this initial LA activation contributes to the main wave polarity.

The terminal segment of the F wave in II, II and aVF also represents a combination of different left and right atrial wavefronts. In CW the negative deflection is the result of concordant activations of the lateral wall of both Atria. These portions of the chambers are both depolarized in an inferior–superior direction by the CS wavefront in the LA, and by the emergence of the isthmus propagation wave in the RA. In CCW the RA wavefront descends from the RA roof along the free wall is

unopposed as the depolarization of the LA is mostly concluded. The resultant electrocardiographic deflection is, therefore, positive both in inferior leads and V1 (yellow arrow in **Fig. 7**).

V1 is also a powerful discriminator between the 2 types of AFL: positive in CCW reflecting a postero-anterior direction of activation, and negative in CW whereby the wavefront mostly propagates in the opposite direction (yellow arrow of **Fig. 8**).

VARIANTS OF ISTHMUS-DEPENDENT ATRIAL FLUTTER

What has been described so far is the typical progression of an activation wave along a well-established flutter circuit. This results in the stereotypical ECG appearance which we recognize as CCW or CW flutter (see **Fig. 5**). This "standard" morphology is present only in 30%of cases as minor changes in the timing of activation of key anatomic structures can alter, subtly or, the ECG appearance of AFL waves (**Fig. 9**). In both flutters, delayed LA activation in the CS or BB connection can alter both the contribution and their timing to LA depolarization vectors. (Ref article in Book I). The CS conduction can be affected by spontaneous pathology or procedures: minor delays will

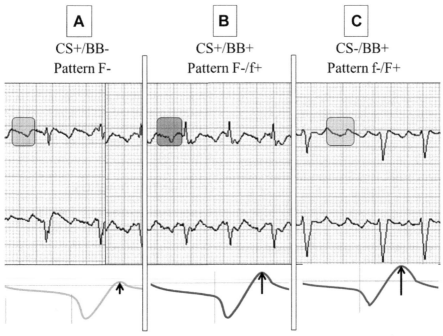

Fig. 9. Isthmus-dependent atrial flutter variants: a schematic representation of the different morphologies of "sawtooth" flutter wave in the inferior leads. The ratio between the negative and the final positive deflection varies from a completely negative (F-) in A, to a mostly positive deflection (F+) in C and an intermediate morphology in B. These changes are due exclusively to the activation of left atrium, that realizes retrogradely from the coronary sinus in A (CS+/BB-) and antero-gradelly from the Bachmann Bundle in C (CS-/BB+); (see text for further details).

go unobserved in CCW flutter (see **Fig. 9**B) while CS conduction block will completely reverse the LA activation and the waveform appearance (see **Fig. 9**C).

Few studies have reported, in a small subset of patients with CCW a shortening of the tachycardia cycle length with subtle ECG changes such as loss of the terminal positive deflection of the flutter in the inferior leads. The authors described, in these cases, a shift of the reentrant circuit to include the IVC bypassing the RA septum and free wall (see Fabio M. Leonelli and colleagues', "Interpretation of Typical and Atypical Atrial Flutters by Precision Electrocardiology Based on Intracardiac Recording," in this issue). The flutter remains isthmus dependent but with a shorter circuit explaining the cl variation.

CW flutter is far less common than the opposite counterpart and therefore fewer detailed observations of ECG variability during this arrhythmia are available.

ATYPICAL ATRIAL FLUTTER
Upper Loop Reentry

Most of the non-IDFL are macro reentrant arrythmias with a circuit bound by incisional or post-RFA scars.

Few exceptions are described and include R and LA flutter circuits delimited by spontaneous scars and an uncommon form of nonisthmus flutter called upper loop reentry (ULR).[10]

In ULR the SVC constitutes the anatomic ring around which the arrythmia rotates thanks to gaps in the continuity of the CT (see Fabio M. Leonelli and colleagues', "Interpretation of Typical and Atypical Atrial Flutters by Precision Electrocardiology Based on Intracardiac Recording," in this issue).

This anatomic structure constitutes a necessary element in typical AFL (see Shumpei Mori and colleagues' article, "Revisiting the Anatomy of the Left Ventricular Summit," in this issue) preventing the short circuit of the posterior and anterior wall wavefronts.

This line of block is probably a combination of anatomic nonconductivity and functional block in response to higher rate of stimulation.

As we have described for LLR, inferior gaps in the line of block can favor, during typical flutter, formation of different smaller circuits.

In ULR the typical CW wavefront of activation shifts from its usual path to a circuit around the SVC rotating around this vein through a small gap in the CT.

In this case, the crista provides, thanks to its inhomogeneous conduction properties, a slow conduction area that allows the perpetuation of a circus movement around the SVC.

LA activation pattern is similar to typical CW flutter, while in the RA 2 wavefronts are generated colliding most often just outside the isthmus. The ECG morphology is, therefore, often undistinguishable from CW flutter.[24]

Scar-Related Flutters

The variables determining the ECG features of scar-related flutters are variable and mostly unpredictable: anatomic location of the "scar," direction of rotation of the reentry, number of active reentrant paths, effects of antiarrhythmic drugs, volume of the chamber, role of the cavo-tricuspid isthmus and the extent of atrial myocyte loss[25],[26],[11] It is, therefore, not surprising that, contrary to isthmus-dependent flutters, the electrographic manifestations of these arrhythmias are not fully understood nor standardized (see **Fig. 6**).

Despite the unpredictable nature of these arrythmias, the determinants of typical and atypical flutter reentrant circuit are fundamentally the same.

Both require a stable reentrant path limited by anatomic and or acquired boundaries. In either circuit exist a segment of tissue, called an isthmus, with slow conduction properties delimited by areas of nonconduction.

Although this may be a simplified model, it is useful in explaining the initiation and maintenance of this arrhythmia and the ECG findings associated with it.

While typical AFL uses to set up determined by RA anatomy, atypical AFL depends on boundaries created by surgical or catheter-based procedures prosthetic material or atrial remodeling due to volume, pressure overload, or long-standing atrial arrhythmias.

DIFFERENTIAL DIAGNOSIS

As previously explained,[27] the diagnosis of supraventricular arrythmia proceeds following a logical step-wise method (**Fig. 10**). In this article, we will focus on the differential diagnosis of SVT and macro-reentrant flutters.

Regular Narrow-Complex Tachycardias

In AFL, when the ventricular rate is sufficiently low (due to an A/V ratio of 4: 1 or higher), the R-R interval is long enough to clearly identify the activation of the atria (see **Fig. 1**A).

More frequently a stable 2: 1 AV ratio is observed and in this situation the flutter wave is buried in the QRS-T and not clearly defined. In

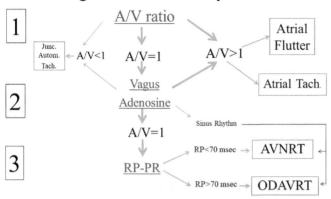

Fig. 10. Flow Chart differentiating Regular Narrow Tachycardias. Three diagnostic steps analyzing, respectively: (1) the basal A/V ratio and the pattern of atrial activation (see also **Fig. 1**), (2) vagal stimulation or adenosine, increasing the A/V ratio better show the pattern of atrial activation and exclude the paroxysmal SVT (AVNRT, ODAVRT) (3) parameters obtained by Electro physiologic study (simple and complex) in case of A/V = 1 despite Vagus-Adenosine (xxxx). See text for further detail.

this case, AFL needs to be differentiated from other supraventricular tachycardias with a regular ventricular rate (see **Fig. 10**).

Any A/V ratio greater than 1 (spontaneous or induced with vagal stimulation or adenosine), clearly excludes an accessory mediated supraventricular tachycardia and makes AVNRT highly unlikely. AT or flutter are both possible. Distinguishing between these 2 arrythmias requires the identification of atrial depolarization in as many leads as possible. A regular oscillatory atrial activation without an isoelectric line, even in a few leads, is highly suggestive of a macro reentrant AFL. The presence of a true isoelectric line (lasting at least 80 msec in all the 12 leads) is more compatible with a focal AT (see **Fig. 1**B).

A "gray zone" in which atypical AFLs can mimic ATs was previously described (see Fabio M. Leonelli and colleagues', "Interpretation of Typical and Atypical Atrial Flutters by Precision Electrocardiology Based on Intracardiac Recording," in this issue).

During prolonged ECG recording (wearable monitors or telemetry) variations of the heart rate can be used for the diagnosis: the warming up and the cool-down phenomena are more typical of non-reentrant atria tachycardias while a constant atrial rate is in keeping with AFL.

RR variations multiple of a basic cycle are more specific for AFL.

Irregular Narrow-Complex Tachycardias

In the presence of supraventricular tachycardia with an irregular RR interval the differential diagnosis includes AF (see **Fig. 1**). In this case, a "total irregularity" orients toward AF while a "regular irregularity" (variable, often recurring AV ratios) strongly suggests AFL; this approach, although indicative, is not diagnostic and needs to be corroborated by the morphology of atrial activation (Flutter, Tachycardia or fibrillation) to reach a final diagnosis.

Multi lead waveform analysis needs to be very accurate in the case of "coarse" AF, at times erroneously defined as "Fibrillo-Flutter," especially when V1 seems to show a well-defined atrial activity (see Fabio M. Leonelli and colleagues', "Interpretation of Typical and Atypical Atrial Flutters by Precision Electrocardiology Based on Intracardiac Recording," in this issue).

Common and Uncommon Form of Typical Atrial Flutter

In the previous paragraphs we have described how, in IDFL, a wavefront can travel the same circuit in 2 opposite directions (CCW or CW) with a very different global atrial activation and 12 lead ECG manifestations. The differential diagnosis between CCW and CW form of isthmic AFL is based on:

a. The pattern of atrial activation in inferior leads:
   i. An asymmetric shape of F wave (slow descending/fast ascending) in CCW AFL (common type) (blue/red arrow in **Fig. 7**)
   ii. Symmetric shape of F wave in CW AFL (uncommon type) (see **Fig. 8**).
b. The polarity of atrial activation compared in inferior leads and in V1:
   i. Same polarity in the CCW AFL (yellow arrow in **Fig. 7**)
   ii. Opposite polarity in CW AFL (yellow arrow in **Fig. 8**).

Typical and Atypical Atrial Flutter

In this approach, the reconstruction of the mechanism of the arrhythmias is based on the interpretation of the ECG waveform morphology (see **Fig. 6**), as well as the knowledge of the patient's clinical history (see Fabio M. Leonelli and colleagues', "Interpretation of Typical and Atypical Atrial Flutters by Precision Electrocardiology Based on Intracardiac Recording," in this issue). Previous scar inducing procedures need to be known in detail; surgical techniques such as atrial approach, use of nonconductive patches, single or bi-atrial involvement, or the extent of ablative procedures (simple PVI, PV or MV linear connections or posterior wall exclusion) are important factors to keep in mind when interpreting an arrhythmia ECG.

The ECG features of typical AFL previously described particularly in the absence of previous interventions make the diagnosis certain.

Some surgeries will be most commonly associated with specific arrhythmias such as CW AFL following ASD repairs.

The arrhythmias become far less predictable following complex CHD repairs or extensive ablations. Unfortunately, a large number of arrhythmias observed nowadays in clinical practice are the consequence of RFA for AF.

The extent of atrial tissue destruction can be gauged by observing the P wave in SR. A low Voltage, wide, notched sinus Pw is in keeping with marked viable tissue loss and likely inter-atrial connection damage.

The mechanism of arrhythmias developing in these settings is difficult to interpret in detail and a stepwise collection of available observations is usually followed Ref Fabio M. Leonelli and colleagues', "Interpretation of Typical and Atypical Atrial Flutters by Precision Electrocardiology Based on Intracardiac Recording," in this issue.

Macro Reentry or Focal Arrhythmia

The distinction between a macro-reentry from a focal arrhythmia (micro-reentrant or automatic) is based on the presence/absence of an isoelectric line (see **Fig. 1**A, B). The absence of an isoelectric line makes a macro-reentry far more likely; the presence of the line can be observed in both cases.

A completely negative lead V1 represents a reliable marker of the RA origin of the flutter. On the contrary, a completely positive or biphasic appearance of this lead with initial positive deflection is more consistent with LA flutters.

Exceptions are frequent and the appearance of CCW IDFL post-AF ablation is worth mentioning. This arrhythmia will have predominantly positive (or biphasic with dominant positive component) inferior leads with a most commonly positive V1. This tachycardia should be considered in patients with post-LA ablation, especially if extensive and if TVIVC isthmus ablation was not performed (see Fabio M. Leonelli and colleagues', "Interpretation of Typical and Atypical Atrial Flutters by Precision Electrocardiology Based on Intracardiac Recording," in this issue). Post-RFA for AF, an LA macro reentry represents more than 50% of the arrhythmias observed. Of these arrhythmias, some are more common than others given the "standardization" of the ablative procedure.

The features of peri-mitral Flutter, both CCW and CW, are the most predictable. The absence of isoelectric line and a predominantly positive P in V1 without precordial transition are present in both rotations.

CW peri-mitral presents with negative inferior leads P waves, positive V1, lead I, and aVL. The absence of precordial transition and a positive lead I distinguishes this macro-reentry from isthmus-dependent CCW AFL.

CCW peri-mitral features positive, notched inferior P waves, a positive P in V1 without precordial transition, and a sharply negative aVL.

Other macro reentrant circuits such as roof-dependent flutter or single PV reentry do not have specific features (See Fabio M. Leonelli and colleagues', "Interpretation of Typical and Atypical Atrial Flutters by Precision Electrocardiology Based on Intracardiac Recording," in this issue).

Postablation micro-reentrant arrythmias are discussed in detail in Fabio M. Leonelli and colleagues', "Interpretation of Typical and Atypical Atrial Flutters by Precision Electrocardiology Based on Intracardiac Recording," in this issue.

Atrial Flutter with Wide QRS Complex

A wide complex in presence of AFL can be associated with the following situations[28]:

- Bundle Branch Bloch: particularly in patients taking AAD for the treatment of AF
- Ventricular tachycardia
- Ventricular preexcitation: in the presence of a manifest accessory pathway, AFL can be conducted to the ventricles with a wide complex tachycardia undistinguishable from ventricular tachycardia.
- Ventricular pacing

In these cases, to reach a definitive diagnosis, the ECG examination needs to be complemented by clinical information or aided by special

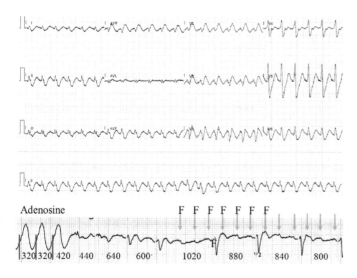

Fig. 11. Aberrant Wide Complex Tachycardia during acute Flecainide therapy: Adenosine for a precision diagnosis of Atrial Flutter and aberrant intraventricular conduction. ECG recording during Flecainide infusion to threat atrial fibrillation; a wide complex tachycardia with a right bundle branch block morphology appears (RR 320 msec, *red lines*). Adenosine infusion (6 mg) reduces heart rate (RR:320→ 440,640,600 1020) and at the same time, the QRS sudden normalize (*Yellow line*). During the longer RR intervals, a clear atrial flutter activity is present (*green arrow*). A stable FF interval of 320 msec confirms the diagnosis of the initial tachycardia in an AFL with a 1:1 A/V ratio and aberrant conduction.

maneuvers. In these difficult situations often the diagnosis requires:

1. Attempts to reduce the ventricular response (vagal maneuvers or Adenosine) to identify AFL and rule out VT (**Fig. 11**).
2. A detailed analysis of QRS morphology using specific algorithms s to identify a ventricular origin (30)
3. Comparison with baseline ECG to identify a similar preexisting wide QRS pattern (see **Fig. 3**, Paolo Compagnucci and colleagues' article, "Atrial Flutter in Particular Patient Populations," in this issue)
4. Trans-oesophageal recording/pacing could also be used to reach a diagnosis

Drug-Induced Atrial Flutter

Class 1C AAD either during acute infusion or chronic administration for the therapy for AF, can generate aberrant wide QRS often impossible to differentiate from VT (see **Fig. 11**).

The widening of the QRS is due to the drug-induced Ventricular sodium-blocking effect more manifest during the tachycardia's high rates.

Furthermore, this class of antiarrhythmic drugs can organize AF into AFL with 1:1 A/V conduction due to their vagolytic effect (in particular when using Flecainide).

In this situation, the impairment of the sodium channel is so marked that the pattern of the QRS can be undistinguishable from a VT.

Providing the patient is clinically stable, vagal maneuvers or adenosine (see **Fig. 11**) can be used to reduce the ventricular rate and help in the diagnosis of aberrant SVT.

SUMMARY

IDFL with its reproducible ECG features has been the prototype of macro-reentrant arrythmias. Backed by extensive and detailed animal and clinical observations, each component of the flutter waveform was analyzed and explained.

Following modifications of atrial substrate induced by surgical and ablative procedures, a crop of new and far more unpredictable macro-reentrant circuits are presently observed in clinical practice.

While the time-honoured principles of reentry remain the same, the ECG manifestations of these new arrhythmias have been far more difficult to interpret.

Furthermore, some of the typical ECG characteristics of IDFL can be modified by extensive LA ablation and some of the macro reentrant circuits generated by the same procedures have ECG presentations similar to typical flutter.

Aided by the advance technologies, many studies have identified features that can be used in the differential diagnosis of these arrhythmias albeit they remain less specific than in typical flutter.

It is, at the present time, impossible to summarize these features in an algorithm useable in the differential diagnosis of macro reentrant flutters.

The clinician is, therefore, left with the task of interpreting electrocardiographic tracings without an established guide.

This difficulty highlights again the importance of a step-wise interpretation of unusual ECG tracings.

In this article, integrated with the other sections of this book, we have focused on the differential diagnosis of macro-reentrant flutters explaining the most typical features of the different arrhythmias.

This was conducted on the belief that ECG identification of the circuit of reentry and the chamber of origin can substantially help in the management of the affected patient.

In the future, further correlations between more refined 3D mapping, histopathology, and basic electrophysiology will continue to provide the information necessary to fully interpret an ECG tracing of these difficult arrhythmias.

We believe that it behooves particularly to the new generation of invasive electro-physiologists to continue the study of these arrhythmias bridging the gap between endocavitary and surface ECG findings.

CLINICS CARE POINTS

- The ECG pattern of atrial activation provides fundamental information on the electrophysiology of atrial flutter.
- The involvement of Cavo-Tricuspid isthmus is easy to identify on the ECG of atrial Flutter.
- The electrophysiology of non-isthmus atrial flutter is extremely complex and the corresponding ECG can be an unreliable tool.
- Atrial Flutter can be effectively cured by trans-catheter ablation but a deep analysis of the ECG should be done first.

DISCLOSURE

A.D. Russo is a consultant for Abbott. All other authors declared no conflict of interest.

REFERENCES

1. Saoudi N, Cosio F, Waldo A, et al. Working group of arrhythmias of the European of cardiology and the north American society of pacing and electrophysiology. A classification of atrial flutter and regular atrial tachycardia according to electrophysiological mechanisms and anatomical bases; a statement from a joint expert group from the working group of arrhythmias of the European society of cardiology and the north American society of pacing and electrophysiology. Eur Heart J 2001;22: 1162–82.
2. Leonelli F, Bagliani G, Boriani G, et al. Arrhythmias originating in the atria. Card Electrophysiol Clin 2017;9:383–409.
3. Lewis T, Drury AN, Iliescu CC. A demonstration of circus movement in clinical flutter of the auricles. Heart 1921;8:341.
4. Ndrepepa G, Zrenner B, Deisenhofer I, et al. Relationship between surface electrocardiogram characteristics and endocardial activation sequence in patients with typical atrial flutter. Z Kardiol 2000;89: 527–37.
5. Guerrero F, Luther V, Sikkel M, et al. Microreentrant left atrial tachycardia circuit mapped with an ultra-high-density mapping system heart rhythm. Case Rep 2017;3:224–8.
6. Brown JP, Krummen DE, et al. Using electrocardiographic activation time and diastolic intervals to separate focal from macro–Re-entrant atrial tachycardias. J Am Coll Cardiol 2007;49:1965–73.
7. Chang S-L, Tsao H-M, Lin Y-J, et al. Differentiating macroreentrant from focal atrial tachycardias occurred after circumferential pulmonary vein isolation. J Cardiovasc Electrophysiol 2011;22:748–55.
8. Paul M, Richardson AW, Obioha-Ngwu O, et al. Josephson variable electrocardiographic characteristics of isthmus-dependent atrial flutter. J Am Coll Cardiol 2002;40:1125–32.
9. Chae S, Oral H, Good E, et al. Atrial tachycardia after circumferential pulmonary vein ablation of atrial fibrillation: mechanistic insights, results of catheter ablation, and risk factors for recurrence. J Am Coll Cardiol 2007;50:1781–7.
10. Chugh A, Latchamsetty R, Oral H, et al. Characteristics of cavotricuspid isthmus–dependent atrial flutter after left atrial ablation of atrial fibrillation. Circulation 2006;113:609–15.
11. Jais P, Shah DC, Haissaguerre M, et al. Mapping and ablation of left atrial flutters. Circulation 2000; 101:2928–34.
12. Wellens HJJ, Gorgels AP. The electrocardiogram 102 years after Einthoven. Circulation 2004;109:652.
13. van Oosterom A. Solidifying the solid angle. J Electrocardiol 2002;35:181–92.
14. Barbato G, Carinci V, Tomasi C. Is electrocardiography a reliable tool for identifying patients with isthmus-dependent atrial flutter? Europace 2009; 11:1071–6.
15. Chan DP, Van Hare GF, Mackall JA, et al. Importance of atrial flutter isthmus in postoperative intra-atrial reentrant tachycardia. Circulation 2000;102:1283–9.
16. Wasmer K, Kobe J, Dechering DG, et al. Isthmus-dependent right atrial flutter as the leading cause of atrial tachycardias after surgical atrial septal defect repair. Int J Cardiol 2013;168:2447–52.
17. Olgin JE, Kalman JM, Saxon LA, et al. Mechanism of initiation of atrial flutter in humans: site of unidirectional block and direction of rotation. J Am Coll Cardiol 1997;29(2):376–84.
18. Yang Y, Varma N, Badhwar N, et al. Prospective observations clin electrophysiological characteristics

intra-isthmus reentry. J Cardiovasc Electrophysiol 2010;21:1099–106.

19. Sasaki M, Kimura O, Horiuchi D. Revisit of typical counterclockwise atrial flutter wave in the ECG: electroanatomic studies on the determinant of the morphology. Pacing Clin Electrophysiol 2013;36:978–87.

20. Milliez P, Allison W, Richardson P. Variable electrocardiographic characteristics of isthmus-dependent atrial flutter. J Am Coll Cardiol 2002;40(6).

21. Medi C, Kalman JM. Prediction of the atrial flutter circuit location from the surface electrocardiogram. Europace 2008;10(7):786–96.

22. Marine JE, Korley VJ, Ngwu O, et al. Different patterns of interatrial conduction in clockwise and counterclockwise atrial flutter. Circulation 2001;104:1153–7.

23. Rodriguez LM, Timmermans C, Nabar A. Biatrial activation in isthmus-dependent atrial flutter. Circulation 2001;104:2545–50.

24. Yan SH, Cheng WJ, Wang LX, et al. Mechanisms of atypical flutter wave morphology in patients with isthmus-dependent atrial flutter. Heart Vessels 2009;24(3):211–8.

25. Fukamizu S, Sakurada H, Hayashi T. Macroreentrant tachycardia in patients without previous atrial surgery or catheter ablation: clinical and electrophysiological characteristics of scar-related left atrial anterior wall reentry. Cardiovasc Electrophysiol 2013;24:404–12.

26. Gerstenfeld EP, Callans DJ, Dixit S. Mechanisms of organized left atrial tachycardias occurring after pulmonary vein isolation. Circulation 2004;110:1351–7.

27. Katritsis DG, Josephson ME. Differential diagnosis of regular, narrow-QRS tachycardias. Heart Rhythm 2015;12(7):1667–76.

28. De Ponti R, Bagliani G, Natale A. General approach to a wide QRS complex. Card Electrophysiol Clin 2017;9:461–85.

Pathophysiology of Typical Atrial Flutter

Yari Valeri, MD[a,b],*, Giuseppe Bagliani, MD[a,b], Paolo Compagnucci, MD[a,b],
Giovanni Volpato, MD[a,b], Laura Cipolletta, MD, PhD[a], Quintino Parisi, MD, PhD[a],
Agostino Misiani, MD[a], Marco Fogante, MD[a,c], Silvano Molini, MD[a],
Antonio Dello Russo, MD, PhD[a,b], Michela Casella, MD, PhD[a,c]

KEYWORDS

- Reentrant arrhythmias • Right atrium • Typical atrial flutter • Inferior vena cava-tricuspid isthmus
- Crista terminalis • Common and uncommon variants • By-stander • Catheter ablation

KEY POINTS

- Typical atrial flutter is a macro-reentry mechanism arrhythmia that walks along precise "rails" delimited by specific anatomic barriers, called isthmuses. The macro reentry circuit is confined in the right atrium.
- Inferior vena cava-tricuspid isthmus median portion is a slow conduction zone and it represents a critical anatomic element of the reentry circuit and arrhythmia maintenance.
- Crista terminalis block during typical atrial flutter is functional and it is also affected by the crista terminalis structural characteristics. Crista terminalis properties proved to be different according to the presence of a clinical atrial flutter.
- During typical atrial flutter the left atrium is a by-stander chamber, but essential in the phenotypic electrocardiogram.

INTRODUCTION: FOCAL AND REENTRANT ARRHYTHMIAS

Electrophysiological mechanisms of arrhythmias can be classified as either focal or reentrant mechanisms.

Focal arrhythmia mechanisms include both the enhanced automatism and triggered activity, which consists of postpotentials developing from membrane potential oscillation. It has been suggested that the seeding of automatic cells expressing HCN channels during embryogenesis might explain the enhanced automaticity of areas other than the sinoatrial node.[1] Focal activity can spread from crista terminalis and tricuspid annulus, in the right atrium, and from pulmonary veins, in the left atrium.[2]

Regarding the reentry mechanism, the study by Alfred Mayer of the causes of rhythmic pulsations in the bell of the medusa suggested that an impulse could circulate in the heart, so it was analyzed in animals and humans.[3] Using a jellyfish, Mayer demonstrated the reentry model and recognized the importance of the relationship between path length, conduction velocity, and the refractory period. He demonstrated that a wave-front traveling in a unidirectional way into a structure of proper size can come back on its track reactivating the now excitable zone. Mayer also postulated that a unidirectional block of conduction is necessary for the reentry.[3,4]

The variability of tachycardia cycle length is an important diagnostic criterion to differentiate automatic and reentrant arrhythmias. A widely variable tachycardia cycle length is highly suggestive of the automatic mechanism, while a flutter-like atrial reentry arrhythmia has a more constant atrial cycle length. During automatic arrhythmias, cycle length

[a] Cardiology and Arrhythmology Clinic, University Hospital "Ospedali Riuniti", Via Conca 71, Ancona 60126, Italy; [b] Department of Biomedical Sciences and Public Health, Marche Polytechnic University, Ancona, Italy; [c] Department of Clinical, Special and Dental Sciences, Marche Polytechnic University, Ancona, Italy
* Corresponding author. Via San Francesco di Villanova, 2, Colli al Metauro 61036, Italy.
E-mail address: yarivaleri1@gmail.com

Card Electrophysiol Clin 14 (2022) 401–409
https://doi.org/10.1016/j.ccep.2022.05.003
1877-9182/22/© 2022 Elsevier Inc. All rights reserved.

variation is associated with exercise, adrenergic stimulation, and it can be observed at the beginning/end of arrhythmia (warming-up and cooling-down phenomena).

BASIC MECHANISM OF REENTRANT ARRHYTHMIAS: THE CORNERSTONE OF MINES LAW

Observing Mayer's study and macro-reentrant atrioventricular tachycardia in humans, Mines postulated the electrophysiological requirement for the genesis of anatomically determined reentry:

- An anatomically determined circuit is required.
- The circuit must be longer than the impulse wave-front length.
- The product between the conduction velocity and the refractory period defines the impulse wave-front length.
- An excitable gap between the wave-front head and its tail is necessary, allowing the repolarization of the tissue.
- A slow conduction area with a short refractory period is necessary for the circuit genesis.[5,6]

Integrating clinical observations with electrocardiogram (ECG) tracings and animal studies, Sir Thomas Lewis first postulated that atrial flutter is based on a right atrium reentry mechanism.[7] The need for a line of block, for the reentry formation, was later postulated and demonstrated by Rosenblueth and Garcia-Ramos.[8] In the anatomically determined circuit, the cardiac chamber anatomy and the scar provide the arrhythmic substrate and determine the reentry pathway. This circuit shows dimensional stability and the presence of an excitable gap. This gap allows an external impulse to enter the circuit, leading to the resetting, entrainment, and interruption of the arrhythmia.[9]

In the meantime, Alessie and colleagues described functional reentry, based on an impulse that travels around a central core of inexcitable tissue, creating an area of block for the impulse's transmission; thein excitability of the central core is due to the continuous bombing and collision of impulses developing from every point of the peripheral ring, keeping the central core in a refractory state. Neither a stable anatomic location nor a constant length is typical of this reentry type, since the area of the circulating movement can change in size, relating to the extension of the central nucleus. Furthermore, there is not an excitable gap: the circuit cannot be interrupted or reset by an external impulse.[10]

In the anatomically determined circuit, the impulse generation frequency depends on the circuit length and on the conduction speed; instead, in the functional determined circuit, it depends on the refractory period: the shorter is the refractory period, the faster the impulse goes: the impulse velocity depends on the availability of excitable tissue; a refractory period reduction will lead the impulse to propagate in a short circuit and the propagation frequency will, therefore, increase.[10]

Through the electromechanical feedback, the atrium tissue distension causes a refractory period prolongation and a conduction time increase, leading to arrhythmia deceleration in an anatomic circuit; instead, it will increase the conduction in a functional reentry.

Both anatomic (or fixed) and functional reentries require tissues with different electrophysiological properties promoting slow conduction and an excitable myocardium ahead of its leading wave-front.

RIGHT ATRIUM AND ATRIAL FLUTTER: THE ANATOMIC AND PHYSIOLOGIC BASES OF A RELATIONSHIP

Typical atrial flutter is characterized by a macro-reentry circuit whose maintenance mechanism may be found in the right atrium. A well-coded relationship between right atrial structures allows reentry circuit formation and maintenance.

The wave-front runs along a stereotyped macro-reentry-circuit located around the tricuspid valve, which isolates it anteriorly; the circuit is posteriorly delimited by crista terminalis, cava veins, coronary sinus orifice, and Eustachian ridge.[11,12] These structures represent anatomic barriers and allow the reentry circuit to self-maintain.

The wave-front runs along precise paths, identified by specific structures, called isthmuses: the inferior vena cava-tricuspid isthmus (CTI), between the inferior vena cava and the tricuspid valve (**Figs. 1** and **2**); the isthmus located between the crista terminalis and the tricuspid valve; the isthmus located between the coronary sinus orifice and the tricuspid valve.

The right atrium reentry circuit occurrence is allowed by the CTI medial portion, which is a fundamental anatomic element (**Fig. 3**); it is delimited by the anterior edge of the inferior vena cava, the Eustachian ridge, and the tricuspid annulus. It is a slow conduction zone and, therefore, it represents a critical element of the reentry circuit: a slow-conduction zone is essential for the self-sustenance of all macro-reentrant circuits.[13] As far as pathophysiology is concerned, the myocardial muscle trabeculation arrangement is disorganized and extremely variable, and therefore it causes a slow conduction area. In fact, the

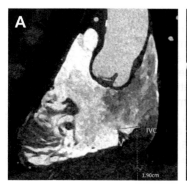 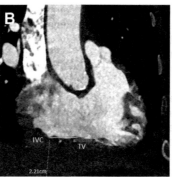 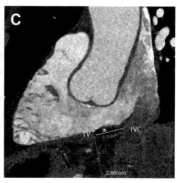

Fig. 1. Inferior vena cava-tricuspid isthmus (CTI) length from cardiac computed tomographic view. The CTI is measured in its middle portion, from the tricuspid valve (TV) to the orifice of the inferior vena cava (IVC). As shown in the figures, CTI length and morphology are variable between people.

terminal muscle bundles of the crista terminalis fan out extending partly anteriorly toward the tricuspid ring and partly upwards, parallel to the tricuspid ring and toward the coronary sinus orifice.[14] The isthmus muscular trabeculation is also separated by thin fibrous tissue areas of variable extension, which also contribute to isthmic conduction slowing.

Muscle trabeculae disorganization determines a slowdown of conduction, as myofibrils conduction in a transverse direction is slower than longitudinal conduction.[15,16] With aging, there is a progressive electrical uncoupling of the side-to-side connections between parallel-oriented atrial fiber groups, while there is no evidence of electrical uncoupling along the fibers' long axis. Therefore, there is the development of extensive collagenous septa that separate small groups of fibers, resulting in a transversal and zigzag course of propagation.[17]

Crista terminalis, Eustachian ridge, and tricuspid annulus are pivotal elements in reentrant circuit establishment and maintenance.

Anatomically, the crista terminalis separates a portion of smooth myocardium, posteriorly, from a portion of nonuniform muscular trabeculation (pectinate muscles), anteriorly; the myocardial strands are arranged perpendicular along the crista terminalis length until, in their final portion, they approach the CTI. During typical atrial flutter, the crista terminalis acts as a barrier and several studies have shown split electrograms along its length.[18–20] The electrical impulse that in a typical atrial flutter reaches the crista terminalis runs anteriorly and posteriorly to the crista. However, only anterior impulse has been demonstrated (with entrainment maneuvers) to belong to the circuit, while the impulse running posteriorly does not

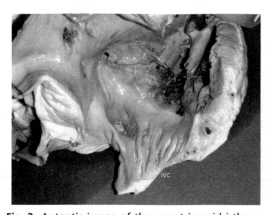

Fig. 2. Autoptic image of the cavo-tricuspid isthmus. Posteriorly it is defined by the Eustachian valve and inferior vena cava (IVC), anteriorly by the tricuspid valve (TV). It can be recognized as the anterior portion of smooth tissue of the isthmus, the tricuspid vestibule; the trabeculate central part of isthmus, that determines a slowdown of conduction, is formed by myocardial bundles by crista terminalis.

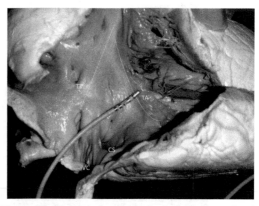

Fig. 3. Koch's triangle anatomic view; the heart is oriented reproducing a right anterior oblique view. An ablation catheter with a 4 mm tip, via the inferior vena cava (IVC), settles into the midseptal area of Koch's triangle. The 2 sides are made, anteriorly, by the hinge of the septal leaflet of the tricuspid annulus (TA) and, posteriorly, by Todaro's tendon (TT). The base of the triangle is represented by the coronary sinus (CS) ostium.

become part of the macro-reentry, and it is subsequently blocked.[21] As demonstrated in multiple studies, the transversal conduction block of crista terminalis during atrial flutter is rate-dependent; therefore, also a functional mechanism of block could be involved.[18–20]

Split electrograms can also be recorded along the length of the Eustachian ridge during typical atrial flutter. Entrainment mapping studies identified that the reentry circuit comprises sites anterior to the Eustachian ridge, whereas posterior sites are excluded.[21,22]

The tricuspid annulus is the anterior barrier of the circuit; activation around the tricuspid annulus can account for 100% of the atrial flutter cycle length[23]; through concealed entrainment, several studies demonstrated that all sites along the length of the tricuspid annulus are within the circuit.

COMMON AND UNCOMMON VARIANTS OF TYPICAL ATRIAL FLUTTER: ONE-WAY PREFERENTIAL CONDUCTION

Typical atrial flutter is a macro-reentry mechanism arrhythmia that, as already explained, walks along precise "rails" delimited by specific anatomic barriers, called isthmuses[24,25] (**Fig. 4**). Through a multipolar catheter around the tricuspid annulus and entrainment maneuvers, it has been demonstrated that macro reentry circuit is confined in the right atrium, with passive activation of the left atrium.[21,26,27]

Using 3-dimensional mapping systems and multipolar catheters around the tricuspid annulus, typical atrial flutter activation mapping shows that the electrical impulse goes downward along the lateral free wall, then through the CTI, after upward the septal wall and, finally, crosses the crista terminalis[28] (**Fig. 5**). Less frequently, the electrical impulse runs across the same circuit (the same "rails") following a reverse direction (clockwise, CW): a caudal-to-cranial direction along the lateral free wall and cranial-to-caudal direction along the interatrial septum.

As already discussed, the CTI is a slow-conduction zone during typical atrial flutter (**Fig. 6**). Furthermore, several studies demonstrated that incremental pacing from the low lateral right atrium and coronary sinus orifice could produce a rate-dependent conduction delay, unidirectional block, and atrial flutter induction at CTI. However, according to some authors, the slowing of isthmus conduction velocity may be demonstrated in all patients, irrespective of history of typical atrial flutter. Instead, according to others, the conduction velocity slowing is present only in patients with clinical or inducible atrial flutter.[13,27,29–31]

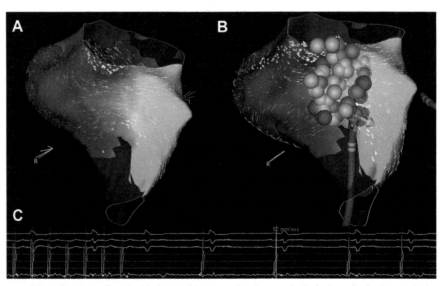

Fig. 4. Accurate identification of critical isthmus (slow conducting region) during clockwise typical atrial flutter using coherent mapping with conduction velocity vectors (CARTO 3 System Version 7 with high-resolution mapping catheter, Biosense Webster Inc.). Dynamic conduction velocity vectors highlight slow conducting areas, represented by thicker conduction velocity vectors, and demonstrate the direction of wave propagation (*A*). Figure (*B*) represents cavo-tricuspid isthmus ablation with Visitag raffiguration: each point represents a radiofrequency pulse (with higher Ablation Index from *red to pink*). Atrial flutter termination can be observed in Figure (*C*); the red potentials are recorded by the coronary sinus electrodes, the white ones by the ablation catheter and the green ones by the surface electrodes.

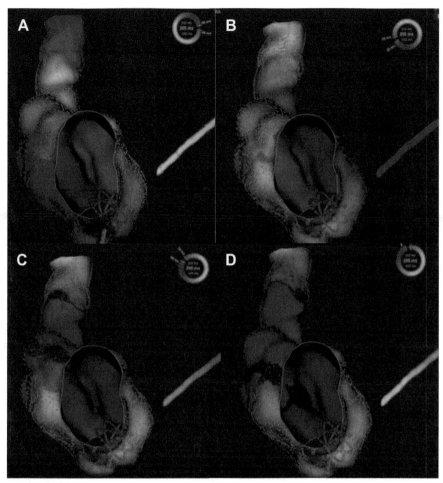

Fig. 5. Typical atrial flutter activation map with ultra-high-density mapping system (Rhythmia©, Boston Scientific). The electrical impulse goes through the cavo-tricuspid isthmus (*A*), then upward the septal wall (*B*), after crosses the crista terminalis (*C*) and finally downward along the lateral free wall (*D*).

Counterclockwise (CCW) atrial flutter is statistically much more frequent than CW atrial flutter; this prevalence is due to preferentially lateral-medial conduction, probably because of the muscle bundles' organization along the CTI. Norishige and colleagues demonstrated that in patients with clinically documented common atrial flutter, CW conduction in the low right atrial isthmus was significantly slower than that in the CCW direction and, when compared with the control subject, only CW conduction was more depressed.[32] Furthermore, after procainamide administration (a drug able to decrease conduction velocity in both directions) CW conduction was preferentially influenced compared with CCW conduction. Similarly, Arenal and colleagues[19] showed that conduction block in crista terminalis is achieved at slower pacing rates from the posterior wall than from the lateral wall: this could explain the crista terminalis role in the greater incidence of CCW atrial flutter.

CRISTA TERMINALIS PHYSIOPATHOLOGY: ANATOMIC AND FUNCTIONAL BLOCK

It has been demonstrated that the atrial flutter reentry circuit is determined by right atrial specific conduction barriers and that the crista terminalis is one of these barriers.[21,33,34] Olgin and colleagues[21,35] suggested that crista terminalis' line of block was fixed and that in patients with atrial flutter microscopic structural abnormalities could be demonstrated in the crista terminalis. However, several subsequent studies have demonstrated that there is no fixed conduction block across the crista terminalis during atrial pacing or induced atrial flutter; therefore, blocks occurring along the crista terminalis are functional in nature.[19,20,24] The crista terminalis rate-dependent conduction block was then demonstrated, suggesting that the line of block during typical atrial flutter is functional. Pacing with longer coupling intervals

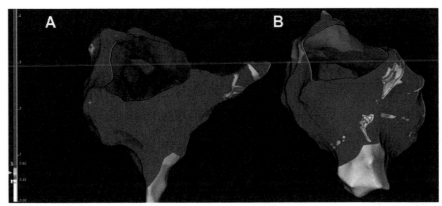

Fig. 6. Wave speed map by the new EnSite Omnipolar Technology, a new color map coded by conduction velocity value giving the value of how fast wave-front is moving. Wave speed map provides a local measurement of how fast or slow the wavefront is traveling on the cardiac surface through a clique. Wave speed is measured in mm/ms or m/s and numeric value can be seen within map metrics. (*A*) Uniform and normal speeds are founded in the cavo-tricuspid isthmus of patients without typical atrial flutter; instead, (*B*) a slow conduction zone con be founded by EnSite Omnipolar Technology in the cavo-tricuspid isthmus of patients with typical atrial flutter.

resulted in a transverse pulse propagation across the crista terminalis; shorter coupling intervals showed split electrograms along the crista, indicating a functional conduction block.[18–20,24] However, in some patients, complete transverse conduction block along the crista terminalis is not achieved and transverse conduction gaps may be found. Some studies demonstrated that during typical atrial flutter the wave-front activation could cross through a gap in the crista terminalis.[36–38] Furthermore, crista terminalis properties proved to be different according to the presence of a clinical atrial flutter. It is suggested that a high degree of block is already present in the crista terminalis of patients with atrial flutter but not in patients without.[20,39] Schumacher and colleagues[18] demonstrated that the longest pacing coupling interval resulting in a complete transverse conduction block at the crista terminalis is significantly longer in patients with atrial flutter. The presence of clinical atrial flutter may thus depend on the conduction properties of the crista terminalis.[20,39]

The functional transverse block along crista terminalis is also conditioned by the structural characteristics of the crista, whose size is greater in the patients with atrial flutter[40,41] (**Fig. 7**). Furthermore, Norishige and colleagues[42] demonstrated that crista terminalis height, width, and area are significantly greater in patients with clinical atrial flutter

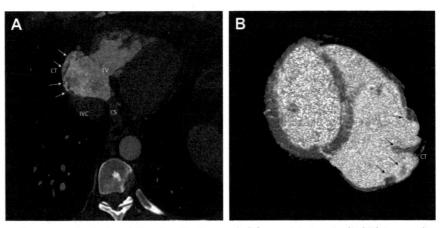

Fig. 7. Nonuniform muscular trabeculation (pectinate muscles) from crista terminalis (CT) in a cardiac computed tomographic view; the myocardial strands are arranged perpendicular along the CT length, in the right atrium lateral wall. The coronary sinus (CS), inferior vena cava (IVC), and tricuspid valve (TV) can also be recognized in the cardiac computed tomographic view (*A*). Figure (*B*) shows 3D volume rendering reconstruction (from cardiac computed tomography) of nonuniform muscular trabeculation from CT.

than in patients without and that crista terminalis inferior portion arborization is more common in patients with clinical atrial flutter. Other structural elements affecting conduction along the crista comprise: the steep slope angle of the crista terminalis on the lateral side[42]; the mismatch between the smooth muscles with small electric capacitance and the pectinate muscle with large electric capacitance[43,44]; and, lastly, histologic changes such as collagen deposition and fibrofatty degeneration and the sparse distribution of gap junction.[15,45,46]

LEFT ATRIUM ROLE DURING TYPICAL ATRIAL FLUTTER: BY-STANDER ELECTROPHYSIOLOGICALLY, ESSENTIAL IN THE PHENOTYPIC ELECTROCARDIOGRAM

During atrial flutter, the left atrium is a by-stander chamber passively activated, and it is not a fundamental circuits component.[47] The left atrium is activated by trans-septal conduction across the coronary sinus, Bachmann's bundle, and fossa ovalis.[47] The 12-lead-ECG flutter wave polarity is mostly determined by left atrium depolarization.[48–50] Primarily, coronary sinus, infero-posteriorly, and Bachmann's bundle, antero-superiorly, represent the 2 main inter-atrial pathways allowing by-stander left atrial activation. Coronary sinus is the major inter-atrial connection during CCW atrial flutter; similarly, Bachmann's bundle during CW atrial flutter and sinus rhythm.[51–53] Through the coronary sinus, which is located in posterior–inferior interatrial septum, the wavefront achieves the left atrium producing caudal-cranial and posterior-to-superior left atrium wall depolarization. When the wavefront crosses along the Bachmann's bundle, situated in the left atrium anterior roof, the left atrium activation proceeds in the opposite direction. Depending on conduction velocity along the inter-atrial structures and upper-to-lower or lower-to-upper left atrium activation, a variable wave-front fusion degree can be obtained, which is reflected in 12-lead-ECG flutter wave polarity.[47] In CCW atrial flutter, the earliest left atrium activation proceeds caudal-cranially from the coronary sinus, inscribing inferior lead negative F wave, until Bachmann's bundle is also activated. Conversely, in CW atrial flutter the earliest left atrium activation proceeds cranium-caudally from the Bachmann's bundle, inscribing positive flutter wave in inferior leads. Hence, left atrium is a by-stander chamber and the macro reentry circuit is confined in the right atrium. CTI block with radiofrequency catheter ablation is the most common and effective therapeutic approach for atrial flutter[54]; it has also been shown that the strategy of combining pulmonary veins isolation + CTI ablation resulted in better long-term arrhythmia-free survival than performing CTI alone in patients with typical flutter, particularly in those aged 55 years.[55]

Lead V1 is also useful to discriminate CCW to CW atrial flutter: a posterior-to-anterior propagation causes V1 positive deflection, while an anterior-to-posterior propagation determines V1's negative polarity. In inferior leads, F wave terminal segment, respectively, in CW or CCW atrial flutter, is negative and positive. The terminal segment polarity, during CW atrial flutter, matches with the inferior-to-superior depolarization of both left (by the coronary sinus wave-front) and right (by the emergence of the CTI) atrium. During CCW atrial flutter, the positive terminal segment is related to the superior-to-inferior right atrium free wall activation.[56] However, 12-lead-ECG peculiar (described above) CCW and CW atrial flutter morphology are infrequent, less than 50% of cases.[56] The right-to-left propagation during atrial flutter may be affected by left atrial disease (ie, left atrial enlargement and fibrosis, coronary sinus catheter ablation...), inducing F wave morphology changes. Coronary sinus or Bachmann's bundle slowing or conduction block may cause different degrees of wave-front fusion in the left atrium and may shift the balance of left atrium activation. Anyway, standard 12-lead-ECG is unlikely to discriminate these variations of dominance.

CLINICS CARE POINTS

- Counterclockwise atrial flutter is more common than clockwise. Catheter ablation is the first-line treatment for both types and the efficacy may be influenced by the anatomical features of the inferior vena cava-tricuspid isthmus.

DISCLOSURE

A.D. Russo is a consultant for Abbott. All other authors declared no conflict of interest.

REFERENCES

1. Kuzmin VS, et Kamensky AA. The molecular and cellular mechanisms of heart pacemaker development in vertebrates. Mosc Univ Biol Sci Bull 2021; 76:147–64.
2. Kistler PM, Chieng D, Tonchev IR, et al. P-Wave morphology in focal atrial tachycardia: an updated

algorithm to predict site of origin. JACC Clin Electrophysiol 2021;7(12):1547–56.

3. Mayer AG. Rhythmical pulsation in scyphomedusae. Carrwgie Inst. Wash.; 1906. Pub. No. 47.

4. Mayer AG. Rhythmical pulsation in scyphomedusae: II. Carwgic Inst. Wash; 1908.

5. Mines GR. On circulating excitations in heart muscles and their possible relation to tachycardia and fibrillation. Trans Roy Soc Gan 1914;8(Ser 3, Sec 4):43.

6. Mines GR. On dynamic equilibrium in the heart. J Physiol 1913;46:349–83.

7. Lewis T, Feil HS, Stround WD. Observations upon flutter and fibrillation: Part II: the nature of auricular flutter. Heart 1920;7:191.

8. Rosenblueth A, Garcia-Ramos J. Studies on flutter and fibrillation. II. The influence of artificial obstacles on experimental auricular flutter. Am Heart J 1947; 33:677–84.

9. Frame LH, Page RL, Hoffman BF. Atrial reentry around an anatomic barrier with a partially refractory excitable gap. A canine model of atrial flutter. Circ Res 1986;58(4):495–511.

10. Allessie MA, Bonke FI, Schopman FJ. Circus movement in rabbit antral muscle as a mechanism of tachycardia. III. The "leading circle" concept: a new model of circus movement in cardiac tissue without the involvement of an anatomical obstacle. Circ Res 1977;41:9–18.

11. Tai C-T, Chen S-A. Conduction barriers of atrial flutter: relation to the anatomy. Pacing Clin Electrophysiol 2008;31(10):1335–42.

12. Jeffrey E, Kalman JM, Lesh MD. Conduction barriers in human atrial flutter: correlation of electrophysiology and anatomy. J Cardiovasc Electrophysiol 1996;7(11):1112–26.

13. Olshansky B, Okumura K, Hess PG, et al. Demonstration of an area of slow conduction in human atrial flutter. J Am Coll Cardiol 1990;16:1639–48.

14. Waki K, Saito T, Becker AE, et al. Right atrial flutter isthmus revisited: normal anatomy favours non-uniform anisotropic conduction. J Cardiovasc Electrophysiol 2000;11:90–4.

15. Spach MS, Miller WT, Dolber PC, et al. The functional role of structural complexities in the propagation of depolarization in the atrium of the dog. Cardiac conduction disturbances due to discontinuities of effective axial resistivity. Circ Res 1982;50:175–91.

16. Spach MS, Josephson ME. Initialing reentry: the role of non-uniform anisotropy in small circuits. J Cardiovasc Electrophysiol 1994;5:182–209.

17. Spach MS, Dolber PC. Relating extracellular potentials and their derivatives in anisotropic propagation at a microscopic level in human cardiac muscle. Evidence for electrical uncoupling of side- to-side fiber connections with increasing age. Circ Res 1986;58: 356–71.

18. Schumacher B, Jung W, Schmidt H, et al. Transverse conduction capabilities of the crista terminalis in patients with atrial flutter and atrial fibrillation. J Am Coll Cardiol 1999;34:363–73.

19. Arenal A, Almendral J, Alday JM, et al. Rate-dependent conduction block of the crista terminalis in patients with typical atrial flutter. Circulation 1999;99: 2771–8.

20. Tai CT, Chen SA, Yu WC, et al. Conduction properties of the crista terminalis in patients with typical atrial flutter: basis for a line of block in the reentrant circuit. J Cardiovasc Electrophysiol 1998;9:811–9.

21. Olgin JE, Kalman JM, Fitzpatrick AP, et al. Role of right atrial endocardial structures as barriers to conduction during human type I atrial flutter. Circulation 1995;92:1839–48.

22. Huang JL, Tai CT, Liu TY, et al. High-resolution mapping around the Eustachian ridge during typical atrial flutter. J Cardiovasc Electrophysiol 2006;17: 1187–92.

23. Nakagawa H, Lazzara R, Khastgir T, et al. Role of the tricuspid annulus and the Eustachian valve/ridge on atrial flutter. Circulation 1996;94:407–24.

24. Matsuo K, Uno K, Khrestian CM, et al. Conduction left-to-right and right-to-left across the crista terminalis. Am J Physiol Heart Circ Physiol 2001;280: H1683–91.

25. Friedman PA, Luria D, Fenton AM, et al. Global right atrial mapping of human atrial flutter: the presence of posteromedial (sinus venosa region) functional block and double potentials: a study in biplane fluoroscopy and intracardiac echocardiography. Circulation 2000;101:1568–77.

26. Cosio FG, Arribas F, Lopez-Gil M, et al. Atrial flutter mapping and ablation. Studying atrial flutter mechanisms by mapping and entrainment. PACE 1996;19: 841–53.

27. Kalman JM, Olgin GE, Saxon LA, et al. Activation and entrainment mapping defines the tricuspid annulus as the anterior barrier in typical atrial flutter. Circulation 1996;94:398–406.

28. Tai C-T, Chen SA. Electrophysiological mechanisms of atrial flutter. J Chin Med Assoc 2009;72(2):60–7.

29. Tai CT, Chen SA, Chiang CE, et al. Characterization of low right atrial isthmus as the slow conduction zone and pharmacological target in typical atrial flutter. Circulation 1997;96:2601–11.

30. Feld GK, Mollerus M, Birgersdotter-Green U, et al. Conduction velocity in the tricuspid valve-inferior vena cava isthmus is slower in patients with type I atrial flutter compared to those without a history of atrial flutter. J Cardiovasc Electrophysiol 1997;8: 1338–48.

31. Lin JL, Lai L, Lin L, et al. Electrophysiological determinant for induction of isthmus dependent counterclockwise and clockwise atrial flutter in humans. Heart 1999;81(1):73–81.

32. Morita N, Kobayashi Y, Ivasaki YK, et al. Pronounced effect of procainamide on clockwise right atrial isthmus conduction compared with counterclockwise conduction: possible mechanism of the greater incidence of common atrial flutter during antiarrhythmic therapy. J Cardiovasc Electrophysiol 2002;13(3):212–22.

33. Frame LH, Page RL, Boyden PA, et al. Circus movement in the canine atrium around the tricuspid ring during experimental atrial flutter and during reentry in vitro. Circulation 1987;76:1155–75.

34. Arribas F, Lòpez-Gil M, Cosio FG, et al. The upper link of human common atrial flutter circuit: definition by multiple endocardial recordings during entrainment. PACE Pacing Clin Electrophysiol 1997;20: 2924–9.

35. Olgin JE, Kalman JM, Lesh MD, et al. Conduction barriers in human atrial flutter: correlation of electrophysiology and anatomy. J Cardiovasc Electrophysiol 1996;7:1112–26.

36. Tai C-T, Huang JL, Lee PC, et al. High-resolution mapping around the crista terminalis during typical atrial flutter: new insights into mechanisms. J Cardiovasc Electrophysiol 2004;15(4):406–14.

37. Schilling RJ, Peters NS, Goldberger J, et al. Characterization of the anatomy and conduction velocities of the human right atrial flutter circuit determined by noncontact mapping. J Am Coll Cardiol 2001; 38:385–93.

38. Chen J, Hoff PI, Erga KS, et al. Global right atrial mapping delineates double posterior lines of block in patients with typical atrial flutter: a study using a three-dimensional noncontact mapping system. J Cardiovasc Electrophysiol 2003;14:1041–8.

39. Hiroshige Y, Misumi I, Fukushima H, et al. Conduction properties of the crista terminalis and its influence on the right atrial activation sequence in patients with typical atrial flutter. Pacing Clin Electrophysiol 2002;25(2):132–41.

40. Mizumaki K, Fujiki A, Nagasawa H, et al. Relation between transverse conduction capability and the anatomy of the crista terminalis in patients with atrial flutter and atrial fibrillation: analysis by intracardiac echocardiography. Circ J 2002;66:1113–8.

41. Ohkubo K, Watanabe I, Okumura Y, et al. Anatomic and electrophysiological differences between chronic and paroxysmal atrial flutter: intracardiac echocardiographic analysis. Pacing Clin Electrophysiol 2008;31:432–7.

42. Morita N, Kobayashi Y, Horie T, et al. The undetermined geometrical factors contributing to the transverse conduction block of the crista terminalis Pacing. Clin Electrophysiol 2009;32(7):868–78.

43. De La Fuente D, Sasyniuk B, Moe GK, et al. Conduction through a narrow isthmus in isolated canine atrial tissue. A model of the WPW syndrome. Circulation 1971;44:803–9.

44. Mendez C, Mueller WJ, Urguiaga X, et al. Propagation of impulses across the Purkinje fiber-muscle junctions in the dog heart. Circ Res 1970;26:135–50.

45. Saffitz JE, Kanter HL, Green KG, et al. Tissue-specific determinants of anisotropic conduction velocity in canine atrial and ventricular myocardium. Circ Res 1994;74:1065–70.

46. Matsuyama TA, Inoue S, Kobayashi Y, et al. Anatomical diversity and age-related histological changes in the human right atrial posterolateral wall. Europace 2004;6:307–15.

47. Rodriguez L-M, Timmermans C, Nabar A, et al. Biatrial activation in isthmus-dependent atrial flutter. Circulation 2001;104(21):2545–50.

48. Ndrepepa G, Zrenner B, Deisenhofer, I, et al. Relationship between surface electrocardiogram characteristics and endocardial activation sequence in patients with typical atrial flutter. Z Kardiol 2000; 89(6):527–37.

49. Okumura K, Plumb VJ, Pagé PL, et al. Atrial activation sequence during atrial flutter in the canine pericarditis model and its effects on the polarity of the flutter wave in the electrocardiogram. J Am Coll Cardiol 1991;17:509–18.

50. Schoels W, Offner B, Brachmann J, et al. Circus movement atrial flutter in the canine sterile pericarditis model. Relation of characteristics of the surface electrocardiogram and conduction properties of the reentrant pathway. J Am Coll Cardiol 1994;23: 799–808.

51. Rodriguez E, Callans DJ, Gottlieb CD, et al. Right atrial activation with coronary sinus pacing: in-sight into patterns of interatrial conduction. J Am Coll Cardiol 1999;33:151A.

52. Roithinger FX, Cheng J, SippensGroenewegen A, et al. Use of electroanatomical mapping to delineate trans-septal atrial conduction in humans. Circulation 1999;100:1791–7.

53. Saoudi N, Nair M, Abdelazziz A, et al. Electrocardiographic patterns and results of radiofrequency catheter ablation of clockwise type I atrial flutter. J Cardiovasc Electrophysiol 1996;7:931–42.

54. Cosio FG, Lopez-Gil M, Goicolea A, et al. Radiofrequency ablation of the inferior vena cava-tricuspid valve isthmus in common atrial flutter. Am J Cardiol 1993;71:705–9.

55. Mohanty S, Natale A, Mohanty P, et al. Pulmonary vein isolation to reduce future risk of atrial fibrillation in patients undergoing typical flutter ablation: results from a randomized pilot study (REDUCE AF). J Cardiovasc Electrophysiol 2015;26(8):819–25.

56. Milliez P, Richardson AW, Obioha-Ngwu O, et al. Variable electrocardiographic characteristics of isthmus-dependent atrial flutter. J Am Coll Cardiol 2002;40:1125–32.

Pathophysiology of Atypical Atrial Flutters

Jacopo Marazzato, MD[a,b], Raffaella Marazzi, MD[a], Lorenzo Adriano Doni, MD[a], Federico Blasi, MD[a,b], Fabio Angeli, MD[b,c], Giuseppe Bagliani, MD[d], Fabio M. Leonelli, MD[e], Roberto De Ponti, MD, FHRS[a,b],*

KEYWORDS

- Atypical atrial flutter • Catheter ablation • Physiopathology • Supraventricular tachycardia

KEY POINTS

- Atypical atrial flutters (AAFLs) are complex supraventricular arrhythmias promoted by macro-reentrant mechanisms. However, differently from typical atrial flutters, the cavotricuspid isthmus plays no role in these atypical arrhythmias.
- If slow conduction caused by atrial scarring and associated with structural heart disease does represent the main pathophysiological hallmark of these complex tachycardias, AAFLs may even occur in apparently healthy subjects.
- To set out the ablation strategy, three-dimensional mapping systems have proved invaluable in helping the cardiac electrophysiologist understand the electrophysiological complexity of these circuits and easily identify and target areas essential for a successful catheter ablation procedure.

INTRODUCTION

Atypical atrial flutters (AAFLs) are complex supraventricular tachyarrhythmias stemming from the right as well as the left atrial chamber and resulting from a variety of pathophysiological mechanisms.[1] However, the cavotricuspid isthmus is excluded in their diagnostic definition[2] and atrial scarring is invariably associated with these complex circuits.[3–6] Although heart surgery[7] and nonsurgical pulmonary vein isolation (PVI)[8] do represent the most common sources of AAFL, these complex atrial arrhythmias may also be encountered in patients with no overt structural heart disease and, therefore, with no apparent reasons for atrial scarring.[9,10] Moreover, despite the implementation of cutting-edge technologies, such as three-dimensional electroanatomic mapping systems and high-density mapping tools, the results of catheter ablation of AAFL are still suboptimal with little role played by antiarrhythmic medications in this setting.[11]

Therefore, to provide more insights into the complex world of AAFL and, thus, to help the cardiac electrophysiologists to better manage these circuits, the clinical scenarios involved in atrial substrate modification and the ensuing pathophysiological and arrhythmogenic mechanisms are thoroughly discussed in this article.

CARDIAC PROCEDURES AND CLINICAL CONDITIONS ASSOCIATED WITH ATYPICAL ATRIAL FLUTTERS

Box 1 summarizes the major clinical scenarios associated with AAFL. As shown in **Box 1**, surgical

a Department of Heart and Vessels, Ospedale di Circolo, Viale Borri, 57, Varese 21100, Italy; b Department of Medicine and Surgery, University of Insubria, Viale Guicciardini, 9, Varese 21100, Italy; c Department of Medicine and Cardiopulmonary Rehabilitation, Maugeri Care and Research Institutes, IRCCS, Via Crotto Roncaccio, 16, Tradate, Varese 21049, Italy; d Cardiology and Arrhythmology Clinic, Marche Polytechnic University, University Hospital "Ospedali Riuniti Umberto I-Lancisi-Salesi", Via Conca 71, Ancona 60126, Italy; e Cardiology Department, James A. Haley Veterans' Hospital, University of South Florida, 13000 Bruce B Down Boulevard, Tampa, FL 33612, USA
* Corresponding author. Department of Heart and Vessels, Ospedale di Circolo, Viale Borri, 57, Varese 21100, Italy
E-mail address: roberto.deponti@uninsubria.it

Card Electrophysiol Clin 14 (2022) 411–420
https://doi.org/10.1016/j.ccep.2022.03.002

atriotomies performed for the correction of congenital heart diseases[3] or acquired mitral valve disorders[12,13] do represent well-acknowledged fertile substrates for non–isthmus-dependent atrial flutter (AFL).[3,14] Moreover, surgical ablation of atrial fibrillation (AF) performed in addition to heart valve surgery seems to boost the hazard of these postsurgical tachycardias,[12,15] and similar observations have been reported for patients undergoing nonsurgical ablation of AF.[16] Independently from the energy source used,[17,18] the incidence of AAFL after nonsurgical PVI greatly varies depending on the chosen ablation strategy: From less than 4% after ostial or antral PVI[19] to 31% for circumferential PVI (i.e., CPVA [circumferential pulmonary vein ablation] technique),[20] especially when further ablation lines are deployed in the left atrium.[8]

However, arrhythmogenic circuits sustaining AAFL have also been mapped and ablated in anatomic areas distantly located from prior atriotomies or ablation lines.[21,22] In this regard, investigating a surgical population by means of three-dimensional electroanatomic mapping systems, Zhou and colleagues showed how nonincisional scars would play an important role in AAFL occurrence[22]; insufficient arterial supply and scarce protection during cardioplegia, surgical trauma,[3] and, not the least, the electroanatomic atrial remodeling progressively occurring after heart surgery may all represent potential sources of atrial scarring beyond surgical atriotomies in these patients.[22] Similar mechanisms seem involved in nonsurgical PVI where arrhythmogenic circuits revolving around the anterior left atrial wall, and distantly located from more posteriorly ablation lines, have been also described.[21]

Interestingly, as the result of overt structural heart disease, atrial scars can also be found in populations naïve to any prior interventional or cardiac surgical procedures. By performing atrial substrate mapping in patients suffering from rheumatic heart disease, John and colleagues recorded vast areas of low atrial voltages as a result of the progressive atrial remodeling occurring in this setting.[23] However, up to 6% of all right-sided AAFL may even occur in patients with no clear evidence of structural heart disease.[24] Electrical silent areas located at the posterior or lateral free wall of the right atrium would explain the arrhythmogenic substrate for most of these cases. In fact, during ongoing tachycardia, the electrical wavefront may revolve around these areas of electrical silence which could be successfully interrupted by radiofrequency (RF) transection of an anatomic area superiorly bounded by the inferior pole of these scars and inferiorly by the inferior vena cava os.[24,25] However, narrow electrical channels or isthmi of remarkably slow conduction may also be found within areas of dense scarring, generally sustaining circuits that could be amenable to effective RF ablation.[24] This would also represent the major arrhythmogenic mechanism in left-sided tachycardias occurring in patients with no overt structural heart disease on account of the crisscrossing of thick epicardial fibers, Bachmann bundle included, which would enhance slow conduction in the common anteroseptal circuits observed in this setting.[24]

A variety of mechanisms may underpin spontaneous scarring in these patients. If "smoldering"

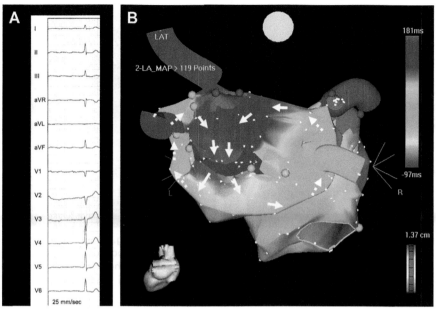

Fig. 1. (*A, B*) Twelve-lead electrocardiogram and activation biatrial mapping in postero-anterior view of AAFL with cycle length of 280 ms in a male patient with no evident heart disease. In (*A*), low-voltage P-waves are evident in both peripheral and precordial leads. In (*B*), the arrhythmia is sustained by two loops around the left and right pulmonary veins and sharing the same critical isthmus located in the postero-lateral left atrium bordered by the area of double potentials (blue and pink dots). This represents the so-called figure-of-eight reentry. The conduction velocity and the bipolar voltage calculated in the critical isthmus were critically low: 26 cm/s and 0.23 ± 0.09 mV, respectively. Tubes represent pulmonary veins; dotted arrows indicate the orientation of the loop in the opposite atrial wall.

structural heart disease may promote chronic stretch of myocardial fibers and unwanted effect of angiotensin II activation, thus leading to scar formation,[25] these complex arrhythmias may also occur in patients with normal atrial size and left ventricular ejection fraction.[24,25] Chronically increased atrial pressure overload in hypertensive patients, occlusion of small atrial branches of epicardial coronary arteries, and isolated inflammation or amyloid infiltration in elderly patients may all be responsible for these circuits even in apparently normal hearts.[9,24] **Figs. 1–3** show two cases of mapping and ablation of a left and right figure-of-eight macro-reentrant circuits, respectively, in patients with no prior surgical/percutaneous interventions nor clear evidence of structural heart disease.

Moreover, as to right-sided circuits, a further mechanism has been described even in the absence of major atrial voltage abnormalities. Different authors[9,24] reported the presence of electrical gaps across lines of double potentials located at the posterior wall of the right atrium and essentially represented by transverse conduction across the crista terminalis. The ensued wide macro-reentrant circuit revolving around the superior vena cava, also known as upper loop reentry,

would be the result of the complex interaction between tissue anisotropy, gap junction distribution, and wavefront curvature,[9] which would all lead to the electrical permeability of this anatomic structure. Likewise, nonuniform anisotropy due to the complex interweaving of myocardial fibers in the interatrial septum[10] would represent a further mechanism of origin of AAFL in perfectly normal hearts.[26]

SUBSTRATE MODIFICATION AND THE ENSUING TACHYCARDIA MECHANISMS IN ATYPICAL ATRIAL FLUTTER

Whatever the underlying heart disease, the described atrial substrate modification may lead to slow-conducting areas that represent the pathophysiological hallmark of AAFL.[8,27,28] In an elegant experimental study conducted on canine hearts, Melby and colleagues showed that anatomic gaps left between ablation lines were associated with slow conduction, and the narrower the gap the slower the conduction velocity.[27] Similar observations were recorded in human beings undergoing both conventional and three-dimensional electroanatomic mapping for post-CPVA AAFL.[8] In this scenario,

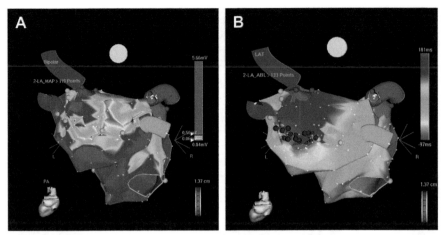

Fig. 2. Voltage (*A*) and activation (*B*) biatrial maps in the same patient as in **Fig. 1**. In (*A*), bipolar voltage mapping identifies a low-voltage area in the posterior wall of the left atrium; the rainbow of colors between red and blue indicates signal amplitude between 0.06 and 0.5 mV. In (*B*), red dots indicate the ablation line connecting the two areas of double potentials. No arrhythmia was inducible after ablation and the follow-up of this patient was uneventful.

Deisenhofer and colleagues showed how slow conduction played a major role in gap-related arrhythmias and, as a further proof of these findings, during mapping of these circuits, up to 60% of tachycardia cycle length was covered by a single fractionated diastolic potential lasting up to 140 ms.[8] Likewise, using three-dimensional electroanatomic mapping systems and a specific setting of the window of interest,[29] it was shown that narrow anatomic areas critical to the tachycardia circuit displayed areas of low bipolar voltages clearly associated with remarkably slow conduction (33 ± 21 cm/s on average)[28] in keeping with prior observations defining slow-conducting areas for conduction velocities smaller than 60 cm/s.[5]

The connection between slow conduction and arrhythmogenesis in AAFL was clarified in studies conducted on animal models[30] and human beings,[3,5–7,29,31] in which reentry proved to be the link between slow conduction and arrhythmogenesis. As shown by Allessie and colleagues in his seminal

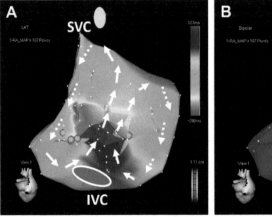
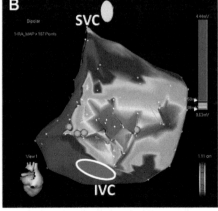

Fig. 3. Activation (*A*) and voltage (*B*) right atrial map in the postero-lateral view in a male patient with no evident heart disease. Similarly to what shown in **Fig. 1**, a figure-of-eight double loop reentry with both loops sharing the same slow-conduction isthmus is present in the right atrium (panel *A*). Arrows indicate a clockwise loop around the tricuspid annulus and a second loop in the posterior region of the right atrium. The small critical isthmus, shared by both loops and measuring 24 mm, is limited by two areas of double potentials (*blue dots*). The conduction velocity measured in the critical isthmus was very low (19 cm/s). Impressively, the bipolar voltage map (*B*) shows very low voltage (red areas) in the postero-lateral wall of the right atrium with mean bipolar voltage of 0.09 ± 0.02 mV in the critical isthmus. IVC and SVC indicate inferior and superior vena cava, respectively.

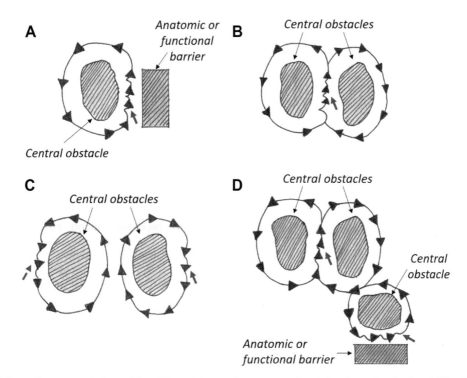

Fig. 4. Schematic representation of the different types of macro-reentrant circuits underpinning AAFLs. Panel (*A*) shows a single loop reentry detouring an area of dense scar (central obstacle) sustained by areas of slow conduction bounded by dense scar and anatomic or functional barriers. In up to 60% of cases, AAFLs show more complex, figure-of-eight circuits with two loops rotating in opposite directions and sharing a common critical isthmus of slow conduction (*B*) or, conversely, revolving around two areas of dense scar as separate circuits as shown in (*C*). Finally, in (*D*), even more complex circuits could be expected in this setting with multiple electrical wavefronts rotating around patchy areas of atrial scars and functional or anatomic barriers promoting different areas of remarkably slow conduction, thus sustaining more reentrant circuits. Tortuous arrows indicated by red arrows indicate areas of slow conduction.

work on rabbits,[30] reentry is essentially represented by the unidirectional conduction block of a premature impulse leading to a one-way electrical wavefront revolving around a central obstacle. Only when the resumption of electrical excitability is fully established at the site of the conduction block, reentry is fully maintained itself in a carousel-like pattern,[30] provided that the anterograde electrical wavefront is slow enough to warrant the reentrant circuit. These findings have also been observed in humans. Kalman and colleagues first proved the reentrant nature of AAFL by conventional mapping in patients with prior history of surgery for congenital heart disease.[7] The authors put forward the existence of narrow anatomic channels clearly associated with concealed entrainment and an unremarkable difference between the postpacing interval and the tachycardia cycle length, as assessed on a roving catheter during pacing maneuvers.[7,31] Furthermore, using three-dimensional electroanatomic mapping systems, Jaïs and colleagues first showed how macro-reentry should be held

responsible for most right-sided and left-sided AAFL[5] successfully treated by RF ablation by targeting narrow channels bounded by areas of double potentials and electrical silence (i.e., <0.05 mV on voltage maps).[5] However, in contrast to other studies,[3,6,8] the authors quite surprisingly reported that slow conduction was not consistently observed at these ablation sites.[5] In fact, in accordance with the available evidence,[3,6,8,28] not only should the critical isthmus be anatomically defined[5] but also regarded as a functional structure associated with low bipolar voltages, fragmented electrograms,[6,31] slow conduction,[28] and a typical mid-diastolic activation during ongoing tachycardia,[7] suggesting that the identification of this critical region is paramount for the understanding of the pathophysiology of these circuits and, therefore, prompting a successful catheter ablation procedure.[29]

Supported by the available evidence in this field, **Fig. 4** displays a schematic representation of the most common macro-reentrant circuits occurring in patients with AAFL.

LOCALIZED REENTRY AND PATHOPHYSIOLOGY OF UNMAPPABLE CIRCUITS

In addition to macro-reentrant circuits, localized reentry has been commonly described in left-sided AAFL occurring after catheter ablation of AF.[8,32,33]

Using conventional mapping, different electrophysiologic criteria have been put forward to define these small circuits as follows: (1) a reentrant circuit diameter $\leq$ 3 cm,[5] (2) the identification of atrial electrograms covering more than 80% of the tachycardia cycle length at the site of earliest activation confirmed by both (3) entrainment maneuvers and (4) a postpacing interval less than 30 ms at the identified site, (5) the recording of a zone of slow conduction, and, finally, (6) the centrifugal electrical activation of the atrium from this area.[32,33] The implementation of three-dimensional electroanatomic mapping systems and high-density mapping tools has further proved the reentrant mechanism underpinning these circuits,[8] which could be as small as 1 cm in diameter[34] with multiple slow-conducting channels along their course.[35] Although limited by the resolution capacity of the employed mapping system, a true focal mechanism should nonetheless be suspected when a centrifugal activation stemming from a unique focus is observed on activation maps. Although cellular uncoupling[36] does promote micro-reentry in most of these cases, triggered activity and enhanced automatism have been also described in this complex scenario.[37,38] Failure to interrupt or modify the tachycardia cycle length by intravenous injection of adenosine bolus may favor the micro-reentrant nature of incredibly small-sized circuits.[37,38]

Finally, in a few cases, the true arrhythmogenic mechanism of these complex atrial arrhythmias cannot be clearly identified. During mapping and ablation of these circuits, some activation maps might not be completed due to spontaneous tachycardia interruption, irregular cycle length of the investigated arrhythmia, change to other morphologies, or degeneration in AF.[5] Careful interpretation of both electrical signals and activation maps during ongoing tachycardia are paramount to clarify the arrhythmia mechanism and set out an effective ablation strategy.

CAVOTRICUSPID ISTHMUS-DEPENDENT AFL WITH AN ATYPICAL ELECTROCARDIOGRAPHIC PRESENTATION: AN UNEXPECTED FINDING

As appraised in both animal models[39] and human beings with isthmus-dependent AFL,[40,41] the dominant flutter wave polarity on 12-lead ECG is clearly associated with the left atrial site of earliest electrical breakthrough during ongoing arrhythmia. Therefore, as observed on surface ECG, a negative sawtooth pattern in the inferior leads with a positive polarity in the right precordial ones is generally expected during typical counterclockwise AFL because of the earliest activation occurring at the infero-posterior atrial region. Conversely, thanks to a more antero-superior left atrial breakthrough involving electrical conduction over the Bachmann bundle, positive and notched flutter waves in the inferior leads with a specular and negative polarity in right precordial ones are commonly recorded during typical clockwise AFL.[40,41] As a result of these findings, in case of any other flutter wave morphology encountered on 12-lead ECG, the arrhythmia should be regarded as AAFL.[2] However, it is worth considering that up to 40% of patients with an atypical electrocardiographic presentation may, in fact, be diagnosed with isthmus-dependent AFL during an electrophysiology study.[42]

Both interatrial conduction block and altered intraatrial electrical activation may explain these findings. During RF catheter ablation of cavotricuspid isthmus in a patient with typical counterclockwise AFL, Zrenner and colleagues[43] reported abrupt modifications of flutter wave morphology observed on the inferior leads, from a typical, predominantly negative, sawtooth pattern to an upright flutter wave polarity. No changes in flutter wave morphology were observed in the right precordial on surface ECG in this patient. As reported by the authors, these ECG changes were recorded when catheter ablation was commenced at a low posteromedial region of the cavotricuspid isthmus, between the tricuspid annulus and the coronary sinus os. Based on the remarkable coronary sinus activation delay observed after RF ablation in this anatomic region together with no reported changes in the right atrial activation sequence nor tachycardia cycle length, the authors concluded that the iatrogenic damage wrought to the coronary sinus musculature would have blocked the lower interatrial connections, thus prompting a different left atrial breakthrough that would have been high enough to reverse the left atrial activation direction and electrocardiographic polarity of the flutter waves. However, not only would debulking of interatrial connections be responsible for an atypical electrocardiographic presentation of cavotricuspid-dependent AFL, but, as observed in both surgical[44] and nonsurgical ablation of AF,[45] altered intraatrial conduction within the left atrium may also cause this unexpected pathophysiological finding.

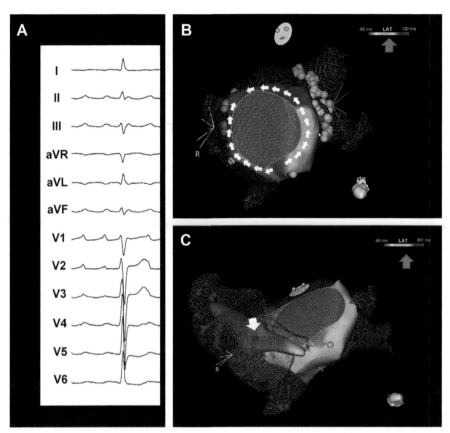

Fig. 5. Twelve lead electrocardiograms (*A*), left atrial activation mapping (*B*), and biatrial activation mapping superimposed to three-dimensional rendering of computed tomography during an isthmus-dependent counterclockwise AFL in a 59-year-old woman with previous history of combined aortic and mitral valve surgery for the correction of rheumatic heart disease. In (*A*), the electrocardiographic pattern resembles the one of an AAFL with positive flutter wave morphology in the inferior and right precordial leads, appearing upon achievement of pulmonary vein isolation performed for concomitant atrial fibrillation. In (*B*), during AFL with cycle length of 360 ms, left atrial activation mapping shows a focal-like activation pattern spreading from the infero-medial left atrium around the mitral annulus and covering only 48% of the flutter cycle length (blue arrow). After continuation of activation mapping into the right atrial chamber (*C*), the flutter activation was reconstructed for greater than 90% (blue arrow) and a clear counter-clockwise peritricuspid loop was identified with a remarkably slow conduction and low atrial voltage in the cavotricuspid isthmus. Radiofrequency energy ablation (red dots) in this region early interrupted the arrhythmia and produced bidirectional block. Patient's anatomy, prior surgery, and ablation were responsible for the atypical electrocardiographic presentation in this patient.

In fact, using three-dimensional electroanatomic mapping systems, Chug and colleagues[45] observed that most patients undergoing mapping of typical counterclockwise AFL after PVI showed different flutter wave morphologies on surface ECG compared with controls with no prior PVI history, spanning from a biphasic morphology to a clearly upright polarity in the inferior leads. As supported by the examination of both biatrial voltage and propagation maps of these circuits, the authors concluded that iatrogenic intraatrial debulking within the left atrium was mainly responsible for an atypical ECG presentation of a typical cavotricuspid-isthmus-dependent AFL. In this regard, on account of these PVI-related low bipolar voltages in the left atrium, the caudocranial atrial activation generally responsible for the well-known sawtooth pattern observed on surface ECG in the typical forms of this arrythmia was clearly overshadowed by the unopposed craniocaudal electrical activation occurring in anterolateral region of the right atrium. This explains the positive flutter wave polarity observed on the inferior leads in patients with prior PVI history. Likewise, negative flutter waves in the inferior leads in patients with clockwise AFL are likely due to an unopposed caudocranial right atrial activation occurring in this setting.

Therefore, prompt recognition of an atypical ECG presentation of a typical cavotricuspid isthmus-dependent AFL is paramount to lower the risk of pointless, time-consuming procedures. In these cases, the use of cutting-edge technologies to carry out proper biatrial mapping is required. Failure to account for more than 50% of the tachycardia cycle length in the left atrial chamber usually implies that the tachycardia circuit is located in the opposite atrial chamber.[45] In a patient with prior history of heart valve surgery, **Fig. 5** shows a case of mapping and ablation of a seeming left-sided AAFL which is, in fact, a cavotricuspid isthmus-dependent arrhythmia.

SUMMARY

Despite the inherent complexity, AAFL share different pathophysiological aspects in common. These circuits are associated with atrial scars and sustained by a slow-conducting area, so-called critical isthmus, which are essential for the tachycardia macro-reentrant circuit. Although atrial scarring is invariably associated with surgical scars and structural heart disease, areas of non-uniform anisotropy bounded by functional and anatomic barriers may well explain the reason why these arrhythmias may even occur in the absence of scar and structural heart disease. Moreover, three-dimensional mapping systems proved to be invaluable in this setting, helping the cardiac electrophysiologist understand the electrophysiological complexity of these circuit and precisely identify areas of electrical silence, double potentials, and low bipolar voltages, which are all paramount to set out the ablation strategy. However, information provided by these systems should properly be interpreted to clarify the arrhythmia mechanism and guide ablation.

CLINICS CARE POINTS

- Accurate evaluation of patients with atypical atrial flutter and no heart disease is needed, as an atrial myopathy can be present.
- Identification of the reentry course and the slow conduction area is essential to understand the tachycardia mechanism and define the most appropriate ablation strategy

- A subset of patients with cavotricuspid isthmus-dependent atrial flutter has an atypical electrocardiographic pattern especially after prior surgical or percutaneous interventions

CONFLICTS OF INTEREST DISCLOSURE

Dr R. De Ponti has received fees for lectures and scientific cooperation from Biosense Webster. None for the other authors. No funding sources to be acknowledged.

REFERENCES

1. Bun SS, Latcu DG, Marchlinski F, et al. Atrial flutter: more than just one of a kind. Eur Heart J 2015;36: 2356–63.
2. Saoudi N, Chairman MD, Cosio F, et al. Classification of atrial flutter and regular atrial tachycardia according to electrophysiologic mechanism and anatomic bases: a statement from a Joint Expert Group from the Working Group of Arrhythmias of the European Society of Cardiology and the North A. J Cardiovasc Electrophysiol 2001;12(7):852–66.
3. Nakagawa H, Shah N, Matsudaira K, et al. Characterization of reentrant circuit in macroreentrant right atrial tachycardia after surgical repair of congenital heart disease. Circulation 2001;103:699–709.
4. Kall JG, Rubenstein DS, Kopp DE, et al. Atypical atrial flutter originating in the right atrial free wall. Circulation 2000;101:270–9.
5. Jaïs P, Shah DC, Haïssaguerre M, et al. Mapping and ablation of left atrial flutters. Circulation 2000; 101:2928–34.
6. Ouyang F, Ernst S, Vogtmann T, et al. Characterization of reentrant circuits in left atrial macroreentrant tachycardia: critical isthmus block can prevent atrial tachycardia recurrence. Circulation 2002;105: 1934–42.
7. Kalman JM, VanHare GF, Olgin JE, et al. Ablation of 'incisional' reentrant atrial tachycardia complicating surgery for congenital heart disease. Circulation 1996;93:502–12.
8. Deisenhofer I, Estner H, Zrenner B, et al. Left atrial tachycardia after circumferential pulmonary vein ablation for atrial fibrillation: incidence, electrophysiological characteristics, and results of radiofrequency ablation. Europace 2006;8:573–82.
9. Tai CT, Huang JL, Lin YK, et al. Noncontact three-dimensional mapping and ablation of upper loop re-entry originating in the right atrium. J Am Coll Cardiol 2002;40:746–53.
10. Marrouche NF, Natale A, Wazni OM, et al. Left septal atrial flutter: electrophysiology, anatomy, and results of ablation. Circulation 2004;109:2440–7.

11. Natale A, Newby KH, Pisanó E, et al. Prospective randomized comparison of antiarrhythmic therapy versus first- line radiofrequency ablation in patients with atrial flutter. J Am Coll Cardiol 2000;35: 1898–904.

12. Marazzato J, Cappabianca G, Angeli F, et al. Ablation of atrial tachycardia in the setting of prior mitral valve surgery. Minerva Cardiol Angiol 2021;69:94–101.

13. Marazzato J, Cappabianca G, Angeli F, et al. Catheter ablation of atrial tachycardias after mitral valve surgery: a systematic review and meta-analysis. J Cardiovasc Electrophysiol 2020;31:2632–41.

14. Markowitz SM, Brodman RF, Stein KM, et al. Lesional tachycardias related to mitral valve surgery. J Am Coll Cardiol 2002;39:1973–83.

15. Gopinathannair R, Mar PL, Afzal MR, et al. Atrial tachycardias after surgical atrial fibrillation ablation: clinical characteristics, electrophysiological mechanisms, and ablation outcomes from a large, multicenter study. JACC Clin Electrophysiol 2017;3: 865–74.

16. Morady F, Oral H, Chugh A. Diagnosis and ablation of atypical atrial tachycardia and flutter complicating atrial fibrillation ablation. Hear Rhythm 2009;6(8 SUPPL):S29–32.

17. Akerström F, Bastani H, Insulander P, et al. Comparison of regular atrial tachycardia incidence after circumferential radiofrequency versus cryoballoon pulmonary vein isolation in real-life practice. J Cardiovasc Electrophysiol 2014;25:948–52.

18. Ciconte G, Baltogiannis G, De Asmundis C, et al. Circumferential pulmonary vein isolation as index procedure for persistent atrial fibrillation: a comparison between radiofrequency catheter ablation and second-generation cryoballoon ablation. Europace 2015;17:559–65.

19. Wasmer K, Mönnig G, Bittner A, et al. Incidence, characteristics, and outcome of left atrial tachycardias after circumferential antral ablation of atrial fibrillation. Hear Rhythm 2012;9:1660–6.

20. Pappone C, Oreto G, Rosanio S, et al. Atrial Electroanatomic remodeling after circumferential radiofrequency pulmonary vein ablation. Circulation 2001; 104:2539–44.

21. Jaïs P, Sanders P, Hsu LF, et al. Flutter localized to the anterior left atrium after catheter ablation of atrial fibrillation. J Cardiovasc Electrophysiol 2006;17: 279–85.

22. Zhou GB, Hu JQ, Guo XG, et al. Very long-term outcome of catheter ablation of post-incisional atrial tachycardia: role of incisional and non-incisional scar. Int J Cardiol 2016;205:72–80.

23. John B, Stiles MK, Kuklik P, et al. Electrical remodelling of the left and right atria due to rheumatic mitral stenosis. Eur Heart J 2008;29:2234–43.

24. Fiala M, Chovančík J, Neuwirth R, et al. Atrial macroreentry tachycardia in patients without obvious structural heart disease or previous cardiac surgical or catheter intervention: characterization of arrhythmogenic substrates, reentry circuits, and results of catheter ablation. J Cardiovasc Electrophysiol 2007;18: 824–32.

25. Stevenson IH, Kistler PM, Spence SJ, et al. Scar-related right atrial macroreentrant tachycardia in patients without prior atrial surgery: electroanatomic characterization and ablation outcome. Hear Rhythm 2005;2:594–601.

26. Kharbanda RK, Özdemir EH, Taverne YJHJ, et al. Current Concepts of anatomy, electrophysiology, and therapeutic implications of the interatrial septum. JACC Clin Electrophysiol 2019;5:647–56.

27. Melby SJ, Lee AM, Zierer A, et al. Atrial fibrillation propagates through gaps in ablation lines: implications for ablative treatment of atrial fibrillation. Hear Rhythm 2008;5:1296–301.

28. De Ponti R, Marazzi R, Zoli L, et al. Electroanatomic mapping and ablation of macroreentrant atrial tachycardia: comparison between successfully and unsuccessfully treated cases. J Cardiovasc Electrophysiol 2010;21:155–62.

29. De Ponti R, Verlato R, Bertaglia E, et al. Treatment of macro-re-entrant atrial tachycardia based on electroanatomic mapping: identification and ablation of the mid-diastolic isthmus. Europace 2007; 9:449–57.

30. Allessie MA, Bonke FIM, Schopman FJG. Circus movement in rabbit atrial muscle as a mechanism of tachycardia. II. The role of nonuniform recovery of excitability in the occurrence of unidirectional block, as studied with multiple microelectrodes. Circ Res 1976;39:168–77.

31. Bogun F, Bender B, Li YG, et al. Ablation of atypical atrial flutter guided by the use of concealed entrainment in patients without prior cardiac surgery. J Cardiovasc Electrophysiol 2000;11:136–45.

32. Sanders P, Hocini M, Jaïs P, et al. Characterization of focal atrial tachycardia using high-density mapping. J Am Coll Cardiol 2005;46:2088–99.

33. Jaïs P, Matsuo S, Knecht S, et al. A deductive mapping strategy for atrial tachycardia following atrial fibrillation ablation: importance of localized reentry. J Cardiovasc Electrophysiol 2009;20:480–91.

34. Luther V, Sikkel M, Bennett N, et al. Visualizing localized reentry with ultra-high density mapping in iatrogenic atrial tachycardia. Circ Arrhythmia Electrophysiol 2017;10:e004724.

35. Frontera A, Mahajan R, Dallet C, et al. Characterizing localized reentry with high-resolution mapping: evidence for multiple slow conducting isthmuses within the circuit. Hear Rhythm 2019;16:679–85.

36. De Groot NMS, Schalij MJ. Fragmented, long-duration, low-amplitude electrograms characterize the origin of focal atrial tachycardia. J Cardiovasc Electrophysiol 2006;17:1086–92.

37. Markowitz SM, Nemirovksy D, Stein KM, et al. Adenosine-insensitive focal atrial tachycardia. evidence for de novo micro-re-entry in the human atrium. J Am Coll Cardiol 2007;49:1324–33.

38. Liu CF, Cheung JW, Ip JE, et al. Unifying algorithm for mechanistic diagnosis of atrial tachycardia. Circ Arrhythmia Electrophysiol 2016;9:e004028.

39. Okumura K, Plumb VJ, Pagé PL, et al. Atrial activation sequence during atrial flutter in the canine pericarditis model and its effects on the polarity of the flutter wave in the electrocardiogram. J Am Coll Cardiol 1991;17:509–18.

40. Ndrepepa G, Zrenner B, Deisenhofer I, et al. Relationship between surface electrocardiogram characteristics and endocardial activation sequence in patients with typical atrial flutter. Z Kardiol 2000;89:527–37.

41. Ndrepepa G, Zrenner B, Weyerbrock S, et al. Activation patterns in the left atrium during counterclockwise and clockwise atrial flutter. J Cardiovasc Electrophysiol 2001;12:893–9.

42. Barbato G, Carinci V, Tomasi C, et al. Is electrocardiography a reliable tool for identifying patients with isthmus-dependent atrial flutter? Europace 2009;11:1071–6.

43. Zrenner B, Ndrepepa G, Karch M, et al. Block of the lower interatrial connections: insight into the sources of electrocardiographic diversities in common type atrial flutter. Pacing Clin Electrophysiol 2000;23:917–20.

44. Akar JG, Al-Chekakie MO, Hai A, et al. Surface electrocardiographic patterns and electrophysiologic characteristics of atrial flutter following modified radiofrequency MAZE procedures. J Cardiovasc Electrophysiol 2007;18:349–55.

45. Chugh A, Latchamsetty R, Oral H, et al. Characteristics of cavotricuspid isthmus-dependent atrial flutter after left atrial ablation of atrial fibrillation. Circulation 2006;113:609–15.

46. Pap R, Kohári M, Makai A, et al. Surgical technique and the mechanism of atrial tachycardia late after open heart surgery. J Interv Card Electrophysiol 2012;35:127–35.

47. Roten L, Lukac P, De Groot N, et al. Catheter ablation of arrhythmias in Ebstein's anomaly: a multicenter study. J Cardiovasc Electrophysiol 2011;22:1391–6.

48. Yap SC, Harris L, Silversides CK, et al. Outcome of intra-atrial re-entrant tachycardia catheter ablation in adults with congenital heart disease: negative impact of age and complex atrial surgery. J Am Coll Cardiol 2010;56:1589–96.

49. Collins KK, Love BA, Walsh EP, et al. Location of acutely successful radiofrequency catheter ablation of intraatrial reentrant tachycardia in patients with congenital heart disease. Am J Cardiol 2000;86:969–74.

50. Chae S, Oral H, Good E, et al. Atrial Tachycardia after circumferential pulmonary vein ablation of atrial fibrillation. mechanistic insights, results of catheter ablation, and risk factors for recurrence. J Am Coll Cardiol 2007;50:1781–7.

51. Mönnig G, Wasmer K, Milberg P, et al. Predictors of long-term success after catheter ablation of atriofascicular accessory pathways. Hear Rhythm 2012;9:704–8.

52. Lyan E, Yalin K, Abdin A, et al. Mechanism, underlying substrate and predictors of atrial tachycardia following atrial fibrillation ablation using the second-generation cryoballoon. J Cardiol 2019;73:497–506.

53. Schaeffer B, Akbulak R, Jularic M, et al. High-density mapping and ablation of primary nonfocal left atrial tachycardia: characterizing a distinct arrhythmogenic substrate. JACC Clin Electrophysiol 2019;5:417–26.

54. Röcken C, Peters B, Juenemann G, et al. Atrial amyloidosis: an arrhythmogenic substrate for persistent atrial fibrillation. Circulation 2002;106:2091–7.

Relationships Between Atrial Flutter and Fibrillation: The Border Zone

Ritesh S. Patel, MD[a], Mohamed Khayata, MD[a],
Roberto De Ponti, MD, FHRS[b,c], Giuseppe Bagliani, MD[d,e],
Fabio M. Leonelli, MD[a,f],*

KEYWORDS

- Atrial flutter • Atrial fibrillation • Line of block • Radiofrequency ablation

KEY POINTS

- Typical atrial flutter (AFL) is a macro reentrant circuit that is dependent on the cavo-tricuspid isthmus in the right atrium, amenable to catheter ablation.
- Atypical atrial flutters are distinct entities observed clinically after interventions on the atria are performed.
- The mechanism of atrial fibrillation (AF) is still not completely understood. The trigger-perpetuator model is generally accepted but the nature of the former is still speculative.
- AF and AFL are closely related by anatomy, substrate, and triggers.
- Catheter ablation of either or both arrhythmia needs to be carefully planned to balance risks, costs, and results.

INTRODUCTION

Atrial flutter (AFL) and fibrillation (AF) have been inextricably linked in the study of Electrophysiology. With astute clinical observation, advanced diagnostic equipment in the Electrophysiology Laboratory, and thoughtful study of animal models, the mechanism and inter-relationship between the 2 conditions have been elucidated and will be reviewed in this article. Though diagnosis and management of these conditions have many similarities, the mechanisms by which they develop and persist are quite unique.

MECHANISMS OF ARRHYTHMIA

Typical Atrial Flutter (Giuseppe Bagliani and colleagues' article, "The history of atrial flutter electrophysiology, from entrainment to ablation: A 100 year experience in the Precision Electrocardiology," elsewhere in this issue)

Typical atrial flutter, also known as cavotricuspid isthmus-dependent flutter, is a macro-reentrant arrhythmia with defined borders including the TV annulus anteriorly and the crista terminalis posteriorly. A macro-reentrant wavefront can travel in this circuit in a clockwise (CW) or counterclockwise

[a] University of South Florida Morsani, College of Medicine, Division of Cardiovascular Diseases, 4202 E Fowler Avenue, Tampa, FL 33620, USA; [b] Department of Heart and Vessels, Ospedale di Circolo, Viale Borri, 57, 21100, Varese, Italy; [c] Department of Medicine and Surgery, University of Insubria, Viale Guicciardini, 9, 21100, Varese, Italy; [d] Cardiology And Arrhythmology Clinic, University Hospital "Ospedali Riuniti", Via Conca 71, 60126, Ancona, Italy; [e] Department of Biomedical Sciences and Public Health, Marche Polytechnic University, Via Conca 71, 60126, Ancona, Italy; [f] James A Haley Veterans Hospital, Tampa, FL, USA
* Corresponding author.
E-mail address: fabio.leonelli@va.gov

Card Electrophysiol Clin 14 (2022) 421–434
https://doi.org/10.1016/j.ccep.2022.06.006

(CCW) direction generating typical ECG patterns. CCW flutter results in a classic "sawtooth" pattern with stable reproducible deeply inverted negative P waves in the inferior leads with a plateau and a terminal positive component of variable amplitude.[1] CW flutter demonstrates an almost mirror image of CCW flutter with positive, slightly notched morphology in the inferior leads on surface ECG.

Atypical Atrial Flutter (Giuseppe Bagliani and colleagues' article, "The history of atrial flutter electrophysiology, from entrainment to ablation: A 100 year experience in the Precision Electrocardiology," Fabio M. Leonelli and colleagues' article, "Interpretation of typical and atypical atrial flutters by precision electrocardiology based on intracardiac recording," elsewhere in this issue)

Noncavotricuspid isthmus flutters are known as "atypical." Their reentrant circuits are more varied and complex as they are bound by other anatomical structures or more often, atrial myocardial scars from prior interventions such as atrial surgery (e.g., congenital heart disease, mitral valve surgery, cardiac transplantation), surgeries to manage AF (Cox Maze procedure), or catheter ablation procedures to manage AF. Rarely, scars can be present without prior atrial manipulation and cause atypical flutters. ECG appearance in atypical atrial flutter is more varied than isthmus-dependent, typical flutters. This is because atypical flutters have less predictable circuits located in either atrium, whereas isthmus-dependent flutters have definite only right-sided reentrant paths.

Atrial Fibrillation

In contrast, the electrocardiographic appearance of AF is small, if not imperceptible, fibrillatory waves with an irregularly, irregular ventricular response. Sometimes, the waves in V1 appear more uniform and regular, confusing the diagnosis of atrial fibrillation (AF) with atrial flutter (usually termed coarse or organized AF) **Fig. 1**.

These profound variations in ECG recording of atrial activity suggest a more complex mechanism of AF initiation and maintenance than that of AFL. Accordingly, clinical emergence and persistence of AF are not, as yet, fully understood although the hypothesis of a trigger/perpetuator model can explain a large number of clinical observations.

Triggers, wavelets, and rotors

Triggers are foci in the atria that discharge usually at very rapid rates leading to the breakdown of organized electrical wavefront propagation into fibrillatory conduction. Seminal observations[2] on the role of ectopic beats in the induction of AF were later confirmed[3] Most AF triggers originate from the PVs due to the unique electrophysiological characteristics of the local myocytes[4] explaining the automatic or triggered activity of these foci. These unique characteristics are probably related to abnormalities in Ca^{2+} handling while the effects of stretch, parasympathetic modulation, and the unusual orientation of the myocytes at the junction between PVs and left atrium favor reentry and make these sites the most likely location of AF triggers.

Though most AF triggers are in the pulmonary venous sleeves, about 20% of triggers are non-PV in origin located in either atria.[5] Single premature contractions, bursts of fast nonsustained AT from focal areas, or more organized rhythms such as atrial flutter were observed to initiate AF. The common denominator of all these different triggers was their ability to induce localized reentry often in areas of natural or acquired anisotropy.[6] Repetitive activation of these areas can lead to persistent reentrant activity expanding to the entire atria inducing AF.

While the role of triggers in the initiation of AF appears to be established, doubts remain on the nature of the perpetuators of the arrhythmia. Postulating a self-perpetuating arrhythmia independent of the initial trigger, Moe and Abildskov[7] hypothesized the existence of wavelets randomly propagating throughout both atria with the course traversed being determined by local refractory periods of nearby atrial tissue. They also suggested that up to 40 wandering wavelets were necessary to sustain AF in computational models. The number of wavelets necessary for the persistence of AF is unclear as Allessie and colleagues[8] later used a canine model to reveal only 4–6 random, wandering wavelets were sufficient to sustain AF. These observations did not resolve the question of whether the wavelets were drivers or simple byproducts of more organized forms of reentry. It is possible that a hidden trigger source is continuously maintaining AF, but current evidence suggests the wavelets are the "daughters" of a more organized albeit random form or reentry such as a "mother rotor."

Moe's multiple wavelet hypothesis requires a random distribution of refractoriness in a circumscribed space inducing a large *local* anisotropy to sustain the reentry. This contrasts with our understanding of how cell-to-cell contact normalizes the APD and refractoriness,[9] suggesting that anisotropy exists in a *large* myocardial volume

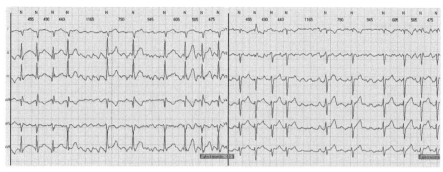

Fig. 1. "Coarse atrial fibrillation." The 12 lead ECG shows a variable degree of atrial organization manifested in irregular waves with variable morphology showing, at times, remarkable uniformity.

and not in microscopic areas as required for the wavelets' hypothesis.

Furthermore, recent evidence based on optic mapping[10] showed that the wavelets were more likely to represent a breakup of a more organized system and not an independent mechanism of the perpetuation of AF. These observations lead to the hypothesis of organized drivers perpetuate AF. A driver can be defined as a localized area of fast and repetitive activation propagating to the surrounding tissue with fibrillatory conduction.[11] The arrhythmic mechanism of a driver is most likely to be reentry either anatomical or functional. The former occurs in areas where fibrosis is present and affects propagation by slowing it and inducing unidirectional block. Anatomical or scar boundaries can create a path of reentry in macro-circuits but often the entire path is contained in a 1–2 mm^2 area of scarred tissue.[12] Despite its small size, a micro-reentry can demonstrate significant structural complexity with areas of fibrosis existing in areas of baseline inhomogeneous conduction, such as in pectinate muscle or regions of a sudden change in fiber orientation like the ostium of the coronary sinus.[13]

In contrast, a stable reentrant circuit may not need a specific anatomical substrate and can be maintained by the nonuniform recovery of excitability in the atrium. In this model, Allessie[14] proposed that the length of the circuit corresponds to the wavelength (conduction velocity x refractoriness) of the circulating impulse. In a functional reentry, there is no gap between its head and tail so that "the head of the circulating wavefront is continuously biting in its own tail of refractoriness"[14] **Fig. 2.**

Continuing the exploration of the concept of functional reentry led to the postulation in animal and human studies of a functional type of reentry, named "rotor" which generates a vortex-like waveform called the "spiral."[15]

The origin of rotors is varied and complex, but to simplify, it can be imagined as the turbulence generated by flowing water when reaches a rock. Similar to water, a wavefront propagating from a source travel in a planar mode until encounter an obstacle. At its edges the wavefront will curve and depending on the excitability and the physical characteristics of the wavefront, it can circumnavigate the obstacle or curve on itself, begin to rotate around its tip beginning a vortex and detach.[16] **Fig. 3.**

This "wave daughter" can continue to spin at a high frequency for a long period of time becoming a source of stimulation while being stationary or meander and possibly reanchor to areas of electrophysiological heterogeneities.

The high frequency of rotor's activation stimulates the surrounding atrial tissue at extremely high rates resulting in fibrillatory conduction. This concept of rotors perpetuating AF was confirmed by observing multiple electrical wave breaks originating from the same reentrant wave (the rotor), leading to fibrillation.

This mechanism has been observed in both atrial and ventricular fibrillation.[17] Further studies mapped, in a perfused sheep heart, the frequency content at different points trying to identify the site of periodic activity with the highest frequency. Multiple narrow band peaks were noted with a single peak of dominant higher activity at the base of the LAA, suggesting the presence of a single source of activation.[2] Jalife and his group visualized the rotors using optic mapping[18] as a vortex rotating CW at the same dominant frequency previously recorded.

As for triggers, animal[19] and human studies[13] have confirmed that the majority of perpetuators of AF are located in the LA. The rapid stimulation propagates to the RA using the physiological interatrial connections[13] where areas of high anatomical complexity, such as the pectinate muscles, when stimulated at high frequency will

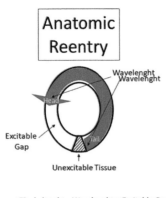

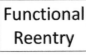

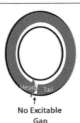

Fig. 2. Anatomic and functional reentry. An Anatomical reentry exists only if its Wavelength is shorter than the circuit and excitable tissue (excitable gap) is in front of the circuit's Head. A Functional reentry has no excitable gap and its Head "bites" the Tail.

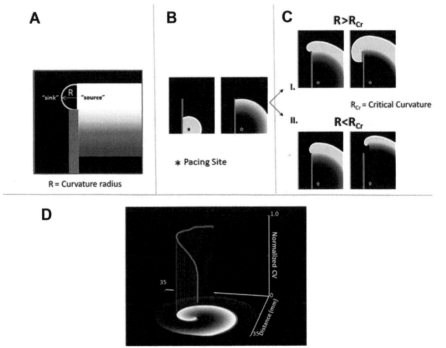

Fig. 3. Mechanism of rotor and spiral wave initiation due to vortex shedding. A: (*A*) stimulus (*B*) has generated a wavefront (*source*) reaching an obstacle with sharp edges (*red line*); at the margin of the red line the wavefront bends "wrapping around" (*white* line) the edge of the obstacle. (*C*): The curvature of the wavefront will determine whether the wave will remain attached to the wavefront (*C I*) and travel around the obstacle or detach (*C II*) and initiate a rotor. Pathophysiological conditions imitating this setting could be areas of scars surrounded by tissue with reduced excitability as in remodeled atria. (*D*): Factors determining the tendency to curve and establish a rotor include the conduction velocity of the spiral of excitation which is lowest at the tip and increases as the curvature is reduced. This is represented by the plot relating curvature distance from the core (*x,y axis*) and conduction velocity (*z axis*). The rotor will pivot and travel along irregular trajectories because of the constant mismatch between the current available (*source*) and need (*sink*) to depolarize tissue in front of the rotor. R: radius Rcr: critical radius of minimum radius of excitation, CV conduction Velocity. (*From* Pandit SV, Jalife J. Rotors and the dynamics of cardiac fibrillation. Circ Res. 2013;112(5):849-862. doi:10.1161/CIRCRESAHA.111.300158; with permission.)

propagate the impulse with fibrillatory conduction to the RA. This hypothesis combining AF triggers and perpetuators which considers rotors the main form of drivers and the LA the main source of both, has received substantial clinical support from human observations. An electrical gradient exists between the atria with the cycle length (CL) of AF almost always shorter in the Left atrium compared to the right atrium (RA),[20] suggesting a higher prevalence of drivers in the LA conducting to the RA. Ablating LA drivers with high frequencies uncovers drivers with longer CL and progressive ablation of these sources leads to SR.[21]

Although rotors have not been clearly identified in humans, some clinical evidence of their role in AF exists. During EP studies, Narayan and colleagues observed a mean of 2.1 focal sources during AF, with over 70% of these being rotors. Ablation of the rotors had improved freedom from AF in follow-up[6] Albeit interesting, these studies have yet to be widely confirmed.

In structurally normal hearts, wave breaks are difficult to sustain.[22] In anatomically or functionally diseased hearts where dynamic changes are occurring from alterations in cellular membrane voltage or calcium inflow, wavefront instability can lead to sustained wave propagation rather than termination of the arrhythmia.[23] Tissue heterogeneity in the diseased heart causes wave-break by the wavefronts encountering areas of long refractory periods. Regardless of their mechanism, rotors could provide the original source of wave-breaks leading to fibrillation.[19] The behavior of the wave breaks originating from the mother rotor can vary depending on the anatomy and electrophysiological properties of the surrounding tissue.[24] If the localized wave-break anchors to an anatomical structure, such as pectinate muscle, it can lead to a monomorphic regular tachycardia similar to atrial flutter.[25] If the rotor is more unstable and unanchored, it can cause clinical AF.[26] Importantly, very rapid pacing can induce rotors in electrophysiology studies, but they cannot be sustained in otherwise normal cardiac tissue. Wave-break can also be the result of source-sink mismatch in the atria if the excitable tissue in front of the wave-break cannot be brought to depolarization threshold. This is what occurs at insertion points of pectinate or papillary muscles, areas of local ischemia, or from drug effects. The equivalent to this variability between regular and disorganized rhythm is the observation on surface ECG or even in intracardiac electrograms of coexisting organized circuits and areas of fibrillation[27] in the atria (**Fig. 4**).

Reentry can also be transient or continuous in different regions of the atria.

FROM ATRIAL FIBRILLATION TO ATRIAL FLUTTER AND VICE VERSA

The existence of a close relationship between AF and AFL was suspected and validated by clinical observation. During EP studies, periods of non-sustained AF often preceded the development of typical AFL[28]; treating AF with class I or III antiarrhythmic drugs (AADs) often converted this fibrillation to typical AFL.[29] Ablating atrial flutter in some of these patients prevented the reoccurrence of AF.[30] Some authors believe typical AFL almost always develops from a previous AF of variable duration.[31] The transition from one to the other arrhythmia can be summarized as a change from an organized rhythm with a stable electrical pathway (atrial flutter), to a rhythm which, regardless of its fundamental mechanism, generates multiple random wavefronts (AF), or vice versa. Despite its profound electrical irregularity, AF maintains some features of a regular rhythm (**Figs. 1** and **4**). The drivers maintaining the arrhythmia, whether rotors or focal sources, have a fundamental periodicity and a basic, albeit shifting, repetitive reentrant path (see above). Evidence that AF electrical activity, defined as chaotic, has periods of organized propagation involving atrial locations of variable extent, comes from many sources.

Analysis of electrical activity using correlation analysis of local activation sequences in the RA,[32] or of local spectral analysis combined with optical mapping in the entire sheep atrium[18] or temporal and spatial phase analysis of ECG waveforms[33] have shown the presence of regional electrical organization of variable size during AF. Though surface ECG does not have the diagnostic resolution of these other techniques, AF appearance on surface ECG still correlates with intracardiac recordings[34] and electrical organization is reflected in some features of the recorded waveforms. On surface ECG, AF classification in fine or coarse[35] or, more granularly, in one of 3 different subtypes,[36] reflects variable degrees of atrial organization (see **Figs. 1** and **4**).

In contrast, atrial flutter is characterized by an organized rhythm with a stable repetitive sequence of activation which results in easily recognizable waveforms on surface ECG. While the difference between these arrhythmias is obvious in extreme cases, there are situations where this distinction is difficult, as AF and AFL can coexist in the same patient with AF localized in some part or the entire atrium while the rest continued to maintain atrial flutter.[37] This situation is favored by the presence of interatrial conduction block dissociating one atrium from the other

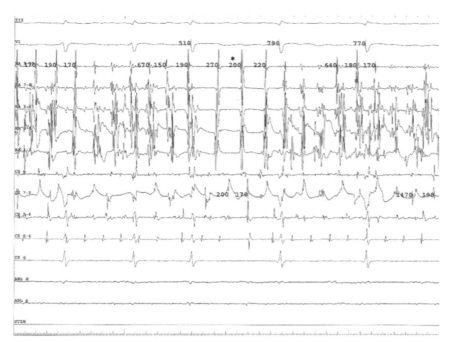

Fig. 4. Intracardiac recording from right atrium (RA), coronary sinus (CS), and superior left pulmonary vein (Abl) showing different degrees of periodic organization. The RA alternated the period of uniformity of CL and endocardial morphology (*) with periods of fibrillatory conduction (*Red* *) Similar observations for the LA (CSp-CSd) with lower Voltage electrograms becoming almost unrecordable near the Pulmonary Vein (Abl).

(**Fig. 5**). In these instances, the surface ECG mostly reflects the RA rhythm regardless of its nature.[37] Further mapping pointed out that the difference between the 3 types of AF was mostly related to RA electrical organization.[36] In studies mapping human AF, some authors[38] have shown more marked disorganized LA activity compared to the RA,[39] where a broad wavefront of organized activity across the RA free wall exists in type I AF. This suggested the presence of a large reentrant circuit rotating around one of the RA anatomical obstacles. Some studies[40] pointed out the favorable relationship between the pectinate muscle of the RA, the naturally occurring anatomical barriers, and the RA shape to suggest that all these factors could explain both the wavefront organization and the preferential craniocaudal activation of the RA free wall.

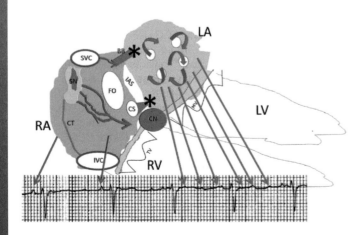

Fig. 5. A rhythm strip shows a well-defined P wave with a regular P-P and stable PR interval. At the same time, an irregular poorly defined rhythm with varying Voltage is evident in a patient who underwent multiple Radio Frequency ablations for AF. The schematic represents the findings of a subsequent intracardiac study. Right atrium (RA) is in SR and conducting (*red lines*) through the AVN (*red circle*) to the ventricles (RV and LV). The interatrial connections (BB and CS) are interrupted (*black asterisks*) following the procedures leaving a disconnected RA in SR and the left atrium (LA) in atrial fibrillation. BB, Bachman bundle; CS, coronary sinus; FO, foramen ovalis; IAS, interatrial septum; IVC, inferior vena cava; MV, mitral valve; SN, sinus node; SVC, superior vena cava; TV, tricuspid valve.

Atrial Fibrillation to Atrial Flutter

The transition of AF to typical AFL can be observed in patients receiving AAD therapy or during RFA for rhythm control of AF. At times, patients without prior history of AFL can spontaneously develop this arrhythmia after being observed to be in AF without any rhythm control administered, suggesting that these arrhythmias may coexist, and their clinical manifestation is favoured by the presence of AADs. Antiarrhythmic drugs modify refractoriness and/or conduction velocity increasing the wavelength rendering the arrhythmia incapable of sustaining itself. For example, using Flecainide will cause reentrant circuits to coalesce and form larger circuits that either terminate due to an excessive prolongation of the wavelength or reorganize into isthmus-dependent AFL.[29] Similarly, reorganization of AF into AFL during RFA is often observed while attempting to manage AF invasively. Here the mechanisms for conversion from one to the other include progressive elimination of fast drivers inducing fibrillatory conduction (see above) allowing sites with longer CLs to be sustained uniformly by both atria. The reentrant path of the resultant flutter may be determined by a variety of factors including the preexisting anatomical boundaries, as in typical AFL, new boundaries created by the ablation lines (inducing left-sided flutters), or small areas of scars sustaining micro-reentrant circuits.[41] Spontaneous conversion of AF to typical AFL is frequently observed during EPS or on telemetry/cardiac monitoring.[28]

This phenomenon underscores the importance of a posterior line of block (LoB) between the 2 vena cavae allowing flutter macroreentry. This LoB can be functional, anatomical, or a mixture of the 2 and regardless its nature, it is one determinant of the reorganization of AF into AFL[42] **Figs. 6 and 7**).

The short CL of AF allows the circulating wavefronts to encounter tissue with different degrees of excitability. Multiple wavefronts encountering a refractory zone can create an area of functional block which can only last a short period, dissolve, and reform at another point.

Lines of block during AF have been described in a few regions of the RA either anteriorly,[43] posteroseptal in the sinus venosus region,[44] but the majority of studies have followed the course of the CT. This anatomical structure (see Giuseppe Bagliani and colleagues' article, "The history of atrial flutter electrophysiology, from entrainment to ablation: A 100 year experience in the Precision Electrocardiology," in this issue) is ideally placed to form a posterior barrier and, thanks to its anisotropic conduction properties

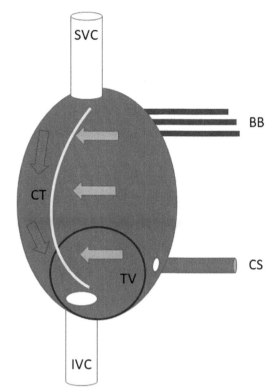

Fig. 6. Schematic representation of the RA and Crista Terminalis (CT). A complete CT is shown preventing a collision between posterior wavefronts of activation (*pink arrows*) and lateral descending wavefronts (*gray arrows*). This situation will favor the reorganization of fibrillatory activity in a stable flutter-like circuit reentry. BB, Bachman bundle CS coronary sinus; CT, crista terminalis; IVC, inferior vena cava; SVC, superior vena cava; TV, tricuspid valve.

(see Fabio M. Leonelli and colleagues' article, "Interpretation of typical and atypical atrial flutters by precision electrocardiology based on intracardiac recording," in this issue), greatly facilitates the creation of a LoB during AF. The fundamental importance of this structure in the AF-AFL relationship cannot be overstated as it prevents the collision between the septal and free wall wavefronts (see Fabio M. Leonelli and colleagues' article, "Interpretation of typical and atypical atrial flutters by precision electrocardiology based on intracardiac recording," in this issue).

The CT presence, length, and location determines the predominance of one or the other arrhythmia. If the line is electrically impermeable it will impede that the septal and free wall wavefronts collide and, as it stretches between the venae cavae, it can function as a separating barrier. It will, therefore, together with the circular TV annulus, create the necessary conditions for a stable AFL. As the LoB shortens due to a change in

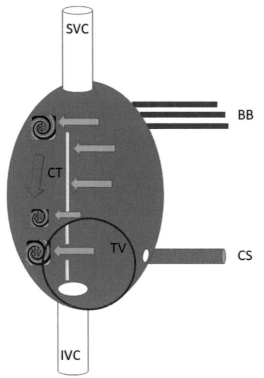

Fig. 7. Schematic representation of the RA and Crista Terminalis (CT). Multiple gaps in the CT are shown allowing a collision between posterior wavefronts of activation (*pink arrows*) and lateral descending wavefronts (*gray arrows*). The collisions of premature beats or during high-rate stimulation will favor the formation of rotors (*red asterisks*) and AF induction. BB, Bachman bundle CS coronary sinus; CT, crista terminalis; IVC, inferior vena cava; SVC, superior vena cava; TV, tricuspid valve.

refractoriness,[42] AFL will degenerate into AF. Areas of slow conduction are also necessary to prolong the CL and stabilize the flutter circuit by slowing its speed of revolution. These regions have been reported to occur naturally at the confluence of the IVC-TV isthmus with the CS-septum[45] where a complex anisotropic fiber arrangement naturally slows the flutter wavefront propagation or low Voltage areas in the posterolateral RA.[46] Presence of scars or atrial dilatation can also constitute a slow conducting substrate reducing the rotation velocity and stabilizing the circuit. In approximately 10–15% of patients, AF is observed to change into mostly typical AFL during IV or oral therapy with class I and III AAD. The conversion is the result of decreased conduction velocity prolonging the reentrant wavelength and favoring the formation of the LoB due to increased refractoriness.[47] It is unclear if these patients are truly a subgroup of patients with AF in whom AFL is the primary arrhythmia and AF is simply a degeneration of the primary arrhythmia. The increased incidence of AF following cavotricuspid isthmus ablation to treat typical AFL suggests the presence of two independent arrhythmia (see later).[47]

Atrial Fibrillation to Atrial Flutter

Premature depolarization and rapid stimulation can be proarrhythmic in any substrate by creating areas of block and slow conduction favoring reentry.[48] Both mechanisms have been observed to convert stable isthmus-dependent AFL into AF, shortening functional block resulting in progressive shortening of the AFL CL before degenerating into AF.[42] When closely mapped in an animal model, conversion of stable typical AFL into AF begins with an acceleration of the flutter rate followed by a beat to beat instability and a shortening or complete loss of the length of the LoB leading to the emergence of frank AF.[42] The AFL rate increase can be mediated by external factors such as a variation in autonomic tone[49] or a change in the components of the macro-reentrant circuit such as an acceleration of propagation through the slow conduction area or a shortening of the reentrant pathway. This latter condition shifts the focus to the CT and its role in establishing and maintaining a stable reentrant circuit. In animals, shortening the length of the posterior LoB by few millimeters decreases the CL of the flutter enough to induce fibrillation.[42]

Atypical flutters or variations of isthmus-dependent flutters in humans are more likely to convert to AF[50] because of the presence of an intrinsically unstable reentrant circuit. The presence of gaps in the CT allows short-circuiting of typical flutter reentrant path[51] by shortening the CL and ultimately predisposing it to degenerate into AF. SVC circular reentry (upper loop reentry) coexisting with isthmus-dependent flutter, not uncommonly observed during EPS (See Fabio M. Leonelli and colleagues' article, "Interpretation of typical and atypical atrial flutters by precision electrocardiology based on intracardiac recording," in this issue), can preexcite the dominant macro-reentry decreasing rotation time and increasing the occurrence of AF. Increasing the rate of stimulation will alter the effective refractory period (ERP) of the atrial myocytes, increase the dispersion of repolarization,[52] and favor induction of a single or multiple reentrant circuits of very short CL.[53] Decreasing CL will induce fibrillatory conduction in the surrounding tissue causing sustained AF. External sources of localized reentry or automatic firing can have the same effect on atrial tissue converting AFL to AF. Single beat[54] or nonsustained runs of ectopic beats from LA or RA sources have been documented to occur in humans during stable AFL[55] and induce AF with a mechanism probably similar to the one described in the animal model.

Remodeling

Regardless of how either arrhythmia is sustained, there is good clinical and experimental evidence of the importance of electrical and structural remodeling in the genesis and persistence of AF.[56] Sustained bouts of AF cause atrial remodeling and AF is the result of the same atrial remodeling it caused, leading to the phrase "Atrial fibrillation begets atrial fibrillation." This process refers to several changes in cellular channel function, induction of cell death due to inflammation and infiltration of fibrosis and adipose tissue as well autonomic remodeling.[41] The end result is the creation of a pro-arrhythmic substrate with shortening of myocytes refractoriness[22] extensive areas of fibrosis generating areas of slow conduction and block and increased automaticity. The effects of neural remodeling lead to an increase in sympathetic and parasympathetic tone contributing to the maintenance of AF in humans.[57] AFL can also reversibly shorten atrial refractoriness[58] in a manner similar to AF, suggesting that remodeling may play a role in their relationship. Shortening the refractory period could have multiple consequences enabling the conversion of AFL to AF. It may increase the likelihood of fibrillatory conduction by favoring the dispersion of the organized flutter wavefront over obstacles such as the pectinate muscle[59] or affect the continuity of the CT block creating shorter reentrant circuits[60] A period of heightened susceptibility to AF following AFL cardioversion[61] or ablation[62] seems to demonstrate the relevance of AFL mediated refractoriness shortening in clinical practice. Furthermore, in an animal model of atrial flutter, the same authors confirmed the electrical remodeling induced by this rhythm and observed a time window of increased susceptibility to AF induction.[63]

Remodeling could be an added factor facilitating both the emergence of ectopic foci discharging bursts or single beats as well as shortening atrial myocytes' refractory period and atrial dispersion of repolarization.

The ectopic focus could generate the burst of rapid atrial activity or a single extra stimulus; AFL could be converted to AF even with a single extra stimulus[55] given the myocytes' electrophysiological changes induced by the combination of remodeling and bursts of rapid firing.

MANAGEMENT OF COMBINED ATRIAL FLUTTER AND ATRIAL FIBRILLATION: IS IT DIFFERENT FROM GUIDELINES?

We have described the close relationship between the mechanisms inducing AF and typical AFL and their reciprocal influence on substrates maintaining these arrhythmia. These observations explain the frequent coexistence of both tachycardia in the same patients and open the question of whether demonstrating one implies the existence of the other. The AFL group consists of multiple different entities (see Fabio M. Leonelli and colleagues' article, "Interpretation of typical and atypical atrial flutters by precision electrocardiology based on intracardiac recording," in this issue) with varied arrhythmic mechanisms, response to drugs, and relation to AF. Several excellent reviews and guidelines detail the management of each one of these arrhythmia.[63] In the following paragraphs we will highlight some unique clinical aspects of AF and typical AFL based on their close relationship discussed in the previous section.

Several clinical similarities and differences exist between AF and AFL in isolation. Both types of arrhythmias are more common in elderly humans who tend to have more comorbidities[64] with patients with AF having higher rates of several comorbidities compared to patients with AFL.[64,65] The latter data was attributed to different degrees of atrial myopathy, endocardial remodeling, and neurohormonal activation among AF group.[65] Previous studies reported higher incidence of mortality among patients with AF compared to patients with AFL[66] and lower incidence of stroke among patients with solitary AFL compared to those with AF.[32]

After diagnosis, 2 facets of management need to be addressed in both arrhythmia. First, both conditions pose a significant thromboembolic risk, with cerebrovascular accident being the most common manifestation. Second, a rate vs rhythm control strategy should be considered, especially if patients have symptoms attributed to their arrhythmia. Given the high success rate and low risk of RFA in patients with AFL, this procedure represents the first line of treatment in isthmus-dependent flutter.[51] For AF the choice is more nuanced and depends on multiple factors. Patient's clinical status, typology of AF, experience, and treating physician's "philosophical" approach to AF will often determine whether the next step will be RFA or AAD. Given the superior outcomes of RFA when compared to AAD, the invasive approach to rhythm restoration is often considered the first line of therapy.[63,67,68]

The close interrelationship between these 2 arrhythmia creates several situations where the *tout court* application of the guidelines may not be optimal. Three groups of patients can be identified: pure AFL, pure AF, or Mixed (where both arrhythmia have been recorded at different times). "Lone AFL" as a unique arrhythmia exists in approximately 30% of patients[69]; in this group, it is likely that an anatomical LoB exists and the set up for a macro-reentry is complete without the necessary functional changes induced by AF. Nevertheless, this is a group at high risk of developing de novo AF, with a risk estimated to be 48% at 5 years.[70] This observation begs the question of whether a prophylactic PVI ablation to prevent future AF is necessary in addition to CTI ablation of AFL in these patients. Following AFL ablation de novo AF has occurred in a variable number of patients estimated between 15%[61] and 80% within 3 years after ablation.[71] This is not surprising considering the shared proarrhythmic substrate and similar triggers for both arrhythmia[72] which explain the AF emergence once AFL is eliminated. The variability of reported AF is accounted for, in part, by the duration and intensity of follow-up and possibly by the presence of AF predating the ablation[73] Furthermore, this wide difference in recurrence rate suggests that the AFL group could be further stratified to identify high-risk patients.

To this end, "lone AFL" patients have been further stratified at the time of ablation by induction or noninduction of AF[74] with, in the former group, a 25–30% chance of developing AF as time progresses versus a 20% in the noninducible. Clinical variables such as previously documented clinical AF are undoubtedly important while loose variables such as BMI, sex, clinical comorbidities, Pw duration, etc. have been suggested as parameters defining high-risk patients but never tested prospectively.[74] Following these findings, PVI at the time of AFL ablation is advocated based on the result of a number of studies showing a decreased incidence of AF recurrence in the AFL + PVI group vs AFL alone ablation from 26.2% to 51.3% at 2 years follow-up.[73,75] This recommendation should be tempered by a study showing that AF recurrence is higher in patients undergoing PVI and AFL ablation than in PVI alone.[47] This study suggests that elimination of PVI triggers may not be sufficient to prevent recurrent AF in patients demonstrating both arrhythmia. The authors speculated that AFL in patients with AF identifies a group with different triggers (RA vs PVI?) or more extensive remodeling with a highly proarrhythmic substrate. Cost/risk analysis[76] also supports the benefit of sequential AF ablation

postponed until the time of its clinical manifestation to spare patients the risks and costs of a possibly unnecessary procedure. The risk of developing AF for patients with lone AFL could be stratified based on some variables grouped into a score (HATCH score[77]). This score was tested and found to be independently associated with new-onset AF after AFL ablation and could be used to identify patients at risk (**Table 1**).

High-risk patients should probably be offered a combined ablation particularly if AF has been demonstrated while the low-risk group should be monitored for possible future AF development.

Anticoagulation should be continued for at least a few months following successful typical flutter RFA. Despite treating the underlying arrhythmia, a prothrombotic atrial myopathy remains, and the specter of developing AF after AFL ablation persists. Clinical evidence shows a reported incidence of 21 strokes per 1000 person-years, mostly in patients who developed AF following RFA for lone AFL.[78] These patients should receive anticoagulation depending on their CHA2DS2-VASc score; new oral anticoagulants, unless contraindicated, should be used to maintain a therapeutic level of the drug. Furthermore, as the occurrence of AF in these patients, increases over time[79] if not anticoagulated, the patient will need an extended, continuous follow-up.

Ablation strategies in patients presenting with AF or both AF and typical AFL can be considered together. Available clinical evidence and previous animal studies, previously discussed, would suggest that AF is probably the precursor of AFL in most patients and both arrhythmia can coexist manifesting themselves at different times and frequency. This is especially true in the "transitional phase" when both arrhythmia are paroxysmal. Progressive remodeling will induce more permanent structural and functional changes promoting the induction and maintenance of AF for longer

Table 1 HATCH score	
Risk Factors	**Points Assigned**
Hypertension	1
Age >75	1
TIA/CVA history	2
COPD	1
Congestive heart failure	2

The HATCH score predicts the risk of progression from paroxysmal to permanent AF. Different points are assigned to the risk factors according to their estimated predictive value. Score >2 indicates higher risk for disease progression.

periods of time rarely reorganizing into typical AFL.[80] The conversion of one into the other, in the early stage of the arrhythmia, is determined by the presence or absence of a posterior LoB as previously described. These patients should be treated as a mixed (AF and AFL) group and both should be addressed at the time of ablation (PVI and CTI isolation).

The coexistence of both arrhythmia, as previously discussed, may be a result of a more expansive pro arrhythmic atrial substrate than AF alone or a marker identifying patients with non-PVI triggers. A single-center study[47] pointed out, as previoulsy mntioned, that the recurrence of AF in the group of mixed arrhythmias was 70% following ablation (PVI and CTI) compared with 30% in the group with only AF treated with PVI. These preliminary findings suggest that AFL may be inducing a more extensive biatrial remodeling generating RA triggers that remain active after PVI and still induce AF even after the removal of LA triggers. These data are not sufficient to support a change of ablative approach in these patients. In the mixed group of arrhythmia, if an AAD rhythm control strategy is preferred to RFA, 10–15% patients with of AF [81] will develop de novo typical AFL. This is likely to be due to the modification of refractoriness induced by the drugs inducing a complete LoB block organizing AF to AFL in this smaller group of patients.[82] The initial approach to these patients was to consider AFL the dominant rhythm at times degenerating into AF. Ablation of isthmus-dependent AFL was proposed as a safer therapy. With time and more evidence, it became obvious that this approach needed to be refined as AF incidence during a follow-up longer than 1 year generally occurred in up to 50% following the initial isthmus ablation.[73] These patients will require therapies directed toward both arrhythmia as previously discussed. De novo evidence of typical AFL following ablation for "lone AF," is observed in less than 10% of patients. This may be due to these patient's inability to form an LoB or elimination of triggers by PVI, suggesting that prophylactic CTI isthmus ablation at the time of RFA for AF in every patient is not warranted. The scourge of atypical AFL occurring as a complication of RFA for AF is disussed elsewhere in this issue (Fabio M. Leonelli and colleagues' article, "Interpretation of typical and atypical atrial flutters by precision electrocardiology based on intracardiac recording,").

SUMMARY AND CLINICS CARE POINTS

AF and AFL are managed similarly and are both reflections of an underlying anatomic and electrophysiological atrial myopathy. Though their clinical courses have significant overlap, their underlying pathophysiology is distinct and interdependent. The interplay between these 2 arrhythmia and their clinical manifestations depends on anatomical structures, arrhythmic triggers, and atrial substrate. Each of these variables is changeable explaining the multifaceted clinical manifestations of these arrhythmia. This close relationship between AF and AFL needs to be understood to better define therapeutic approaches to their management.

Overall, fastidious risk factor modification and surveillance are required whenever a patient is diagnosed with either AF or AFL as these 2 conditions are intertwined and can recur despite improvements in ablative therapies. They represent a continuum of how atrial disease can manifest in clinical practice and will remain an area of intense cardiovascular research for years to come.

CLINICS CARE POINTS

- AF and AFL are distinct arrhythmias often transitioning spontaneously or under the effect of AAD or during RFA.
- This coexistence informs the arrythmias' clinical management.
- AFL is often considered a more "benign" arrythmia than AF as possibly carries less risk of thromboembolic events and can be "cured" with a uncomplicated highly effective RFA.
- In patients presenting with typical AFL 30% will have pure AFL (lone group) and close to 50% will manifest AF (mixed group) during follow up.
- In the mixed group the risk of stroke is as high as AF counterpatrts. Patients converting from AF to AFL duirng AAD loading should be considered within the mixed group. The likelihood of conversion to AF increases with higher HATCH score or AF inducibility at the time of ablation.
- Simultaneous CTI and PVI is recommended in the mixed group.
- In the lone group PVI should be postponed if and when AF is manifested.
- Following CTI ablation anticoagulation should either be continued in high CHAD score patients or follow up should be close and prolonged.

DISCLOSURE

RDP has received fees for lectures and scientific cooperation from Biosense Webster. All other authors declared no conflict of interest.

REFERENCES

1. Zipes DP, Jalife J, Stevenson WG. Cardiac electrophysiology: from cell to bedside: seventh edition. Circulation 2017. https://doi.org/10.1161/01.cir.0000146800.76451.65.

2. Haïssaguerre M, Jais P, Shah DC, et al. Spontaneous initiation of atrial fibrillation by ectopic beats originating in the pulmonary veins. N Engl J Med 1998;339:659–66.

3. Wu TJ, Liang KW, Ting CT. Relation between the rapid focal activation in the pulmonary vein and the maintenance of paroxysmal atrial fibrillation. Pacing Clin Electrophysiol 2001;24:902–5.

4. Ehrlich JR, Cha TJ, Zhang L, et al. Cellular electrophysiology of canine pulmonary vein cardiomyocytes: action potential and ionic current properties. J Physiol 2003;551:801–81.

5. Yamaguchi T, Tsuchiya T, Miyamoto K, et al. Characterization of non-pulmonary vein foci with an EnSite array in patients with paroxysmal atrial fibrillation. Europace 2010;12:1698–706.

6. Nattel S. New ideas about atrial fibrillation 50 years on. Nature 2002;415:219–26.

7. Moe GK, Rheinboldt WC, Abildskov JA. A computer model of atrial fibrillation. Am Heart J 1964;67:200–20.

8. Allessie MA, Lammers WEJEP, Bonke FIM, et al. Experimental evaluation of Moe's multiple wavelet hypothesis of atrial their role in atrial fibrillation. In: Zipes DP, Jalife J, editors. Cardiac electrophysiology and arrhythmias. Orlando: Grune and Stratton; 1985. p. 265–75.

9. Lesh MD, Pring M, Spear JF. Cellular uncoupling can unmask dispersion of action potential duration in ventricular myocardium. A computer modeling study. Circ Res 1989;65:1426–40.

10. Chen J, Mandapati R, Berenfeld O, et al. Dynamics of wavelets and their role in atrial fibrillation in the isolated sheep heart. Cardiovasc Res 2000;48:220–32.

11. Hansen BJ, Csepe TA, Zhao J, et al. Maintenance of atrial fibrillation: are reentrant drivers with spatial stability the key? Circ Arrhythm Electrophysiol 2016;9:e004398.

12. Spach MS, Dolber PC. Relating extracellular potentials and their derivatives to anisotropic propagation at a microscopic level in human cardiac muscle. Evidence for electrical uncoupling of side-to-side fiber connections with increasing age. Circ Res 1986;58:356–71.

13. Hansen BJ, Zhao J, Csepe TA, et al. Atrial fibrillation driven by micro-anatomic intramural re-entry revealed by simultaneous sub-epicardial and sub-endocardial optical mapping in explanted human hearts. Eur Heart J 2015;36:2390–401.

14. Allessie MA, Bonke FI, Schopman FJ. Circus movement in rabbit atrial muscle as a mechanism of tachycardia. III. The "leading circle" concept: a new model of circus movement in cardiac tissue without the involvement of an anatomical obstacle. Circ Res 1977;41:9–18.

15. Winfree AT. Scroll-shaped waves of chemical activity in three dimensions. Science 1973;181:937–9.

16. Cabo C, Pertsov AM, Davidenko JM, et al. Vortex shedding as a precursor of turbulent electrical activity in cardiac muscle. Biophys J 1996;70:1105–11.

17. Bagliani G, Della Rocca DG, De Ponti R, et al. Ectopic beats: insights from timing and morphology. Card Electrophysiol Clin 2018. https://doi.org/10.1016/j.ccep.2018.02.013.

18. Davidenko JM, Kent PF, Chialvo DR, et al. Sustained vortex-like waves in normal isolated ventricular muscle. Proc Natl Acad Sci U S A 1990;87:8785–9.

19. Mandapati R, Skanes A, Chen J, Berenfeld O, Jalife J. Stable microreentrant sources as a mechanism of atrial fibrillation in the isolated sheep heart. Circulation 2000;101:194–9.

20. Lazar S, Dixit S, Marchlinski FE, Callans D et alii Presence of Left-to-Right Atrial Frequency Gradient in Paroxysmal but Not Persistent Atrial Fibrillation in Humans Circulation. 2004;110:3181–3186.

21. Hocini M, Nault I, Wright M, et al. Disparate evolution of right and left atrial rate during ablation of long-lasting persistent atrial fibrillation. J Am Coll Cardiol 2010;55:1007–16.

22. Wijffels MC, Kirchhof CJ, Dorland R, et al. Atrial fibrillation begets atrial fibrillation. A study in Awake Chronically Instrumented Goats. Circulation 1995;92(7):1954–68.

23. Platonov PG, Mitrofanova LB, Orshanskaya V, et al. Structural abnormalities in atrial walls are associated with presence and persistency of atrial fibrillation but not with age. J Am Coll Cardiol 2011;58:2225–32.

24. Derakhchan K, Li D, Courtemanche M, et al. Method for simultaneous epicardial and endocardial mapping of in vivo canine heart: application to atrial conduction properties and arrhythmia mechanisms. J Cardiovasc Electrophysiol 2001;12:548–55.

25. Skanes AC, Mandapati R, Berenfeld O, et al. Spatiotemporal periodicity during atrial fibrillation in the isolated sheep heart. Circulation 1998;98:1236–48.

26. Gray RA, Jalife J, Panfilov AV, et al. Mechanisms of cardiac atrial fibrillation. Science 1995;270:1222–3.

27. Cox JL, Canavan TE, Schuessler RB, et al. The surgical treatment of atrial fibrillation II. Intraoperative electrophysiologic mapping and description of the electrophysiologic basis of atrial flutter and atrial fibrillation. J Thorac Cardiovasc Surg 1991;101:406–26.

28. Watson RM, Josephson ME. Atrial flutter. I. Electro-physiologic substrates and modes of initiation and termination. Am J Cardiol 1980;45:732–40.

29. Wang Z, Pagé P. Nattel S Mechanism of flecainide's antiarrhythmic action in experimental atrial fibrilla-tion. Circ Res 1992;71(2):271–8.

30. Reithmann C, Hoffmann E, Spitzlberger G, et al. Catheter ablation of atrial flutter due to amiodarone therapy for paroxysmal atrial fibrillation. Eur Heart J 2000;21:565–72.

31. Waldo AL, Feld GK. Inter-relationships of atrial fibril-lation and atrial flutter mechanisms and clinical im-plications. J Am Coll Cardiol 2008;51:779–86.

32. Botteron GW, Smith JM. Quantitative assessment of the spatial organization of atrial fibrillation in the intact human heart. Circulation 1996;93:513–8.

33. Narayan SM, Feld GK, Hassankhani A. Bhargava V quantifying intracardiac organization of atrial arrhyth-mias using temporospatial phase of the electrocardio-gram. J Cardiovasc Electrophysiol 2003;14:971–81.

34. Konings KTS, Kirchhof CJHJ, Smeets JRLM, et al. High-density mapping of electrically induced atrial fibrillation in humans. Circulation 1994;89:1665–80.

35. Nelson RM, Jenson CB, Davis RW. Differential atrial arrythmias in cardiac surgical patients. J Thorac Cardiovsc Surg 1969;58:581–7.

36. Wells JL, Karp RB, Mac Lean WAH, et al. Character-ization of atrial fibrillation in man: studies following open heart surgery. Pacing Clin Electophysiol 1978;1:426–38.

37. Horvath G, Goldberger JJ, Kadish AH. Simultaneous occurrence of atrial fibrillation and atrial flutter. J Cardiovasc Electrophysiol 2000;11:849–58.

38. Roithinger FX, Sipphnsgrohnewegen A, Karch MR, et al. Organized activation during atrial fibrillation in man; endocardial and electrocardiographic manifes-tations. J Cardiovasc Electrophysiol 1998;9:451–61.

39. Jais P, Haissaguerre M, Shah DC, et al. Regional disparities of endocardial atrial activation in parox-ysmal atrial fibrillation. PACE 1996;19:1998–2003.

40. Rosenblueth A, Garcia-Ramos J. Studies on flutter and fibrillation. II. The influence of artificial obstacles on experimental auricular flutter. Am Heart J 1947; 33:677–84.

41. Shimizu A, Nozaki A, Rudy Y, et al. Onset of induced atrial flutter in the canine pericarditis model. J Am Coll Cardiol 1991;17:1223–34.

42. Ortiz J, Niwano S, Abe H, et al. Mapping the conver-sion of atrial flutter to atrial fibrillation and atrial fibril-lation to atrial flutter insights into mechanisms. Circ Res 1994;74:882–94.

43. Uno K, Kumagai K, Khrestian C, et al. New insights regarding the atrial flutter reentrant circuit in the canine sterile pericarditis model. J Am Coll Cardiol 1997;229:254A,. abstract.

44. Friedman PA, Luria D, Fenton AM, et al. Global right atrial mapping of human atrial flutter: the presence of posteromedial (Sinus Venosa Region) functional block and double potentials. A study in biplane fluo-roscopy and intracardiac echocardiography. Circu-lation 2000;101:1568–77.

45. Huang JL, Tai C-T, Lin Y-J, Huang B-H, et al. Sub-strate mapping to detect abnormal atrial endocar-dium with slow conduction in patients with atypical right atrial flutter. J Am Coll Cardiol 2006;48(3):492–8.

46. Tai CT, Chen SA, Chiang CE, et al. Characterization of low right atrial isthmus as the slow conduction zone and pharmacological target in typical atrial flutter. Circulation 1997;96:2601–11.

47. Moreira W, Timmermans C, Wellens HJJ, et al. Can common-type atrial flutter be a sign of an arrhythmo-genic substrate in paroxysmal atrial fibrillation? Clin-ical and ablative consequences in patients with coexistent paroxysmal atrial fibrillation/atrial flutter. Circulation 2007;116:2786–92.

48. Kumar S, Kalman JM, Sutherland F, et al. Atrial fibril-lation inducibility in the absence of structural heart disease or clinical atrial fibrillation. Critical depen-dence on induction protocol, inducibility definition, and number of inductions. Circ Arrhythmia Electro-physiol 2012;5:531–6.

49. Bettoni M, Zimmermann M. Autonomic tone varia-tions before the onset of paroxysmal atrial fibrillation. Circulation 2002;105:2753–9.

50. Yang Y, Mangat I, Glatter KA, et al. Mechanism of conversion of atypical right atrial flutter to atrial fibril-lation. Am J Cardiol 2003;91:46–52.

51. Yang Y, Cheng J, Bochoeyer A, et al. Atypical right atrial flutter patterns. Circulation 2001;103:3092–8.

52. Yu WC, Chen SA, Lee SH, et al. Tachycardia-induced change of atrial refractory period in hu-mans: rate dependency and effects of antiar-rhythmic drugs. Circulation 1998;97:2331–7.

53. Matsuo K, Tomita Y, Khrestian CM,Waldo AL. A new mechanism description of the electrophysiologic ba-sis of atrial flutter and atrial of sustained atrial fibril-lation: studies in the sterile pericarditis fibrillation. J Thorac Cardiovasc Surg 1991;101:406–26. model. Circulation 1998;98:I-209, abstract.

54. Schuessler RB, Grayson TM, Bromberg BI, et al. Cholinergically mediated tachyarrhythmias induced by a single extrastimulus in the isolated canine right atrium. Circ Res 1992;71:1254–67.

55. Hsieh MH, Tai CT, Tsai CF, et al. Mechanism of spon-taneous transition from typical atrial flutter to atrial fibrillation: role of ectopic atrial fibrillation foci. PACE 2001;24:46–52.

56. Moe GK, Abildskov JA. Atrial fibrillation as a self-sustaining arrhythmia independent of focal discharge. Am Heart J 1959. https://doi.org/10.1016/0002-8703(59)90274-1.

57. Ajijola OA, Wisco JJ, Lambert HW, et al. Extracar-diac neural remodeling in humans with cardiomyop-athy. Circ Arrhythm Electrophysiol 2012;5:1010–116.

58. Sparks PB, Jayaprakash S, Vohra JK, et al. Electrical remodeling of the atria associated with paroxysmal and chronic atrial flutter. Circulation 2000;102: 1807–13.

59. Wu TJ, Yashima M, Xie F, et al. Role of pectinate muscle bundles in the generation and maintenance of intra-atrial reentry: potential implications for the mechanism of conversion between atrial fibrillation and atrial flutter. Circ Res 1998;83:448–62.

60. Schumacher B, Jung W, Schmidt H, et al. Transverse conduction capabilities of the crista terminalis in patients with atrial flutter and atrial fibrillation. J Am Coll Cardiol 1999;34:363–73.

61. Franz MR, Karasik PL, Li C, et al. Electrical remodeling of the human atrium: similar effects in patients with chronic atrial fibrillation and atrial flutter. J Am Coll Cardiol 1997;30:1785–92.

62. Philippon F, Plumb VJ, Epstein AE, et al. The risk of atrial fibrillation following radiofrequency catheter ablation of atrial flutter. Circulation 1995;92:430–5.

63. 2020 Guidelines for Management of Atrial Fibrillation ESC Clinical Practice Guideline 20 Aug 2020) (2019 AHA/ACC/HRS Focused Update of the 2014 AHA/ACC/HRS Guideline for the Management of Patients With Atrial Fibrillation: A Report of the American College of Cardiology/American Heart Association Task Force on Clinical Practice Guidelines and the Heart Rhythm Society in Collaboration With the Society of Thoracic Surgeons Circulation Volume 140, Issue 2, 9 July 2019; Pages e125–e15.

64. Nabar A, Rodriguez LM, Timmermans C, et al. Effect of right atrial isthmus ablation on the occurrence of atrial fibrillation: observations in four patient groups having type I atrial flutter with or without associated atrial fibrillation. Circulation 1999;99(11):1441–5. https://doi.org/10.1161/01.CIR.99.11.1441.

65. Wazni O, Marrouche NF, Martin DO, et al. Randomized study comparing combined pulmonary vein-left atrial junction disconnection and cavotricuspid isthmus ablation versus pulmonary vein-left atrial junction disconnection alone in patients presenting with typical atrial flutter and atrial fibrillat. Circulation 2003. https://doi.org/10.1161/01.CIR.0000101684.88679.AB.

66. Waldo AL, Cooper TB. Spontaneous onset of type I atrial flutter in patients. J Am Coll Cardiol 1996. https://doi.org/10.1016/S0735-1097(96)00223-9.

67. Glover BM, Chen J, Hong KL, et al. Catheter ablation for atrial flutter: a survey by the European heart rhythm association and Canadian heart rhythm society. Europace 2016;18:1880–5.

68. Turgam MK, Musikantow D, Whang W, et al. Assessment of catheter ablation or antiarrhythmic drugs for first-line therapy of atrial fibrillation. A meta-analysis of randomized clinical trials. JAMA Cardiol 2021; 6(6):697–705.

69. Granada J, Uribe W, Chyou PH, et al. Incidence and predictors of atrial flutter in the general population. J Am Coll Cardiol 2000;36:2242–6.

70. Halligan S, Maurer M, Munger T, et al. Risk and predictors of subsequent atrial fibrillation in patients presenting with typical atrial flutter [abstract]. Circulation 2001;104:II714.

71. Pokushalov E, Romanov A, Corbucci G, et al. Ablation of paroxysmal and persistent atrial fibrillation: 1-year follow-up through continuous subcutaneous monitoring. J Cardiovasc Electrophysiol 2011;22: 369–75.

72. Morton JB, Byrne MJ, Power JM, et al. Electrical remodeling of the atrium in an anatomic model of atrial flutter relationship between substrate and triggers for conversion to atrial fibrillation. Circulation 2002; 105:258–64.

73. Maskoun W, Pino MI, Ayoub K, Llanos OL, et al. Incidence of atrial fibrillation after atrial flutter ablation. JACC Clin Electrophysiol 2016;2:682–90.

74. Da Costa A, Romeyer-Bouchard C, Zarqane-Sliman N, et al. Impact of first line radiofrequency ablation in patients with lone atrial flutter on the long term risk of subsequent atrial fibrillation. Heart 2005;91:97–8.

75. Luria DM, Hodge DO, Monahan KH, et al. Effect of radiofrequency ablation of atrial flutter on the natural history of subsequent atrial arrhythmias. J Cardiovasc Electrophysiol 2008;19:1145–50.

76. Gula LJ, Skanes AC, Klein GJ, et al. Atrial flutter and atrial fibrillation ablation - sequential or combined? A cost-benefit and risk analysis of primary prevention pulmonary vein ablation. Heart Rhythm 2016;13: 1441–8.

77. Chen X, Bai R, Deng W, et al. HATCH score in the prediction of new-onset atrial fibrillation after catheter ablation of typical atrial flutter. Heart Rhythm 2015;12:1483–9.

78. Tomson TT, Kapa S, Bala R, et al. Risk of stroke and atrial fibrillation after radiofrequency catheter ablation of typical atrial flutter. Heart Rhythm 2012;9: 1779–84.

79. Healey JS, Connolly SJ, Gold MR, et al. Subclinical atrial fibrillation, and the risk of stroke. N Engl J Med 2012;366:120–9.

80. Kim AM, Olgin JE, Everett TH. Role of atrial substrate and spatiotemporal organization in atrial fibrillation. Heart Rhythm 2009;6:S1–7.

81. Falk RH. Proarrhythmic responses to atrial antiarrhythmic therapy. In: Falk RH, Podrid PJ, eds. Atrial fibrillation: mechanisms and management. New York: Raven Press.

82. Schumacher B, Jung W, Lewalter T, et al. Radiofrequency ablation of atrial flutter due to administration of class IC antiarrhythmic drugs for atrial fibrillation. Am J Cardiol 1999;83:710–3.

Interpretation of Typical and Atypical Atrial Flutters by Precision Electrocardiology Based on Intracardiac Recording

Fabio M. Leonelli, MD[a,b,]*, Roberto De Ponti, MD, FHRS[c,d],
Giuseppe Bagliani, MD[e,f]

KEYWORDS

- Atrial flutter • Typical atrial flutter • Atypical atrial flutter • Isthmus-dependent atrial flutter
- Scar-related flutter • Electrocardiogram • Macroreentry • Microreentry

KEY POINTS

- Despite its limitations, electrocardiogram (ECG) continues to be the first approach to every arrhythmia. This is particularly true in the case of atrial flutters (AFL) where the initial classification of isthmus- and nonisthmus-dependent flutters is based on ECG criteria.
- This classification also defines the reentrant circuit, which in one case is well understood while in the other remains often speculative and requires intravascular recording and electroanatomic mapping for the final diagnosis.
- Many AFLs presenting in clinical practice arise as a complication of radiofrequency ablation procedures for atrial fibrillation. ECG interpretation of this subset of nonisthmus-dependent flutters requires a detailed knowledge of cardiac anatomy, basic electrocardiology, the type of ablation performed, and potential consequences.
- No diagnostic ECG criteria have been developed for postablation flutters, but several features suggest some specific reentrant mechanisms. Diagnosis of these arrhythmias rests on intracardiac electrophysiology study.

ELECTROCARDIOGRAM IN ATRIAL FLUTTERS: ADVANTAGES AND LIMITATIONS

The definition of reentry and the description of atrial flutter (AFL) as a macroreentrant arrhythmia is one of the brilliant pages in the history of electrophysiology (EP).

Initial observations on circus movement[1] were later recreated in animal studies[2] and followed by description in patients[3] using basic equipment for endocardial simulation and signal recording.[4]

As technology improved, the quality and the number of endocardial recordings increased from less than 100 in the late 1990s to several hundred

[a] Cardiology Department, James A. Haley Veterans' Hospital, University of South Florida, 13000 Bruce B Down Boulevard, Tampa, FL 33612, USA; [b] University of South Florida FL 4202 E Fowler Avenue, Tampa, FL 33620, USA; [c] Department of Heart and Vessels, Ospedale di Circolo, Viale Borri, 57, Varese 21100, Italy; [d] Department of Medicine and Surgery, University of Insubria, Viale Guicciardini, 9, Varese 21100, Italy; [e] Cardiology And Arrhythmology Clinic, University Hospital "Ospedali Riuniti", Via Conca 71, Ancona 60126, Italy; [f] Department of Biomedical Sciences and Public Health, Marche Polytechnic University, Via Conca 71, Ancona 60126, Italy
* Corresponding author. Cardiology Department, James A. Haley Veterans' Hospital, University of South Florida, 13000 Bruce B Down Boulevard, Tampa FL 33612.
E-mail address: fabio.leonelli@va.gov

Card Electrophysiol Clin 14 (2022) 435–458
https://doi.org/10.1016/j.ccep.2022.05.004
1877-9182/22/© 2022 Elsevier Inc. All rights reserved.

in the most recent reports allowing a more detailed reconstruction of the reentry. To this, 3-dimensional representation of the arrhythmia, so-called electroanatomic mapping, has added a clear visual representation of arrhythmic concepts. Electrophysiology (EP) maneuvers, first of all entrainment, and detailed analysis of electrograms, continue to be the backbone of arrhythmia mechanism definition. It became possible with time to reconstruct faithfully the entire macro- and microreentrant circuit defining areas of slow or no conduction.

In particular, these tolols allowed a more cohesive view of all the components of typical and atypical flutter's circuit describing multiple nontypical circuits differing in size, location, and boundaries.

The advent of high-density intracardiac mapping has shown the limitations of previous ECG-based classification of AFLs and focal tachycardias,[5] and there is now a general agreement that the final diagnosis of most AFLs rests on the analysis of intracardiac recordings and ablation of the hypothesized arrhythmia circuit.

This is particularly obvious when dealing with scar-related arrhythmias following surgical or ablative procedure to treat atrial fibrillation (AF) and the uncertainty in differentiating microreentry from AT.

The role of the ECG, which was dominant at the time of the initial classification, has progressively diminished in importance because of the limitations in the information provided by of a standard 12 lead ECG. Nevertheless, given its low cost, ubiquitous equipment and still considerable diagnostic accuracy, the ECG remains one of the most used tool in cardiology.

To improve the diagnostic power of this tool, several modifications have been reported, from the use of 3 leads in orthogonal planes,[6] to multi lead ECG recording.[7]

Despite these new advances, correlating intracardiac findings with ECG morphology has always been the most useful method to explain electrocardiographic tracings. Thanks to the detailed intracardiac information generated during an EPS, this correlation has greatly improved the ECG ability to understand the mechanism and classify many nontypical arrhythmias.

INTRACARDIAC AND ELECTROCARDIOGRAM RECORDINGS IN TYPICAL FLUTTER
Definition of Typical and Atypical Atrial Flutter

Before detailed intracardiac recording, electroanatomical mapping, and pacing maneuvers had

become commonly used to understand the arrhythmia mechanism and origin, ECG morphology was used to define the mechanism of arrhythmias.[5] Although this continues to be valid in typical flutter originating in a healthy atrium, most flutters observed now are scar-related and require a detailed analysis of the ECG waveforms and correlation with intracardiac findings. Thanks to its remarkable uniform ECG morphology, CL stability, and unvarying reentrant path, typical AFL is promptly recognized at first look (**Fig. 1**). The terms typical or isthmus-dependent are used interchangeably since a group of electrophysiologists described the isthmus between tricuspid valve (TV) and inferior vena cava (IVC) as an obligatory part of the macroreentry, a necessary area of slow conduction and unidirectional block.[8] The crista terminalis (CT) posteriorly and the Tricuspid Valve-Inferior Vena Cava (TV-IVC) isthmus anteriorly were subsequently demonstrated to be the boundaries defining the reentrant path.[9] A different posterior line of block at the level of the sinus venosa region was suggested by some authors,[10] but in general this has been discounted in favor of the CT.

The TV-IVC isthmus role allowed a definition of the flutters into 2 groups: isthmus-dependent AF (IDFL) or typical when this isthmus was a necessary component of the circuit and NIDFL (nonisthmus-dependent AF) when the isthmus was not required to maintain the arrhythmia. With the advent of RFA, this preprocedural differentiation became clinically useful, as ablation of the TV-IVC isthmus, a relatively straightforward procedure, had consistent excellent results.[11]

During these early studies, 2 possible directions of the reentry around the TV, using the same path, were reported and termed typical clock (CW) and counterclockwise (CCW) flutter.[12] Activation of the R and LA, and consequently the ECG tracing, were markedly different in these 2 flutters[5] even though, in both cases, the TV/IVC isthmus was an obligatory part of the reentrant circuit.

Typical Atrial Flutter

Counterclockwise isthmus-dependent atrial flutter

In CCW flutter, by far the most common form, the wavefront exits the isthmus at the septal junction ascends the RA septum and the posterior wall and descendeds this chamber's antero-lateral wall. (**Fig. 2**)The CT functions as an anatomic/functional barrier protecting the anticlockwise TV rotation from short-circuiting wavefronts. The electrocardiographic pattern of typical CCWID flutter waves is easily recognizable: the FL wave is predominantly negative in the inferior leads (sawtooth) and V6 while positive in V1. Intracardiac mapping has shown what these ECG features depend on (**Fig. 3**A, B):

1. The period of isthmus conduction occurs at a time of minimal or no left atrium (LA) depolarization and determines the plateau.
2. Two distinct wavefronts of activation occur in the right atrium (RA), an initial inferosuperior activation followed by a superoinferior activation inscribing the sawtooth pattern.
3. Two wavefronts collision occur, one at the posterior atrium along the IVC and one in the inferior anterolateral atrium.
4. LA activation occurs mostly in a superoinferior and postero-anterior direction.

Variations in the sequence, timing, and direction of depolarization of these main wavefronts can change subtly or drastically the appearance of the FL wave.[13]

The slow return to baseline characterizing the AFL plateau is possibly caused by the depolarization of the small muscle mass of the isthmus[14] generating a low V vector. Prolongation of isthmus conduction, as often observed in failed isthmus ablations, will markedly prolong this AFW's component without altering the typical sawtooth wavefront.

Intracardiac recording also demonstrated that LA, despite not being part of the reentrant circuit, greatly contributes to the morphology of the flutter wave.[15] The impulse exiting the septal isthmus will immediately engage the coronary sinus (CS) and proceed proximal to distal, creating an inferosuperior activation of the posterior LA wall. Approximately 30 to 35 milliseconds later, the septal wavefront will reach the Bachman bundle (BB) and generate a second wavefront of activation proceeding superoinferiorly and merging with the initial one. Biatrial activation is often synchronous, with a similar direction of activation generating the large negative and positive components of the FLW.

In particular, any modification in interatrial connections (eg, delay in CS engagement, faster septal or BB conduction, or LA enlargement) could alter, at times radically, the FLW morphology.[16] More subtle ECG changes have also been explained by intracardiac mapping. The voltage of the terminal positive deflection represents an unopposed superoinferior vector, and its ECG variability has been associated with depolarization of the lateral wall of an enlarged LA[17] or delayed activation of RA lateral wall.[18]

Clockwise isthmus-dependent FL In CW flutter the wavefront of activation exits the isthmus at its lateral insertion, and the RA lateral wall and septum are depolarized in a direction opposite to the CCW flutter (**Figs. 4** and **5**). The CW FLW's features, on 12-lead ECG, a prominent notching (see **Fig. 4**) on the inferior leads between 2 mostly positive deflections attributed to cranio-caudal activation of the septum (first notch) and superoinferior depolarization of the LA (second notch). The intervals between peaks correspond, according to some authors, to the interatrial conduction time.[16]

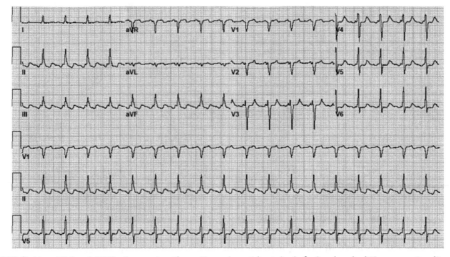

Fig. 1. CCW flutter 12 lead ECG. A saw-tooth pattern is evident in inferior leads (Giuseppe Bagliani and colleagues' article, "Electrocardiographic Approach to Atrial Flutter: Classifications and Differential Diagnosis," in this issue). Predominant polarity of Fl wave is positive in lead I, inferior leads, and V6. In V1 and aVR, the polarity is positive. Notching is present on the positive dome of the inferior leads, representing interatrial conduction time according to some authors.[16]

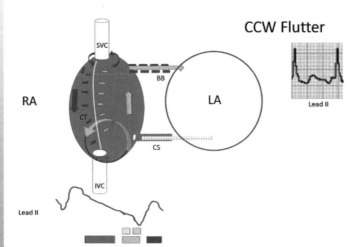

Fig. 2. CCW isthmus-dependent flutter schematic representation. Major RA vectors are depicted in red (isthmus activation), yellow (septal wall), green checkered (inferior LA wall via CS), purple (anterolateral RA wall) and green solid (superior LA via BB). The circular arrow describes the CCW wavefront rotation around the TV and the CT, blocking and preventing the wavefronts form short-circuiting the circuit. Septal wavefront turns inferiorly after passing behind the SVC.[22] BB, Bachman bundle; CCW, counterclockwise; CS, coronary sinus; CT, crista terminalis; LA, left atrium; RA, right atrium; TV, tricuspid valve.

As the BB is engaged before the CS, the LA in CW flutter is activated as in sinus rhythm (SR) and therefore inscribes a similar vector, predominantly negative in V1 and positive in V6 and left lateral limb leads. Compared with CCW flutter, LA activation appears to be less uniform with variable fusion between BB and CS activation times.[16]

Variants of Typical Atrial Flutter

Mechanism of variations

The difference between recording and analysis of intracardiac potentials and surface ECG observations becomes obvious when attempting to understand the cause of morphology and cycle length (CL) variations occurring during an otherwise stable IDFL. The ECG recording of atrial activity during a stable AFL will appreciably change only if there is a change in LA activation and synchronized septal RA wall depolarization. Modification of the RA anterolateral wall activation is more subtle and usually goes undetected.[7] Shifts in the arrhythmia's path can occur and be manifested only by CL variations while a typical ECG suggestive of IDFL remains unchanged. On the contrary, even minor shifts within the reentrant circuit changes are, readily observed by intracardiac recording/mapping, and several variations of

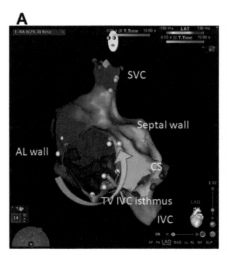
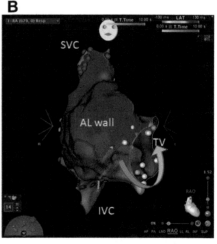

Fig. 3. CCW isthmus-dependent flutter electroanatomical map in left lateral projection (*A*) and right lateral projection (*B*). Colorimetric representation of wavefront progression timed against a fixed reference recording. Red color represents earliest activation, purple latest. Note the CCW rotation around the TV with head (*red*) and tail (*purple*) propagation fronts meeting on the RA lateral wall. This picture explains the circularity of the macroreentry and the progression of activation from the isthmus ascending along the septal wall and descending along the anterolateral RA wall. AL, anterolateral; CS, coronary sinus; IVC, inferior vena cava; SVC, superior vena cava; TV, tricuspid valve.

isthmus-dependent flutters have been described using these techniques. These variations are usually caused by a change in one of the circuit boundaries shifting the reentry path. If isthmus (anterior boundary) dependency of the flutter is maintained, change can only occur at the CT (posterior boundary) level. Early intracardiac recordings along the CT showed, in SR, a marked anisotropic transverse delayed conduction in this structure.[19] At higher rates of stimulation, functional block is added to the anatomic delay, creating a longer posterior barrier more marked in patients with spontaneous AFL than in normal subjects[9,20]

Although this concept of fixed/functional block is generally accepted, the extent of the CT block has not been completely resolved. If there are no breakthroughs along the CT from IVC to superior vena cava (SVC),[21] the flutter is more likely to remain a typical CCW or CW. In the case, of a solid CT in CCW flutter, the posterior propagation wavefront crosses to the anterior wall by passing behind the SVC[22] (see **Fig. 2**). In CW, the wavefront progresses superiorly on the anterolateral RA wall and crosses in front of the SVC to proceed posteriorly toward the septal insertion of the isthmus[22] (see **Fig. 5**). Complete CT block is present in a few cases while gaps are observed in most CTs, most commonly at the point of connection with the SVC or along the inferior CT[22,23] (**Figs. 6** and **7**).

Counterclockwise lower loop reentry

The RA is composed of anatomic structures ideally set up to favor the establishment of a macroreentrant circuit, the IDFL being the most frequently observed (see **Fig. 6**). The IVC can also establish a possible reentrant circuit with its circular path limited anteriorly by the isthmus. In typical CCW AFL, this potential circuit remains inactive because of the collision, in the posterior wall, of 2 wavefronts traveling in opposite direction around this vein (see **Fig. 6**).

The inferior CT prevents short-circuiting of the established path; in the presence of gaps in this

region,[23] the posterior wavefront proceeds laterally, bypassing the IVC, and generates 2 wavefronts, one directed superiorly and the second anteriorly to enter the IVC/TV isthmus. The first wavefront will collide with the inferiorly directed activation of the lateral wall, while the second will perpetuate the tachycardia along a different, shorter albeit isthmus-dependent, circuit (see **Fig. 5**).

Concealed entrainment and termination without reinduction of the flutter following IVC-TV isthmus ablation confirmed the previously described interpretation of these findings aptly named lower loop reentry (LLR).[24] Conversion from LLR to CCW flutter can occur spontaneously when the breakthrough along the inferior CT disappears. This suggests that, at least this area, represents a functional more than a fixed anatomic barrier, and shorter refractory period and oscillation of action potential duration during tachycardia could change the degree of conduction block.[24]

Oscillation of the flutter CL becoming shorter during LLR and lengthening when returned to the typical circuit will be observed during intracardiac and surface recordings. The morphology of the flutter wave remains mostly unchanged, but the terminal positive deflection becomes less marked, possibly because of a reversal of RA lateral wall activation.[24]

Atypical Flutters

The implication of this definition is that the TV IVC is not a necessary component of the reentrant circuit. The RA and LA reentrant circuit of these flutters is determined by different boundaries, and therefore a dissimilar ECG from typical AFL is recorded. Because the possible combinations of boundaries and resultant circuits can be numerous, the ECG becomes less typical of 1 specific type of flutter, and the diagnosis depends exclusively on intracardiac recordings and anatomic mapping. The boundaries sustaining these tachycardias include mostly anatomic

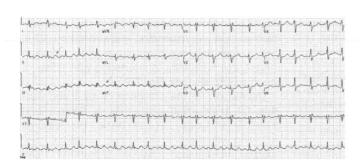

Fig. 4. CW flutter 12-lead ECG. Predominant polarity of FI wave is positive in lead I, inferior leads, and V6. In V1 and aVR, the polarity is negative. Notching (*blue arrows*) is present on the positive dome of the inferior leads, representing interatrial conduction time according to some authors.

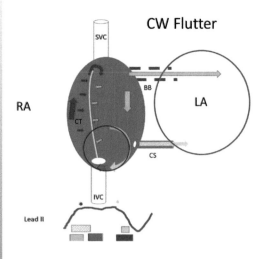

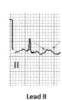

CW Flutter

Lead II

Fig. 5. CW isthmus-dependent flutter schematic representation. Major RA vectors are depicted in red (isthmus activation), yellow (septal and posterior wall) Green checkered (inferior LA wall via CS), purple (Antero-lateral RA wall), and green solid (superior LA via BB). The function of the CT as described in **Fig. 1**: the antero-lateral wall wavefront reaches the anteroseptal region passing in front of the SVC.[22] The circular arrow describes the CW wavefront rotation around the TV. The 2 blue arrows identify the 2 notches. BB, Bachman bundle; CCW, counterclockwise; CS, coronary sinus; LA, left atrium; RA, right atrium; TV, tricuspid valve.

Lower loop reentry

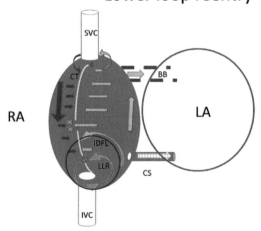

Fig. 6. CCW isthmus-dependent flutter and lower loop reentry schematic representation. Major RA vectors are depicted in yellow (septal wall), green checkered (inferior LA wall via CS), purple (anterolateral RA wall), and green solid (superior LA via BB). The function of the CT as described in **Fig. 1**: the anterolateral wall wavefront reaches the anteroseptal region passing behind the SVC.[22] The circular yellow arrow describes the CCW wavefront rotation around the TV (IDFL), while the smaller circular orange arrow represents the wavefront rotating around the IVC/TV isthmus (LLR). The CT is represented as noncontinuous line with a mid and inferior gap. A wavefront from the septal activation (*orange arrow*) traverses the CT but collides (*green crosses*) with an anterior wavefront (*purple arrow*). More inferiorly, the CT gap allows a short-circuiting of the CCW reentry and establishes an LLR, which, having a shorter path, will emerge.

structures or scars and at least in 1 reported series an area of functional block on the RA free wall.[25]

Upper loop reentry

Although the combination of CT and isthmus is an ideal set up for a reentrant path, the RA, with its varied morphology, offers other possible variations to this typical pathway (see **Fig. 7**; **Fig. 8**). The SVC is a semicircular anatomic obstacle that could create an independent circuit providing its wavelength is sufficiently long and the reentrant waveform is protected from extraneous collisions.

The SVC constitutes the upper turnaround point in typical AFL, anteriorly in CW flutter and posteriorly in CCW flutter.[26] The gap existing between the upper reach of the CT and the SVC determines whether an independent reentry can be sustained around this vein, often simultaneously with an isthmus-dependent flutter.[27] A wavefront breaking through a higher CT gap could anticipate RA free wall activation, reversing the typical caudocranial direction of activation of at least part of the RA free wall and septum.[23] Presence or absence of CT gaps and their locations will determine whether only the typical CCW reentrant circuit is present or 2 different competing loops are present sharing the IVC-TV isthmus (see **Fig. 7**B). If the 2 arrhythmias coexist, an ascending wavefront from IDFL and descending wavefront from ULR collide in the RA free wall without interfering with either of the main circuits (see **Fig. 7**B)

The reason for the presence of gaps and variable CT conduction properties is unclear and probably includes several basic EP features including wavefront direction and curvature, gap-junction expression, tissue anisotropy, and source-sink relations.[26] The result is an

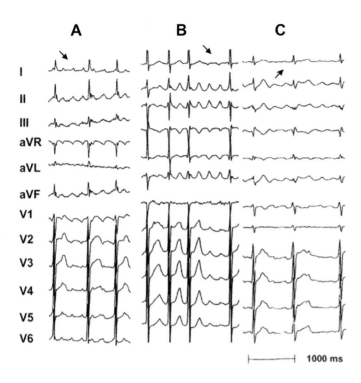

Fig. 7. Comparison between CW AFL (*A*) and upper loop reentry (*B*, *C*). Prominent positive polarity in lead I in CW flutter (*A arrow*) compared with flat or negative in ULR (*B*, *C arrows*). The inferior lead morphology is similar in both reentrant circuits. BB, Bachman bundle; CCW, counterclockwise; CS, coronary sinus; IDFL, isthmus-dependent AFL; LA, left atrium; LLP, lower loop reentry; RA, right atrium; TV, tricuspid valve; ULR, Upper Loop Reentry. (*From:* Yuniadi Y, Tai CT, MD, Lee KT, Huang BH, Lin YC, Higa S, Liu TY, Huang JL, Lee PC, MD, Chen SAA New Electrocardiographic Algorithm to Differentiate Upper Loop Re-Entry From Reverse Typical Atrial Flutter J Am Coll Cardiol 2005;46:524.)

inhomogeneous conduction across the CT facilitating unidirectional block, particularly during fast stimulation and oscillatory variation of its refractory properties.

Main LA and RA septum activation remain, at first sight, similar in ULR and CW flutter (see **Figs. 5** and **7**B). The overall 12-lead ECG shows, in ULR, less positive flutter waves in the inferior leads and negative V1 not dissimilar from a typical CW circuit (see **Fig. 7**A).

A detailed ECG analysis (**Fig. 7**) suggests that lead I could help in differentiating these 2 entities. A negative or flat wave polarity was more consistent with ULR, while a positive polarity of more than 0.07 milliseconds was consistent with CW flutter.[28]

The authors explained the finding by the different timing of activation of the LA and RA free wall in CW flutter and ULR. In the former, the LA activation occurs after the RA free wall is completely activated (see **Fig. 5**). In the latter (see **Fig. 7**A, B), it occurs at the same time and concurrently with interatrial septum. These wavefronts, similar to SR, are leftward and inferiorly directed, generating a positive deflection in lead I. In ULR, the RA free wall and LA activation occur simultaneously, canceling each other and inscribing a flat P wave in lead I.

A coexistence of typical flutter and ULR was observed, in 1 study, in more than half of the

patients with an apparent isthmus-dependent AFL. Paradoxic delayed capture during pacing from a different site within the circuits demonstrated the presence of 2 functioning reentrant loops.[27] As the reentry shifts from competing loops, the CL varies, and the instability of the circuit increases. This favors the degeneration of these flutters into AF, particularly in the presence of numerous breakthroughs generating multiple collision sites. The occurrence of these reentrant circuit variations is difficult to quantify, but it varies from 10% in the largest series[23] to 50% in a smaller study.[27] Lower and upper loop reentries demonstrate the importance of the CT as a posterior barrier in the genesis and maintenance of RA flutters; the length, site, and number of CT breaks have different consequences on the reentrant circuit path and on the ECG morphology.

Scar-Related Atrial Flutter: Introduction

Scars can be defined as island of tissue of variable size where mixtures of fibrous tissue and surviving myocytes are combined. These areas demonstrate profoundly altered electrophysiological properties such as delayed or no conduction[29]

Scarring is the result of myocardial death for any reason and is frequently observed following surgical or ablatives atrial procedures. The hemodynamic effects of scarring on atrial contraction are

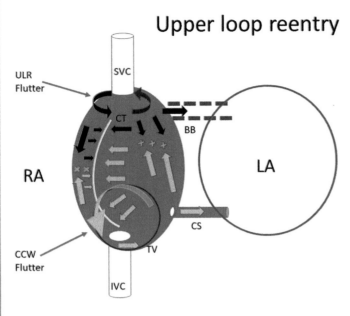

Upper loop reentry

Fig. 8. Two AFLs (*black and yellow arrows*) are simultaneously present: ULR is represented by black arrows circulating around the IVC and propagating inferiorly along the postero-lateral and septla wall. The BB is activated by the same circuit. Major CCW (*yellow arrows*) vectors are depicted as in **Fig. 5** caudo-cranial along the septal wall and inferior LA wall via CS, the circular yellow arrow representing TV activation that continues in the IVC-TV isthmus and up to the antero-lateral wall. The CT is fully continent inferiorly but has a large gap in front of the SVC, allowing a reentry around this vein (*black arrows*). The anterolateral wall is activated as a fusion between a superior wavefront from the ULR and an inferior from the CCW flutter. Septal and antero-lateral lines of collision (*green crosses*) are shown between craniocaudal wavefronts from ULR (*black arrows*) and caudocranial CCW flutter (*yellow arrows*).

LA is activated as usual from BB and CS, but the timing of propagation along these 2 connections is not sequential as it depends on 2 (ULR and CCW flutters) unrelated macroreentrant circuits.[25] BB, Bachman bundle; CCW, counterclockwise; CS, coronary sinus; IDFL, isthmus-dependent AFL; LA, left atrium; LLP, lower loop reentry; RA, right atrium; TV, tricuspid valve.

generally less prominent than electrical consequences. Patches of nonconduction and strategically located islands of slow conduction can constitute respectively boundaries and isthmuses of macroreentrant circuits.[30]

Surgical incisions will often provide a proarrhythmic substrate resulting in variable arrhythmia location, mechanism, and circuit. Postsurgical atrial arrhythmias have been observed for any procedure aimed directly at one or both atria, or when the atria serve only as an access portal as in lung[31] and heart transplant.[32]

Spontaneous atrial scarring can also constitute an arrhythmic substrate and appears to have a predilection for specific RA and LA sites.[33,34] Fibrosis probably is, in these cases, the end result of several different noninterventional pathologies such as infection, hypertension, and ischemia. These etiologies are uncommon compared with RA or LA surgical or ablative procedures that have, after the advent of radiofrequency ablation (RFA) to treat AF, become the most common causes of scar-related arrhythmias.

Scar-related atrial flutter: substrate and mechanism

Postprocedural atrial scarring was, for many years, observed mostly after repair of congenital or acquired heart defects or cardiac surgery requiring cardio-pulmonary bypass. More

recently, the substrates involved in atrial fibrillation have become the target of surgical procedures and later of catheter-based ablation made possible by considerable technology advances. Any procedure that destroys tissue will be followed by scarring and create a proarrhythmic substrate.

This was initially observed in repaired atrial or ventricular congenital heart disease (CHD), where the likelihood of developing scar related flutters is related to patient's age, complexity of surgical reconstruction, and remodeling following unphysiological hemodynamic conditions.[35] The more complex the surgery, often including extensive biatrial reconstruction, the higher the number of intricate atriotomy scars and widely distributed surgical material. These areas can easily become part of a reentrant circuit, the stability of which will depend on a fine balance of multiple factors including path length, delayed conduction, and unidirectional block.

This explains the uncommonly high number of adults with treated complex CHD developing right atrial arrhythmias that can be, on long follow-ups, as high as 100% as is the case following Fountain procedure.[36,37] Catheter-based RFA for AF is a more standardized technique complicated by more predictable arrhythmias. Even in this less invasive procedure, the relationship between complexity of ablation and likelihood of subsequent arrhythmias, holds true.

In any case, given the intricacy and variability of scar-related arrhythmias, a full understanding of their electrophysiological mechanism has been possible only after the advent of new technologies. Electro-anatomical mapping and improved electrogram resolution, combined with standard EP techniques, have allowed detail descriptions of many reentrant circuits.

Despite the large number of arrhythmias observed following scar inducing procedures, some generalizations are possible. Reentry is the dominant mechanism with a minority of arrhythmias due to automaticity/triggered activity.[38,39] The reentrant circuit can be contained in a miniscule amount of tissue (microreentry) or in a larger well-defined path (macroreentry). The distinction between these 2 entities is not completely agreed upon.[40]

In general in a macroreentrant circuit, an isthmus of tissue between 2 nonconductive boundaries is always present.[41] The isthmus generally has a slow velocity of propagation accounting for the long CL often observed in these arrhythmias. At times, an isthmus can be used by 2 independent circuits,[42] creating a reentrant figure of 8. Not uncommonly, macroreentrant circuits shift from one to another circuit spontaneously or more commonly during rapid pacing or delivery of a single extra stimulus. A microreentry contains an entire reentrant circuit in a small amount of tissue, often at the border zone or embedded in a larger scar. The requirements for reentry are met in miniature, with a miniscule isthmus of slow conduction between nonconductive boundaries.[43]

Microreentry cannot be distinguished from automatic ATs using only an anatomic mapping, as both will appear as centrifugal single areas of activation; local entrainment, adenosine response, and detailed electrogram analysis of the circuit are necessary. The causal connection between these nonreentrant arrhythmias and scarring or the atrial remodeling before or after the procedure is unclear.

Scar-Related Right Atrium Flutters

Nonprocedure-related scars

Uncommonly, scar-related flutters occur in patients not exposed to atrial ablation or surgery (**Figs. 9** and **10**). A few patients were described with flutters due to posterolateral scars extending from CT to tricuspid anulus.[33]

In every patient of this group, both isthmus-dependent and -independent arrhythmias rotating around the scar were observed. In this flutter the ECG morpholoyg is non typical with negative flutter waves both in the inferior leads and V1 to V6 and isoelectric or positive wave in leads I and aVL.

Flutters Related to Surgical Scars and Radiofrequency Ablation

The RA often constitutes the initial surgical access to the other cardiac chambers, and it is a convenient way to provide venous access during circulatory bypass. Most resultant RA surgical scars, due to these procedure, are located in the anterior wall and the septum and not infrequently become the substrate of macroreentry.[44] Furthermore, the RA anatomy predisposes this chamber to develop spontaneous isthmus-dependent flutter, and this propensity is accentuated by the addition of new surgically induced barriers.[45]

Following atrial septal repair, for example, CW isthmus-dependent flutter is the most common[46] arrhythmia observed. This type of flutter, rarely observed to occur spontaneously in the general population, is much more common in patients with previous scars, most commonly after ASD or even nonsurgical RA scars.[33] CW flutter is frequently observed even following complex repairs such as the Mustard/Senning procedure,[47] stressing again the RA propensity to develop isthmus-dependent flutters.

The reason why the uncommon form of isthmus-dependent flutter is observed is possibly related to the site of origin of the triggering stimulus and its relationship with the slow conduction area determining the direction of unidirectional block and flutter rotation.[48] The only surgical procedure where isthmus flutter is rarely observed is the Fontan operation, where complex, mostly incisional tachycardias, represent the majority of postprocedural arrhythmias observed.[49] Although numerous studies describe the intracardiac recordings and electro-anatomical mapping of arrhythmias following CHD repair surgery, no systematic ECG description of these varied and unusual tachycardias exists in literature.

Intraisthmus Reentry

Intraisthmus reentry is an uncommon arrhythmia originating along the Eustachian ridge either close to the septum or in the middle-anterior CTI.[50] In most cases, it is associated with spontaneous or ablation induced isthmus scars. The circuit is probably confined within the isthmus, but it is not isthmus dependent as it is often observed following successful typical flutter ablation with documented isthmus conduction block[50]. In a minority of cases, the isthmus scarring occurs in the

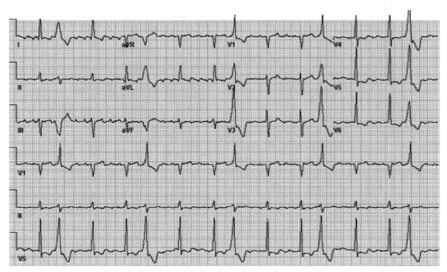

Fig. 9. 12-lead ECG of spontaneous scar related RA flutter. Predominant polarity of Fl wave is positive in lead III, becoming biphasic in lead aVF, and negative in lead II. Low voltage in precordial leads with positive/flat polarity. Lead I and aVL are clearly negative. An isoelectric line is present. This combination suggests a LA tachycardia, possibly focal.

context of extensive areas of septal RA idiopathic fibrosis. Because it is more commonly a micro-reentry, intraisthmus reentry can be differentiated by AT located in the same area only by mapping, entrainment maneuvers, and recognition of areas of fragmented electrograms (EGMs), which are often a necessary part of the circuit.

ECG is in keeping with typical CCW flutter in over 80% of cases and more uncommonly shows an atypical pattern with positive inferior flutter waves in the inferior leads and V1. Morphology shifts from typical CCW to CW, and more atypical waveforms were observed without a change in arrhythmia CL.[51]

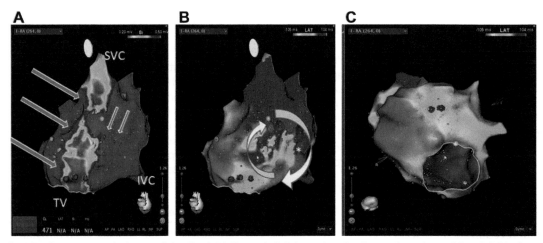

Fig. 10. Electroanatomical map of the **Fig. 9** RA flutter in left lateral projection and craniocaudal LAO (*A*) Voltage map shows a color-coded representation from very low/absent voltage (*red*) to normal (*purple*). An area of low or absent voltage (*arrows*) extending from SVC to TV on the anteroseptal wall is shown. (*B*) Colorimetric representation of wavefront progression timed against a fixed reference in the CS. Red color represents earliest activation, purple latest. The flutter rotates on the posterior RA wall (*yellow arrow*) with a channel in the inferoposterior wall (*white asterisk*). More septally, the red wavefront is less defined with a serpiginous propagation between scars. (*C*) Note the TV activation without a clear meeting point between a head (*red*) and tail (*purple*) propagation fronts as shown in **Fig. 3**B. In this case, the TV is passively activated by the posterior circuit. CS, coronary sinus; IVC, inferior vena cava; LAO, left anterior oblique; SVC, superior vena cava; TV, tricuspid valve.

Intracardiac mapping is inconsistent with the ECG appearance in 40% of patients when inferior dominant negative flutter waves were observed despite a CW activation of the RA. The authors suggested that given the vicinity of the arrhythmia exit site to the CS os, an early engagement of this structure and RA septum could generate a dominant caudo-cranial activation in both chambers.

Scar-Related Left Atrium Flutters

Nonprocedure-related scars

The LA is not predisposed to develop de novo reentrant arrhythmias and a nonscarred, normal chamber is rarely the source of spontaneous macro reentry.

A few cases of nonscar-related flutter[51] were reported involving the L side of the interatrial septum where the reentrant circuit rotated in CW or CCW direction, around the fossa ovalis with the R superior PV posteriorly, and the MV ring anteriorly constituting the anatomic/functional barriers.

A defined scar was not identified, and the main promoter of this spontaneous flutter was felt to be either a myopathy or the effect of antiarrhythmic drugs (AADs) slowing of atrial conduction.

The ECG features of this arrhythmia were flat P waves in most leads with, in the inferior leads, a hint of positivity in CCW and negativity in CW flutter. V1 was prominent with a direction similar to the inferior leads. The authors explained the finding by a rapid, early activation from the LA septum to the RA using both the BB and the CS, resulting in a cancellation of the RA superior and inferior vectors.[51]

Most LA macroreentrant flutters are caused by procedure related scars, with rare reports of spontaneous scars of unknown etiopathology, including every LA wall, septum, and roof.[52] With the aid of electro-anatomic mapping during EP studies, slow or blocked propagation within the scars has been documneted and found to be similar to post procedural scars creating an ideal reentry set up. Concomitant use of Anti Arrythmic Drugs (AAD) appears to favor the emergence of these flutters by further slowing myocardial propagation.[34]

The number of circuits varied from single to multi loop macroreentry, and in a few cases, a single small area of critical slow conduction was observed maintaining a microreentry.[42] Anterior wall scars were more likely to induce a figure-of-8 reentry circulating around the MV and the scar above this valve. A common isthmus with slow conduction existed between these 2 circuits,[53] often becoming the target of successful ablation.[53]

Paucity of cases, variety of scar extent and location, different macroreentrant circuits, and nonuniform patient population prevent any attempt to formulate a systematic approach to the electrocardiographic interpretation of these flutters' mechanism or location.

Flutters Related to Surgical Scars and Radiofrequency Ablation

Surgery

The LA is not often a target for CHD surgery, and most LA surgical procedures involve repair or replacement of the MV. In this procedure, the RA is cannulated, and the LA is accessed using different approaches to expose the MV leaving behind scars in the RA and/or LA, causing arrhythmias at a later stage.[54]

These arrhythmias are, in most cases macroreentry circuits mostly related to previous atriotomies or cannulation sites and show different degree of complexity likely related to the extent and number of incisional scars.[54] Rarely, areas of low voltage away from surgical suture lines have been found to be the substrate for reentry. This, as previously mentioned, suggests the presence of a nonincisional myopathic process observed in the RA and LA, and possibly caused by ischemia, trauma, or mechanical stresses pre- and postoperatively.

Post-MV repair/replacement tachycardias are infrequent compared with arrhythmias following catheter-based or surgical corrective procedures to treat AF. In these cases, the LA is the initial and often the sole target of these ablations or surgical incisions aimed at eliminating triggers or modifying atrial tissue perpetuating AF.

Atrial arrhythmia surgery to treat AF (maze procedure), which initially established the feasibility of this approach[55] is rarely performed today according to the original description because of its complexity and invasiveness. The use of radiofrequency energy to complete the atrial set of lines required in the maze has improved its completion time, and it is not uncommonly used as adjunct to other cardiac surgery in patients with atrial fibrillation[56]

AT and macroreentrant flutters have been documented following either a cut-and-saw or radiofrequency maze. In both cases, the circuits develop in areas of incomplete lesions most commonly observed at PV-atrial interface or PV to mitral ring lines, the latter serving as a substrate for perimitral flutters.[56] Loss of viable tissue by reducing P wave voltage makes a reliable diagnosis of the arrhythmia difficult and, at times, even impedes the differentiation between AF and AFL.[57]

Radiofrequency ablation

The increased incidence of AF coupled with rapid technological advances has rendered catheter-based AF ablation safer and more accurate and has allowed more aggressive approaches in the treatment of every type of AF. PVI isolation, the initial standard procedure in the AF treatment, became a wide atrial circumferential ablation (WACA) soon complemented by lines connecting the R and L upper ablation areas. Preventive MV perimetral flutter lines, isolation of the posterior LA wall or the appendage, and ablation of fragmented atrial tissue were frequently added, reducing the viable LA tissue, in some cases, to less than 50%.[58] The reentrant circuits are strongly related to the extent of the ablation and presence of gaps in the ablation lines.[59]

Appraoch to Scar related Flutters: Electrophysiology Study

A strategic approach to these arrythmias[60] includes an initial differentiation between focal and macroreentrant arrhythmias during an EPS. Assessment of the arrhythmia CL suggests the presence of an automatic mechanism in the presence of repetitive short bursts of arrhythmia or a CL variability in excess of 15% of the basic rate.

A stable CL is shared by macro- and microreentry. Analysis of the sequence of activation of strategically located fixed or rowing catheters, response to entrainment maneuvers, and construction of electroanatomic maps is used to distinguish between these 2 mechanisms of the arrythmia.[61] Macroreentry will appear as a continuously propagating waveform around a fixed obstacle with an early and late wavefront. A focal tachycardia will demonstrate a focal point of origin with centrifugal activation. Differentiation between microreentry and focal AT requires further detailed mapping of the site of origin.

Demonstration of continuing electrical activity slowly propagating for more than 75% of the arrhythmia cycle length in an area of less than 3 cm of diameter was considered diagnostic of microreentry. The absence of these features was consistent with focal AT.[62]

Every area targeted by ablation resulting in a scar can be the substrate of a reentrant circuit,[63] but given the standardization of AF ablation procedures, few macroreentrant circuits are observed in most cases. The most common macroreentrant flutters following RFA for AF are, in order of frequency, perimitral, roof-dependent, septal, and less commonly IDFLs.[62] The factors determining the preferential emergence of 1 type of macroreentry instead of another are unknown with the exception of roof lines, which have been found to favor the development of perimitral flutters.[64] They, as a group, represent

between 56%[62] and 85%[39] of postablation arrhythmias. Most focal ATs are microreentry, usually located in the LA in the vicinity of incomplete ablation lines, creating areas of slow conduction.[38,65] Typical sites include the LAA, septum, or PV-atrial junction, specifically at the superior LPV or anterior to the RPVs, possibly because of catheter instability or thickness of the tissue at these sites.[66]

Electrocardiogram Recognition of Scar-Related Atrial Flutter

The effects of scars on the electrocardiogram in SR

Compared with the refined technologies used during an EPS, the ECG has the only advantages of being noninvasive, easily performed, and inexpensive (**Figs. 11–14**). Analysis of a 12-lead ECG is nevertheless useful as it can help in identifying the mechanism and localize the site of origin of the. Understanding these characteristics will help in planning the most appropriate procedure and guiding the initial mapping strategy.

A diagnostic reconstruction of the mechanism of a supraventricular arrhythmias based on an ECG tracing depends on the analysis of the different vectors composing it. Understanding the contribution of each arrhythmia vector requires beat-to-beat stability, uniform cardiac conduction, known anatomic and functional boundaries, and a stable propagation path. This is present in IDFL as the reentrant path is fixed and predictable and allows interpretations of the typical AFL and its variations. (Giuseppe Bagliani and colleagues' article, "The history of atrial flutter electrophysiology, from entrainment to ablation: A 100 year experience in the Precision Electrocardiology," in this issue.)

Atrial scarring, on the contrary, can modify, at time extensively, all these parameters, creating new boundaries and areas of slow conduction and decreasing the amount of viable tissue contributing to the electrical vectors. This variability and the complexity of scar-related arrhythmias explain the small number of published detailed reviews of their ECG morphology and the absence of validated interpreting algorithms.

Extensive ablation has an effect on sinus P waves, which are more likely to show a lower voltage and particularly a decreased LA component. This may be reflected by a lower or absent negative component in V1, a negative-only component at aVL or an undetectable Pw after extensive RA and LA ablation during a maze procedure.[67] In these cases, it is likely that sinus interatrial and intra-atrial propagation are profoundly altered, and a considerable mass of viable

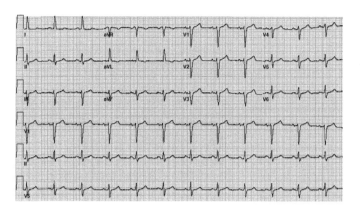

Fig. 11. 12-lead ECG showing normal sinus rhythm with normal voltage P wave and borderline interatrial delay.

tissue has been replaced by electrically inert myocardium (see **Figs. 12–14**). Although, in general, the function of the LA is maintained, these extreme cases have been accompanied by mechanical LA standstill[68] (see **Fig. 14C**).

ELECTROCARDIOGRAM APPROACH TO ATYPICAL ATRIAL FLUTTER

An atypical AFL is defined as an arrhythmia with ECG features differing from typical isthmus-dependent flutter (**Table 1**). An approach to the former should include identification of the chamber of origin, mechanism, and detailed localization.

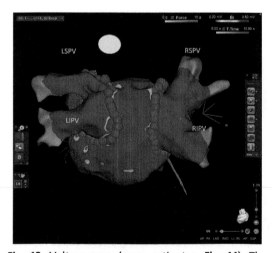

Fig. 12. Voltage map (same patient as **Fig. 11**). The posterior LA map shows an overall normal voltage with evident 4 pulmonary veins isolatED following wide area circumferential ablation (*red dots*). LIPV, left inferior pulmonary vein; LSPV, left superior pulmonary vein; RSPV, right superior pulmonary vein.

Identifying the Chamber of Origin

In order to identify the chamber of origin, it is necessary to recognize the atrial activity during the arrhythmia. This may be difficult, as often the voltage of this wave is small (defined as a maximal voltage ≤ 0.1 mV, in any of the 12 leads), or it can be hidden by the ST-T complex.

The only parameter that appears to have some consistent value in this initial step is V1 polarity, with a positive (completely positive or biphasic with second component negative) F-wave present in up to 90% of L atrial arrythmias[42,69] and a negative F-wave identifying a right origin albeit with less predictive power.[25]

This is because of the posterior location of the LA within the thorax and a predominant postero-anterior vector generated by LA arrhythmias and an opposite vector in RA tachycardias. Isoelectric P wave in V1 is nonspecific.[70] Other leads such as aVL, I, and aVR used in nonscarred atria to localize the origin of the arrythmia[70] are far less useful after ablation.

Arrhythmia Mechanism

Differentiating ATs from macro reentrant atrial flutter (MRAF) is useful in preprocedural planning given the different success rates and risk of complications. Review of all the available ECGs can lead to valuable insights. Observing the mode of arrhythmia initiation, for example, can distinguish between AT and MRAF; the former often begins with a P wave like the rest of the arrhythmia, while the latter is usually initiated by a PAC of different morphology.

P wave duration should reflect the focal or the macroreentrant nature of the arrhythmia. This measurement can be done more accurately using orthogonal ECG helpful in detecting precisely the timing, duration of every atrial waveform, and the

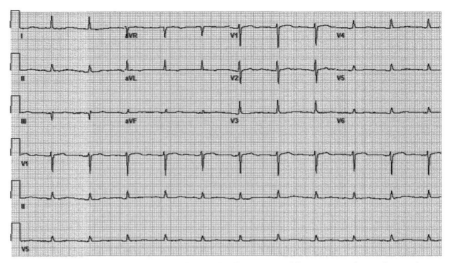

Fig. 13. 12-lead ECG showing normal sinus rhythm with almost invisible P wave of very low voltage.

arrhythmia's CL.[71] In a small patient's cohort, these authors claimed a 90% sensitivity and specificity for their combined index to separate macroreentry flutters from ATs. The mechanism of AT, reentry vs non-reentry, can also be helped by observing CL stability, as previously mentioned.

Defining the Pw also identifies the isoelectric line. This line corresponds to a period of unrecordable electrical activity and has, traditionally, be used to distinguish between AT and macroreentry.[5] Given the AT single site of origin and its centrifugal activation, a rapid biatrial depolarization will be followed by a period of electrical silence, the duration of which is determined by the arrhythmia's CL.

Macroreentry creates a continuous activation wavefront spreading over both chambers, inscribing in the ECG an undulating wave (**Fig. 15**; see **Fig. 17**). If a protected, electrically silent isthmus bound by nonconductive tissue is present in a macroreentry, the period during which the wavefront propagates through this structure could, if sufficiently long, correspond to an isoelectric line in the 12-lead ECG.[72]

This is not uncommon in a scarred atrium. Isoelectric lines of less than 80 milliseconds were noted in approximately 30% of the total arrhythmias, more commonly in focal AT (47% vs 23%), but this parameter could not be used to reliably establish the arrhythmia's mechanism.[62]

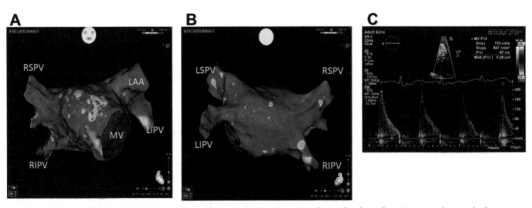

Fig. 14. Voltage Mal (same patient as **Fig. 13**). LA voltage maps in sinus rhythm showing a color-coded representation from very low/absent voltage (*red*) to normal (*purple*) in anterior (*A*) and posterior projection (*B*). The figures show an almost complete absence of voltage in the entire LA except for small surviving areas of electrical activity. This is the results of previous MA annuloplasty, 3 RFAs, and remodeling following previous longstanding persistent AF. (*C*) Mitral inflow contemporary to the voltage maps shows a normal E wave and absent A wave, suggestive of a complete loss of LA mechanical function. CS, coronary sinus; IVC, inferior vena cava; LAO, left anterior oblique; MV, mitral valve; SVC, superior vena cava; TV, tricuspid valve.

Table 1
Electrocardiogram characteristics of most common post PVI arrhythmias

General Findings		
P-P > 15% variation		Nonreentrant FAT
No isoelectric line all leads[a]		Macroreentrant flutter
Precordial Leads		
V1	Positive or +/−	RA arrhythmia
	Negative or −/+	LA arrhythmia
	M shaped	LPV FAT
Precordial leads transition	Yes:+ V1 to −V6	CCW TVIVC flutter
	No:+ without transition	CCW MV flutter
	NO: + with small initial-lateral leads	CW MV flutter
Inferior Leads		
	Negative	Inferior FAT
	Positive	CCW TV IVC after ablation
	Positive With early negative notch	CW MV

The table lists electrocardiogram findings characteristic of the most common post PVI arrhythmias. As an algorithm cannot be constructed, the arrythmias are color coded to better identify all the features most likely associated with them.

Abbreviations: CCW, counter clock wise; FAT, focal atrial tachycardia; LA, left atrium; LPV, left pulmonary vein; MV, mitral valve; R, right atrium; TV IVC, tricuspid valve inferior vena cava.

[a] Isoelectric line ≥ 80 msec.

Furthermore, the presence of an isoelectric line was directly correlated with the voltage of the sinus Pw, being more frequently observed in patients with a PV less than 0.1 mV. Absence of an isoelectric line, on the other hand, was more common in macroreentry (78%) but was also observed in ATs (22%) as described in some rare cases[73] because of slow propagation through a scarred atrium.

MACROREENTRANT FLUTTERS

As previously mentioned, the 3 most common macroreentrant circuits, following RFA for AF, are roof-dependent, perimetral, and TVIVC isthmus-dependent. They constitute most of the arrhythmias observed after catheter-based or surgical ablation AF ablation[39,62,74]

Roof-Dependent

Roof-dependent flutter uses a circuit rotating around the ablated PVs, almost exclusively RPVS, possibly because the larger anatomic size of the circuit, and involves the LA roof with 2 possible directions of rotation, most commonly posteroanterior (PA) or less commonly anteroposterior (AP).

Some authors[62] could not find specific features differentiating this arrhythmia for other reentrant circuits. Other authors constructed an algorithm using CS activation time as a first step followed by analysis of the polarity of inferior leads

assessed by using a specifically timed P wave interval.[75] The purpose of this stepwise approach was to distinguish PA and AP roof-dependent flutters from the CW and CCW perimitral reentry.

In this report, the ECG of a PA roof-dependent flutter was characterized by positive P in the inferior leads positive across the precordial leads, particularly in V1 and V2 with a reduced voltage in lateral precordial leads. Lead aVL was always negative, while Lead I morphology was less uniform.

An AP rotation showed the opposite pattern with negative P waves inferiorly, positive in I and aVL, and V1 to V2 transitioning to flat/negative in V3. The ECG morphology of PA roof flutter was similar to CCW perimitral flutter, and the AP to CW and CS activation was necessary to distinguish one form the other. No single or combination of unique ECG features without CS recordings could distinguish roof flutter from other scar-reentrant tachycardias.

Perimitral Flutter

Perimitral flutter, practically never observed in unscarred LA, rotates around the MV (see **Fig. 15**; **Fig. 16**). Scars preventing wavefront extinction (roof scars) or restricting the reentrant path (PVI) are necessary to make this arrhythmia sustainable.

The usefulness of ECG analysis in correctly identifying this circuit of reentry and its direction of rotation varies among the authors (see

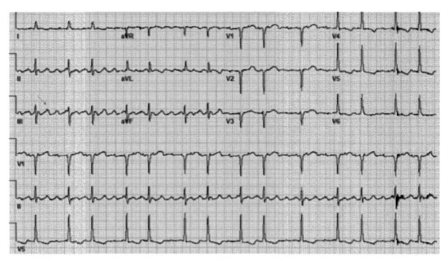

Fig. 15. Perimitral flutter 12-lead ECG showing AFL with 3:1, 2:1 block. An isoelectric line is present in V1 but continuous in the inferior leads. Polarity is biphasic (+/−) in V1 and predominantly positive in the inferior leads. aVL is predominantly negative. Notching is present on inferior leads on the ascending limb (*blue arrow*). P wave remains positive without transition across the precordial leads (clearly visible in V5). The pattern is highly suggestive of perimitral flutter with CCW rotation.[39,68]

Fig. 15). Lead V1 is positive or biphasic (+/−) in every PMF identifying the L atrium as the chamber of origin. Two features were found, when present, to be specific for PMF by a group of researchers.[62]

First, an early negative notch on the positive ascending limb of inferior leads was associated with a CW mitral valve with a 77% predictive value. Second, the absence of a precordial transition with negative or negative/positive F waves from V2 to V6 was reported in 30% of PMF and in 3% of other arrhythmias, with a 82% positive and 97% negative predictive value (see **Fig. 15**).

Different reports characterize the usefulness of the peripheral leads in identifying this flutter's direction of rotation. Although a group of investigators found them unreliable,[62] others[65] have found a mostly positive inferior polarity and predominant negativity in I and aVL in CCW perimitral flutter; the opposite pattern is more often associated with CW flutter. The latter group of authors also reports an absence of isoelectric line in every PMF.

Typical atrial flutter following radiofrequency ablation or ablation for AF

IDFL constitutes less than 20% of arrhythmias following RF[76] or surgical mini-maze[77] for AF and is, in most cases, CCW. The ECG presentation of this arrhythmia differs from the typical patterns in up to 85% of cases.[78] The chest leads continue to have the typical CCW pattern,[70] following RFA with a positive P wave in V1 followed by a gradual transition across the precordial leads to a negative V6.[76]

A typical sawtooth pattern, highly specific when it occurs spontaneously, is present in less than 30% of cases following ablation for AF despite an unaffected RA reentry circuit. In most patients, the typical sawtooth morphology in the inferior leads is replaced by an upright wave and a negative flutter wave in aVL.[76,78]

These changes are difficult to explain by ECG analysis, as it often combines features of CW flutter (positive inferior leads) with a left origin of the arrhythmia (aVL), suggesting an atypical LA reentrant circuit. These findings highlight the relevance of LA depolarization for the morphology of the flutter wave.

Because the LA is a bystandard component of the ID flutter circuit, a change in its activation will not affect the arrhythmia CL but will greatly alter the ECG appearance. The shift from a dominant superior (BB) to inferior (CS) propagation of LA depolarizing wavefront is usually the consequence of a shift or delay in timing of engagement of 1 of these 2 interatrial connections.

A reversal in the sequence of RA septum/free wall will switch time of engagement of CS or BBB profoundly modifying the ECG morphology of the flutter.[79] BB and CS propagation time was unchanged by the ablation and propagation to the LA occurred, as expected, mostly via the CS.[79]

Biatrial mapping, voltage recording, and entrainment of these arrhythmias suggest that this pattern was caused by a large destruction of LA with a marked diminution of LA voltage. This would leave tissue the craniocaudal RA activation

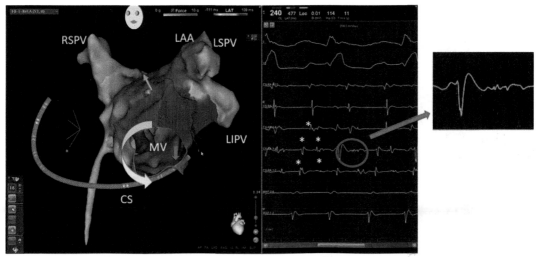

Fig. 16. Perimitral flutter: electroanatomic map and intracardiac electrograms of LA in an LAO projection with caudocranial tilt (same patient as **Fig. 15**). Timing of wavefront progression is shown with red being earliest and purple latest. A head (*red*)/tail (*purple*) collision is shown on the anterior wall in keeping with a rotation around the MV (*yellow arrow*). On the right side, EMGs recorded from the CS catheter are displayed with fragmentation (*blue arrow* and enlargement) and split potentials (*white asterisks*). The flutter rotates in CCW direction. CS, coronary sinus; IVC, inferior vena cava; LAO, left anterior oblique; LIPV, left inferior pulmonary vein; LSPV, left superior pulmonary vein; MV, mitral valve; RSPV, right superior pulmonary vein; SVC, superior vena cava; TV, tricuspid valve.

unopposed, resulting in positive/biphasic ECG in the inferior leads and unopposed right-to-left depolarization vector.[79] In other cases, an isoelectric line, a biphasic or a multicomponent low V uninterpretable wave were observed[78] in the inferior leads.

Timing and extent of RFA procedure may affect the ECG pattern the inferior leads, requiring a more extensive debulking and more time between RFA and the emergence of the flutter.

Three different macroreentrant arrhythmias (see **Figs. 4** and **15**): CW IDFL, CCW perimitral, and postablation CCW IDFL can present with a pattern of positive FL waves in the inferior leads (**Table 1**). The morphology of the flutter wave in postablation CCW IDL varies from biphasic with a narrow negative and a predominant positive component to fully

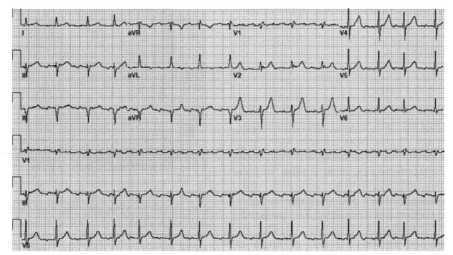

Fig. 17. 12-lead ECG showing AFL with 2:1 block. An isoelectric line is present in every lead, most clearly in V1. Polarity is biphasic (+/−) in V1 with a characteristic M shape and negative in aVL. The pattern is consistent with LIPV.

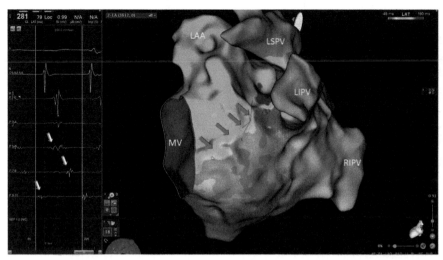

Fig. 18. Electroanatomic map and intracardiac electrograms of LA in a posterolateral projection (same patient as **Fig. 17**). Timing of wavefront progression is shown with red being earliest and purple latest. An early focal site emerges from the LIPV and expands preferentially inferiorly and posteriorly with a uniform delay on the anterior wavefront (*blue arrows*). On the left side, EMGs recorded from a multipolar catheter at the site of earliest activation shows fragmented electrograms (*white arrows*), spanning almost the entire tachycardia cl, suggesting the presence of a microreentry.

positive.[65] Notching, particularly evident in the inferior leads (see **Figs. 4** and **15**), is a feature of CCW perimitral and spontaneous CW flutter.

The similarity in ECG tracings despite different direction of rotation was explained by the comparable septal activation in the first two and the effect of ablation on LA vectors. Differentiating among these flutters will also require an analysis of the entire 12-lead tracing. CCW IDFL will maintain a positive V1 in most cases, together with a positive aVL. V1 and aVL are predominantly negative in the other 2 flutters.

Possibly the most sensitive/specific parameters is the absence of precordial transition always present in perimitral but not in peritricuspid flutter (see **Table 1**).[16,62,65]

AT: Localize the Origin

The incidence, in the largest series,[62,65] of focal ATs after RFA for AF is around 40%, most being microreentrant. Some ECG criteria were suggested to differentiate macroreentry from focal AT[80] but not confirmed by other studies. In general, CL variability suggests an automatic origin, while the presence of an isoelectric line is less specific, being present in 30% to 50% of AT patients[62]

P wave morphology, used to identify the mechanism and localize the site of origin of nonscar-related ATs,[81] has a variable reported predictivity.[62,65] Some authors[65] observed a good correlation between Pw in scar-related ATs and the Pw

observed in spontaneous or pacing induced premature beats originating around the PVs[82]

According to this group, a positive morphology across the entire precordium with a typical M shape in V1 was often consistent with tachycardias originating from LPVs. A negative Pw in aVL and an isoelectric line in lead I were the features most commonly observed for this site of origin.

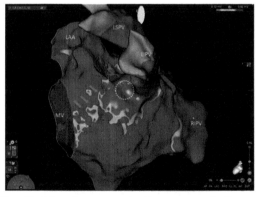

Fig. 19. LA voltage map in the same projection as **Fig. 18** (same patient as **Fig. 17**). Red areas indicate scars inside the LPVs and the RIPV. Just below the LIPV, some EGMs are recorded surrounded by scar. This is the area where the microcircuit was mapped (*white dotted circle*) and later successfully ablated. Also note an incomplete LIPV-MV ablation line of low V below the LIPV (*blue arrows*) explaining the delay noted in this area in the previous activation map.

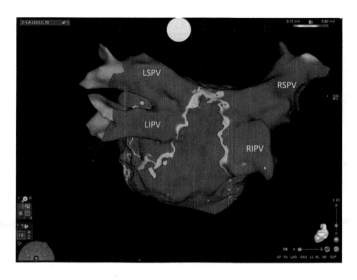

Fig. 20. Voltage map of LA posterior wall demonstrating isolation of the 4 PVs. (same patient as **Fig. 17**). The microreentry did not appear to be associated with PV reconnection but with the profound modification of the substrate induced by the ablation. CS, coronary sinus; IVC, inferior vena cava; LAO, left anterior oblique; LIPV, left inferior pulmonary vein; LSPV, left superior pulmonary vein; MV, mitral valveRSPV, right superior pulmonary vein; SVC, superior vena cava; TV, tricuspid valve.

Lead I was found to be able to discriminate between RPV (positive) and LPV (flat/negative). Despite disagreement, some observations are consistent across the largest published studies (see **Table 1**).[62,65,75] A positive polarity in the inferior leads was nonspecific, as it was observed in up to 81% of cases regardless of the source of the arrhythmia.

A uniformly positive polarity across the precordial leads, often with a typical M shape in V1, was observed in most ATs originating in the LPVs (**Figs. 17–20**). In the same study,[39] a focal tachycardia from the RPV presenteds with a late-peaking positivity in V1 and throughout the precordium and a positive component in lead I with a flat/biphasic aVL (**Figs. 21** and **22**).

Negative inferior leads were uncommon (approximately 20% of cases) but, when present, they predicted an inferior origin of these centrifugal ATs, most commonly from the inferior left atrium or CS.[62,65] ATs originating in the LAA seem to have a more reproducible ECG patterns with a positive P in V1 and the inferior leads, negative in aVL and I.[83]

In summary, there is no accepted diagnostic ECG algorithm when presented with an organized atrial arrhythmia following RFA for AF. This is mostly because of the unpredictable path followed by the macro reentrant arrhythmias and the effects of extensive scarring on atrial

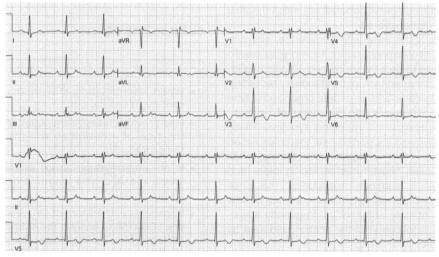

Fig. 21. 12-lead ECG showing an atrial tachycardia with 2:1 block. A long (>200 milliseconds) isoelectric line is present in all 12 leads. P wave polarity is fully positive in V1 and across the precordium, with a clear slow ascending branch. It is positive in I and inferior leads and predominantly positive in aVL with a small initial negative notch. This pattern suggests an RSPV focal AT.

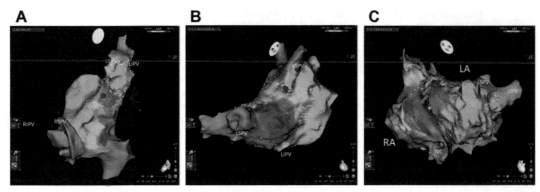

Fig. 22. Focal tachycardia electroanatomic map of LA superoposterior (*A*) and superoanterior (*B*) view. A focal activation beginning in the roof side of the RSPV (*A*) preferentially spreads anteriorly (*B*). The L and R atrial progress of activation is shown in (*C*) with superior septal activation (*blue arrow*) at the BB level to activate the RA septum (*asterisk*) and proceed superiorly and inferiorly (same patient as **Fig. 21**).

propagation. ECG features that are consistent in more than 1 large series of observations are reported in **Table 1**.

SUMMARY

Unraveling the mechanism of AFL is one of the most successful endeavors achieved by a large group of scientists and clinicians (Giuseppe Bagliani and colleagues' article, "The history of atrial flutter electrophysiology, from entrainment to ablation: A 100 year experience in the Precision Electrocardiology," in this issue). The initial astute observations in animal models were confirmed in patients by ECG observations using a simple technology unchanged over the course of decades. As recording systems improved, supported by safer invasive procedures and progressively larger computer capabilities, initial theories were fully demonstrated.

As often is the case with knowledge, answers lead to more questions waiting for more advanced technologies to be fully addressed. The limited information provided by mostly stationary recording catheters became a trove of data organized in time and space sequences with the advent of 3-dimensional electroanatomic mapping systems. These technologies also supported new therapies aimed at treating more complex arrhythmias, with catheter-based procedures replacing older and more invasive surgical procedures. The price paid for this progress was the occurrence of new and more intricate arrhythmias, frequently occurring as a complication of the scarring induced by the ablation.

The complexity of these new arrhythmias originating in altered substrates, limits the use of the time-honored ECG recordings. Routine 12-lead tracings, often diagnostic in the case of spontaneously occurring AFLs, showed limitations when dealing with variable, unpredictable patterns of reentry as observed in this new crop of scar-related flutters. Despite its shortcomings, ECG has endured and remains an obligatory test in every patient presenting with arrhythmias. Furthermore, thanks to few painstakingly conducted and detailed studies, some correlations between ECG waveform morphology and patterns of reentry have been established.

Study of an electrocardiographic tracing, always based on a deep knowledge of anatomy and vector analysis, nowdays requires a detailed understanding of the effects of RFA on a chamber already remodeled by preexisting AF. Modern technology has therefore widened the usefulness of an old tool in a clear demonstration of the validity of the precision electrocardiology concept.

CLINICS CARE POINTS

- When interpretating ECG of Atypical AFLs consider if the patient:
- Had previous invasive therapies; if so review the type of intervention and the details of the procedure.
- Is on antiarrhythmic drugs as they can increase the AFL cycle length and change its reentrant path.
- In patients with history of PVI, review a baseline ECG in SR to analyze the morphology and Voltage of the P wave; these observations can clarify the atrial (mostly LA) scar burden and possible interatrial delays.
- Consider isthmus dependent flutter in patients with recurrent arrythmias following

PVI. Be aware of the different ECG morphology of this arrythmia following LA interventions.

- Despite its varied presentations, some characteristic features in atypical AFL can help in identifying the location and the type of reentrant circuit.

DISCLOSURE

R.D. Ponti has received fees for lectures and scientific cooperation from Biosense Webster. All other authors declared no conflict of interest.

REFERENCES

1. Mines GR. On circulating excitations in heart muscle and their possible relation to tachycardia and fibrillation. Trans R Soc Can 1914;8:43–53.
2. Lewis T, Drury AN, Iliescu CC. A demonstration of circus movement in clinical flutter of the auricles. Heart 1921;8:341.
3. Wells JL, MacLean WA, James TN, et al. Characterization of atrial flutter. Studies in man after open heart surgery using fixed atrial electrodes. Circulation 1979;60(3):665–73.
4. Wellens HJ. Forty years of invasive clinical electrophysiology: 1967-2007. Circ Arrhythm Electrophysiol 2008;1(1):49–53.
5. Saoudi N, Cosío F, Waldo A, et al. Working Group of Arrhythmias of the European Society of Cardiology and the North American Society of Pacing and Electrophysiology. A classification of atrial flutter and regular atrial tachycardia according to electrophysiological mechanisms and anatomical bases; a statement from a joint expert group from the working group of arrhythmias of the European Society of Cardiology and the North American Society of Pacing and Electrophysiology. Eur Heart J 2001;22: 1162–82.
6. Kahn AM, Krummen DE, Feld GK, et al. Localizing circuits of atrial macro-reentry using ECG planes of coherent atrial activation. Heart Rhythm 2007;4(4): 445–51.
7. Sippens-Groenewegen A, Lesh MD, Roithinger FX. et al. Body surface mapping of counterclockwise and clockwise typical atrial flutter: a comparative analysis with endocardial activation sequence mapping. J Am Coll Cardiol 2000;35:1276–87.
8. Olgin J, Kalman J, Fitzpatrick A, et al. The role of right atrial endocardial structures as barriers to conduction during human type I atrial flutter: activation and entrainment mapping guided by intracardiac echocardiography. Circulation 1995;92: 1831–48.

9. Olgin JE, Kalman JM, Lesh MD. Conduction barriers in human atrial flutter correlation of electrophysiology and anatomy. J Cardiovasc Electrophysiol 1996;7:1112–26.
10. Friedman PA, Luria D, Fenton AM, et al. Global right atrial mapping of human atrial flutter: the presence of posteromedial (sinus venosa region) functional block and double potentials: a study in biplane fluoroscopy and intracardiac echocardiography. Circulation 2000;101:1568–77.
11. Perez FJ, Schuber CM, Parvez B, et al. Long-term outcomes after catheter ablation of cavo-tricuspid isthmus dependent atrial flutter. Circ Arrhythmia Electrophysiol 2009;4:393–400.
12. Kail J, Glascock D, Kopp D, et al. Characterization and catheter ablation of the antidromic form of typical atrial flutter. Circulation 1995;92:I–84. Abstract.
13. Yan SH, Cheng WJ, Wang LX, Chen MY, et al. Mechanisms of atypical flutter wave morphology in patients with isthmus-dependent atrial flutter Heart Vessels 2009;24:211–8.
14. Allessie MA, Lammers WJEP, Bonke IM, et al. Intra atrial reentry as a mechanism for atrial flutter induced by acetylcholine and rapid atrial pacing in the dog. Circulation 1984;70:123–35.
15. Okumura K, Plumb VJ, Page PL, et al. Atrial activation sequence mapping during atrial flutter in the canine pericarditis model and its effects on the polarity of the flutter wave in the electrocardiogram. J Am Coll Cardiol 1991;17:509–18.
16. Ndrepepa G, Zrenner BI, Deisenhofer M, et al. Relationship between surface electrocardiogram characteristics and endocardial activation sequence in patients with typical atrial flutter. Z Kardiol 2000;89: 527–37.
17. Kalman JM, Olgin JE, Saxon LA, et al. Electrocardiographic and electrophysiologic characterization of atypical atrial flutter in man: use of activation and entrainment mapping and implications for catheter ablation. J Cardiovasc Electrophysiol 1997;8: 121–44.
18. Saoudi N, Nair M, Abdelazziz A, et al. Electrocardiographic patterns and results of radiofrequency catheter ablation of clockwise type I flutter. J Cardiovasc Electrophysiol 1996;7:931–42.
19. Spach MS, Miller WT, Geselowitz DB, et al. The discontinuous nature of propagation in normal canine cardiac muscle. Evidence for recurrent discontinuities of intracellular resistance that affect the membrane currents. Circ Res 1981;48:39–54.
20. Tai CT, Chen SA, Chen YJ. et al. Conduction properties of the crista terminalis in patients with typical atrial flutter: basis for a line of block in the reentrant circuit. J Cardiovasc Electrophysiol 1998;9:811–9.
21. Tai CT, Huang JL, Lee PC, et al. High resolution mapping around the crista terminalis during typical

atrial flutter: new insights into mechanisms. J Cardiovasc Electrophysiol 2004;15:406–14.

22. Yang Y, Cheng J, Bochoyer A, et al. Atypical right atrial flutter patterns. Circulation 2001;103:3092–8.

23. Zhang S, Younis G, Hariharan R, et al. Lower loop reentry as a mechanism of clockwise right atrial flutter. Circulation 2004;109:1630–5.

24. Cheng J, Cabeen WR Jr, Scheinman MM. Right atrial flutter due to lower loop reentry mechanism and anatomic substrates. Circulation 1999;99(13): 1700–5.

25. Kall JG, Rubenstein DS, Kopp DE, et al. Atypical atrial flutter originating in the right atrial free wall. Circulation 2000;101:270–9.

26. Shimizu A, Nozaki A, Rudy Y, et al. Onset of induced atrial flutter in the canine pericarditis model. J Am Coll Cardiol 1991;17:1223–34.

27. Fujiki A, Nishida K, Sakabe M, et al. Entrainment mapping of dual-loop macroreentry in common atrial flutter: new insights into the atrial flutter circuit. J Cardiovasc Electrophysiol 2004;15:679–85.

28. Yuniadi Y, Tai CT, et al. A new electrocardiographic algorithm to differentiate upper loop Re-entry from Reverse typical atrial flutter. J Am Coll Cardiol 2005;46:524–8.

29. Rutherford SL, Trew ML, Sands GB, et al. High-resolution 3-dimensional reconstruction of the infarct border zone: impact of structural remodeling on electrical activation. Circ Res 2012;111:301–11.

30. Long Huang JL, Tai C-T, Lin Y-J, et al. Substrate mapping to detect abnormal atrial endocardium with slow conduction in patients with atypical right atrial flutter. J Am Coll Cardiol 2006;48:492–8.

31. Azadani PN, Kumar UN, Yang Y, et al. Frequency of atrial flutter after adult lung transplantation. Am J Cardiol 2011;107:922–6.

32. Thajudeen A, Stecker E, Shehata M,, et al. Arrhythmias after heart transplantation: mechanisms and management. J Am Heart Assoc 2012;1: e001461.

33. Stevenson IH, Kistler PM, Spence SJ,, et al. Scar-related right atrial macroreentrant tachycardia in patients without prior atrial surgery: electroanatomic characterization and ablation outcome Heart. Rhythm 2005;2:594–601.

34. Fukamizu S, Sakurada H, Hayashi T. et al. Macroreentrant atrial tachycardia in patients without previous atrial surgery or catheter ablation: clinical and electrophysiological characteristics of scar-related left atrial anterior wall reentry. Cardiovasc Electrophysiol 2013;24:404–12.

35. Ávila P, Oliver JM, Gallego P, et al. Natural history and clinical predictors of atrial tachycardia in adults with congenital heart disease. Circ Arrhythm Electrophysiol 2017;10:e005396.

36. Quinton E, Nightingale P, Hudsmith L, et al. Prevalence of atrial tachyarrhythmia in adults after Fontan operation. Heart 2015;101:1672–7.

37. Wu MH, Lu CW, Chen HC, et al. Arrhythmic burdens in patients with tetralogy of Fallot: a national database study. Heart Rhythm 2015;12:604–9.

38. Gerstenfeld EP, Callans DJ, Dixit S, et al. Mechanisms of organized left atrial tachycardias occurring after pulmonary vein isolation. Circulation 2004;110: 1351–7.

39. Chae S, Oral H, Good E, et al. Atrial tachycardia after circumferential pulmonary vein ablation of atrial fibrillation: mechanistic insights, results of catheter ablation, and risk factors for recurrence. J Am Coll Cardiol 2007;50:1781–7.

40. Latcu DG, Bun S-S, Viera F, et al. Selection of critical isthmus in scar-related atrial tachycardia using a new automated ultra-high resolution mapping system. Circ Arrhythm Electrophysiol 2016;9:e004510. https://doi.org/10.1161/CIRCEP.116.004510.

41. Nakagawa H, Shah N, Matsudaira K, et al. Characterization of reentrant circuit in macroreentrant right atrial tachycardia after surgical repair of congenital heart disease: isolated channels between scars allow "focal" ablation. Circulation 2001;103: 699–709.

42. Jaïs P, Shah DC, Haissaguerre M, et al. Mapping and ablation of left atrial flutters. Circulation 2000; 101:2928–34.

43. Ng FS, Guerrero F, Luther V, et al. Microreentrant left atrial tachycardia circuit mapped with an ultra-high-density mapping system Heart Rhythm Case. Rep 2017;3:224–8.

44. Roberts-Thomson KC, Kalman JM. Right septal macroreentrant tachycardia late after mitral valve repair: importance of surgical access approach Heart. Rhythm 2007;4:32–6.

45. Chan DP, Van Hare GF, Mackall JA, et al. Importance of atrial flutter isthmus in postoperative intra-atrial reentrant tachycardia. Circulation 2000;102:1283–9.

46. Wasmer K, Kobe J, Dechering DG, et al. Isthmus-dependent right atrial flutter as the leading cause of atrial tachycardias after surgical atrial septal defect repair. Int J Cardiol 2013;168:2447–52.

47. Collins KK, Love BA, Walsh EP, et al. Location of acutely successful radiofrequency catheter ablation of intra atrial reentrant tachycardia in patients with congenital heart disease. Am J Cardiol 2000;86:969–74.

48. Olgin JE, Kalman JM, Saxon LA, et al. Mechanism of initiation of atrial flutter in humans: site of unidirectional block and direction of rotation. J Am Coll Cardiol 1997;29(2):376–84.

49. Lukac P, Pedersen AK, Mortensen PT, et al. Ablation of atrial tachycardia after surgery for congenital and acquired heart disease using an electroanatomic mapping system: which circuits to expect in which substrate? Heart Rhythm 2005;2:64–72.

50. Yang Y, Varma N, Badhwar N, et al. Prospective observations in the clinical and electrophysiological characteristics of intra-isthmus re-entry. Cardiovasc Electrophysiol 2010;21:1099–106.

51. Marrouche NF, Natale A, Wazni OM, et al. Left septal atrial flutter: electrophysiology, anatomy, and results of ablation. Circulation 2004;109:2440–7.

52. Fiala M, Chovancik J, Neuwirth R, et al. Atrial macro reentry tachycardia in patients without obvious structural heart disease or previous cardiac surgical or catheter intervention: characterization of arrhythmogenic substrates, reentry circuits, and results of catheter ablation. J Cardiovasc Electrophysiol 2007;18:824–32.

53. Jhang J, Tang C, Zhang Y, et al. Electroanatomic characterization and ablation outcome of non-lesion related left atrial macroreentrant tachycardia in patients without obvious structural heart disease. J Cardiovasc Electrophysiol DOI:10.1111/j.1540-8167.2012.02426

54. Markowitz SM, Brodman RF, Stein KM, et al. Lesional tachycardias related to mitral valve surgery. J Am Coll Cardiol 2002;39:1973–83.

55. Cox JL, Jaquiss RD, Schuessler RB, et al. Modification of the maze procedure for atrial flutter and atrial fibrillation. II. Surgical technique of the maze III procedure. J Thorac Cardiovasc Surg 1995;110:485–95.

56. Gillinov AM, McCarthy PM. Advances in the surgical treatment of atrial fibrillation. Cardiol Clin 2004;22: 147–57.

57. Park HE, Kim K-H, Kim K-B, et al. Characteristics of P wave in patients with sinus rhythm after maze operation. J Korean Med Sci 2010;25:712–5.

58. Takahashi Y, O'Neill MD, Hocini M, et al. Effects of stepwise ablation of chronic atrial fibrillation on atrial electrical and mechanical properties. J Am Coll Cardiol 2007;49:1306–14.

59. Wasmer K, Mö nnig G, Bittner A, et al. Incidence, characteristics, and outcome of left atrial tachycardias after circumferential antral ablation of atrial fibrillation. Heart Rhythm 2012;9:1660–6.

60. Knecht S, Veenhuyzen G, O'Neill M, et al. Atrial tachycardias encountered in the context of catheter ablation for atrial fibrillation part II: mapping and ablation. PACE 2009;32:528–38.

61. Jais P, Matsuo S, Knecht S,, et al. A deductive mapping strategy for atrial tachycardia following atrial fibrillation ablation: importance of localized reentry. J Cardiovasc Electrophysiol 2009;20:480–91.

62. Pascale P, Roten L, Shah A,, et al. Useful electrocardiographic features to help identify the mechanism of atrial tachycardia occurring after persistent atrial fibrillation ablation. J Am Coll Cardiol 2018;4:33–45.

63. Jais P, Sanders P, Hsu L-F, et al. Flutter localized to the anterior left atrium after catheter ablation of atrial fibrillation. J Cardiovasc Electrophysiol 2006;17: 279–85.

64. Hocini M, Jais P, Sanders P, et al. Techniques, evaluation, and consequences of linear block at the left atrial roof in paroxysmal atrial fibrillation: a prospective randomized study. Circulation 2005;112: 3688–96.

65. Gerstenfeld E, Dixit S, Bala R, et al. Surface electrocardiogram characteristics of atrial tachycardias occurring after pulmonary vein isolation Circ. Arrhythm Electrophysiol 2013;6:481–90.

66. Mesas CEE, Pappone C, Lang CCE, et al. Left atrial tachycardia after circumferential pulmonary vein ablation for atrial fibrillation: electroanatomic characterization and treatment. J Am Coll Cardiol 2004;44: 1071–9.

67. Shrestha S, Chen O, Greene M, et al. Change in P wave morphology after convergent atrial fibrillation ablation. Indian Pacing Electrophysiol J 2016; 16(1):3–7.

68. Jonathan Buber J, Luria D, Sternik L, et al. . Morphological features of the P-waves at surface electrocardiogram as surrogate to mechanical function of the left atrium following a successful modified maze procedure. Europace 2014;16;578–86.

69. Bochoeyer A, Yang Y, Cheng J, et al. Surface electrocardiographic characteristics of right and left atrial flutter. Circulation 2003;108:60–6.

70. Medi C, Kalman JM. Prediction of the atrial flutter circuit location from the surface electrocardiogram. Europace 2008;10(7):786–96.

71. Brown JP, Krummen DE, Feld GK, et al. Using electrocardiographic activation time and diastolic intervals to separate focal from macro–re-entrant atrial tachycardias. J Am Coll Cardiol 2007;49:1965–73.

72. Shah D, Sunthorn H, Burri H, et al. Narrow, slow-conducting isthmus dependent left atrial reentry developing after ablation for atrial fibrillation: ECG characterization and elimination by focal RF ablation. J Cardiovasc Electrophysiol 2006;17:508–15.

73. Lee JM, Turner I, Agarwal A, et al. An unusual atrial tachycardia in a patient with Friedreich ataxia. Europace 2011;13(11):1660–1.

74. Huo Y, Schoenbauer R, Richter S, et al. Atrial arrhythmias following surgical AF ablation: electrophysiological findings, ablation strategies, and clinical outcome. J Cardiovasc Electrophysiol 2014;25:725–38.

75. Casado Arroyo R, Latcu DG, Maeda S, et al. Coronary sinus activation and ECG characteristics of roof-dependent left atrial flutter after pulmonary vein isolation. Circ Arrhythm Electrophysiol 2018; 11:e005948. https://doi.org/10.1161/CIRCEP.117. 005948.

76. Chugh A, Latchamsetty R, Oral H, et al. Characteristics of cavotricuspid isthmus–dependent atrial flutter after left atrial ablation of atrial fibrillation. Circulation 2006;113:609–15.

77. Gopinathannair R, Mar PL, Afzal MR, et al. Atrial tachycardias after surgical atrial fibrillation ablation: clinical characteristics, electrophysiological mechanisms, and ablation outcomes from a large, multicenter study. J Am Coll Cardiol EP 2017;3:865–74.

78. Chyou JY, Hickey K, Diamond L, et al. Atypical electrocardiographic features of cavo tricuspid isthmus-dependent atrial flutter occurring during left atrial fibrillation ablation. Ann Noninvasive Electrocardiol 2010;15:200–8.

79. Ashino S, Watanabe I, Okumura Y, et al. Change in atrial flutter wave morphology—insight into the sources of electrocardiographic variants in common atrial flutter. PACE 2007;30:1023–6.

80. Chang S-L, Tsao H-M, Lin Y-J, et al. Differentiating macroreentrant from focal atrial tachycardias occurred after circumferential pulmonary vein isolation. J Cardiovasc Electrophysiol 2011;22:748–55.

81. Kistler PM, Kurt C, Roberts-Thomson KC, et al. P-wave morphology in focal atrial tachycardia: development of an algorithm to predict the anatomic site of origin. J Am Coll Cardiol 2006;48:1010–7.

82. Rajawat YS, Gerstenfeld EP, Patel VV, et al. ECG criteria for localizing the pulmonary vein origin of spontaneous atrial premature complexes: validation using intracardiac recordings. Pacing Clin Electrophysiol 2004;27:182–8.

83. Yamada T, Murakami Y, Yoshida Y, et al. Electrophysiologic and electrocardiographic characteristics and radiofrequency catheter ablation of focal atrial tachycardia originating from the left atrial appendage. Heart Rhythm 2007;4:1284–91.

Typical Atrial Flutter Mapping and Ablation

Francesco Notaristefano, MD[a],*, Gianluca Zingarini, MD[a], Claudio Cavallini, MD[a], Giuseppe Bagliani, MD[b,c], Roberto De Ponti, MD[d,e], Fabio M. Leonelli, MD[f,g]

KEYWORDS

- Typical atrial flutter • Entrainment pacing • Electro-anatomic mapping • Trans-catheter ablation

KEY POINTS

- The common atrial flutter is a re-entrant arrhythmia in which the cavo-tricuspid isthmus (CTI), the interatrial septum, the roof of the right atrium, and the crista terminalis are involved in the circuit of re-entry.
- The entrainment of the flutter circuit by pacing was a necessary step in the ablation procedure and identified CTI as the optimal site for ablation.
- Electroanatomic mapping techniques can now be used to reconstruct the re-entrant path and identify the CTI before ablation.

HISTORY OF TYPICAL ATRIAL FLUTTER MAPPING AND ABLATION

Typical Atrial Flutter Electrophysiology: From Focal Activity to Re-entry

At present, typical atrial flutter (TAFL) is considered the prototype of re-entrant arrhythmias but for several decades the underlying mechanism was unclear.

In the 1950s, Scherf and coworkers[1] conducted several experiments in the canine model to demonstrate the ectopic and focal origin of atrial flutter (AFL). The application of aconitine on the atrial appendage tip could easily induce sustained AFL and sinus rhythm could be restored by clamping or cooling this region. AFL persisted in the isolated auricular region and on the removal of the clamping, the arrhythmia recurred in the whole atrium. These phenomena were judged inconsistent with re-entry and were considered the proof of the focal mechanism.

Early in 1925 Lewis in his pioneering work postulated that AFL was sustained by re-entry and he proposed that the path of the circuit was moving around the venae cavae or around the sinus node. According to Lewis's theory, two conditions were necessary for the perpetuation of the circular movement of the wavefront:

1. The presence of a central anatomic obstacle and
2. The wavelength of the impulse had to be shorter than the length of the pathway allowing for a fully excitable gap.

More than 50 years later in the canine model, Boineau and coworkers[2] made fundamental observations demonstrating that re-entry was the mechanism of AFL as proposed by Lewis. In a dog with spontaneous type 1 (counterclockwise) and type 2 (clockwise) AFL they confirmed not only the circular movement of the impulse but

[a] Cardiovascular Disease Department- Arrhytmology, University of Perugia, Piazza Menghini 1, Perugia 06129, Italy; [b] Cardiology And Arrhythmology Clinic, University Hospital "Ospedali Riuniti", Via Conca 71, Ancona 60126, Italy; [c] Department of Biomedical Sciences and Public Health, Marche Polytechnic University, Via Conca 71, Ancona 60126, Italy; [d] Department of Heart and Vessels, Ospedale di Circolo, Viale Borri, 57, Varese 21100, Italy; [e] Department of Medicine and Surgery, University of Insubria, Viale Guicciardini, 9, Varese 21100, Italy; [f] Cardiology Department, James A. Haley Veterans' Hospital, University of South Florida, 13000 Bruce B Down Boulevard, Tampa, FL 33612, USA; [g] University of South Florida FL, 4202 E Fowler Avenue, Tampa, FL 33620, USA
* Corresponding author.
E-mail address: not.francesco@gmail.com

Card Electrophysiol Clin 14 (2022) 459–469
https://doi.org/10.1016/j.ccep.2022.06.007

also the presence of a slow conduction zone close to the crista terminalis. Both type 1 and type 2 AFL shared the same slow conduction zone and the artificial ligation of this area could make inducible even dogs without spontaneous AFL at baseline.[2]

In the same period, in the isolated rabbit atrial myocardium, Allessie and coworkers[3] showed that a premature atrial beat could induce a circular movement tachycardia without the need for an anatomic unexcitable structure. In the so-called "leading circle movement" theory the length of the circuit could change according to the electrophysiological properties of the tissue and no fully excitable gap was present given the similarity between the wavelength and the pathway length. This model did not seem to fit the observed AFL because the variability of the leading circle circuit could not explain the highly reproducible electrocardiogram (ECG) presentation of the arrhythmia.

In addition, the electrophysiological studies in humans had already confirmed the presence of a wide excitable gap through atrial stimulation during atrial flutter (AF) that could reset or terminate the tachycardia.

Those seminal findings completed the modern triad explaining re-entrant arrhythmias and consisted of

1. unidirectional block
2. slow conduction
3. presence of an unexcitable area and this theory was ready for the demonstration in human AFL.

Disertori and coworkers[4] performed invasive electrophysiological studies in patients with spontaneous typical AFL. In their study, they positioned recording electrodes at the low right atrial paraseptal region, high right atrium (HRA), and lateral right atrial wall and introduced timed premature stimulations from different right atrium (RA) sites. The findings demonstrated the re-entrant mechanism of the TAFL and further supported the probable anatomic circuit of the arrhythmia.

Despite the accurate study the exact pathway of the re-entry could not be precisely mapped but the temporal relationship between the three mapped atrial sites strongly suggested an entirely right atrial macro re-entry.

Typical Atrial Flutter Re-entrant Circuit Identification and Ablation

The characterization of the AFL macro re-entrant circuit was further elucidated by endocardial recordings and also by intraoperative epicardial mapping.[5]

In two patients with typical AFL, Klein and coworkers[5] reconstructed the re-entrant circuit recording the first endocardial activation at the coronary sinus (CS) ostium. Then the activation wavefront proceeded from low to high along the septum to reach first the HRA and later the lateral wall. From there it returned to the starting point, whereas before the left atrium had been passively activated. The epicardial map confirmed these findings.

During AFL when the CS region was refractory, an extra stimulus from the HRA advanced the next atrial activation confirming the presence of a wide excitable gap. When pacing was delivered from the CS ostium all the subsequent recording points were ordinately captured and the postpacing interval was equal to the arrhythmia cycle length. In addition, both the activation pattern during the extra stimulus and the surface F-wave on the ECG were identical to the AFL suggesting a macro re-entrant circuit.

This study added another important piece to the puzzle of the AFL pathway by identifying an anatomic narrow region with slow conduction velocity bounded by the tricuspid valve (TV) ring, the ostium of the CS, and the inferior vena cava. Epicardial cryoablation of this region during cardiac surgery successfully prevented AFL recurrences in both patients.

Further studies recorded, in the same low posterior-septal area, fragmented potentials in keeping with a region of slow conduction.

Endocardial fulguration from a mapping catheter was successfully delivered at this site and in seven out of eight patients AFL was not inducible anymore.[6] Fulguration had several limitations, such as the risks of heart block, constant interruption of the arrhythmia, and damage to a relatively wide area of the myocardium.

Feld and coworkers[7] recorded low amplitude fragmented potentials and a long stimulus-F wave during entrainment in the posterior septal region between inferior vena cava and tricuspid annulus, whereas in the region around the CS ostium concealed entrainment with short stimulus-F wave interval was demonstrated. The former represented a slow conductive isthmus and the latter the circuit exit site, which was successfully targeted with discrete radiofrequency ablation. Radiofrequency ablation in this area carried a significant risk of complications, such as an atrioventricular (AV) block, and the success rate was variable.

Taking into account the limitation of this approach, Cosio and coworkers[8] proposed to deliver a linear set of radiofrequency lesions from the tricuspid annulus to the inferior vena cava to create a line of block for the activation wavefront. The isthmus between the tricuspid annulus and the inferior vena cava was a relatively safe anatomic area for ablation because it was far from the AV node. The line of the block at this site prevented the impulse to reach the septal area of slow conduction usually located more septally; targeting the isthmus appeared to be both for counterclockwise and clockwise common AFL.

In a cohort of 200 patients, Fischer and coworkers,[9] 1 year later, demonstrated that an anatomical approach to creating a linear ablation across the cavo-tricuspid isthmus (CTI) was more effective compared with the mixed anatomic and electrophysiological approach, which targeted signals in three different regions (1—area between inferior vena cava and tricuspid annulus, 2—area between tricuspid annulus and CS ostium, and 3—area between CS ostium and inferior vena cava).

Since then the region between the inferior vena cava and the tricuspid annulus has become the target of AFL ablation and it has been referred to as CTI.

TYPICAL ATRIAL FLUTTER MAPPING

Typical AFL can be reproduced in the electrophysiology laboratory using programmed stimulation from the RA with high sensitivity and specificity. Typical AFL can be induced in more than 90% of patients with a clinical history of this arrhythmia and in less than 10% of those without documented AFL.[10] Despite that successful induction can be achieved in the majority of patients, however, several attempts are often required. Among 10 patients with a history of typical AFL, Olgin and coworkers[11] could induce the arrhythmia in every patient but only 6.2% of pacing attempts were successful similar to the 5.2% of attempts inducing AF.

The site of pacing can influence the probability of AFL induction but different studies have provided conflicting results.

Josephson's group identified the HRA as the most effective pacing site, whereas Olgin and coworkers did not find a significant difference between trabeculated (superior and inferior crista terminalis) and smooth (septal and posterior) RA.[11,12] This discrepancy may be explained by the exclusion from Olgin's cohort of patients with transient AF or atypical flutter before stable typical AFL and by the absence of pacing from the CS ostium.

Despite not having demonstrated the superiority of one site over the others for AFL initiation Olgin and coworkers found that specific sites were related to clockwise or counterclockwise wavefront propagation. In their study, 90% of clockwise and 100% of counterclockwise AFLs were induced from the trabeculated and from the smooth atrium, respectively.[11]

Across all the mentioned studies burst pacing and double atrial extra stimuli have been demonstrated to be superior to single atrial extra stimulus at inducing AFL but burst pacing resulted in a higher rate of AF induction.

AFL induction is characterized by a sudden endocardial beat-to-beat activation change, which is the result of a unidirectional block in the area delimited by the inferior vena cava, the Eustachian ridge, the CS ostium, and the tricuspid annulus. This unidirectional block site has been described in the same anatomic region both for clockwise and counterclockwise AFL. The same shared pathway can explain the similar cycle length when both rotations are observed in the same patient.

In some instances, the unidirectional block at the isthmus may be preceded by a Wenckebach type block or transient atrial fibrillation in the Koch triangle.

The reproducible induction of this stable arrhythmia is an important and specific feature of AFL because it allows to do a complete mapping to achieve a definite diagnosis. Diagnostic pacing maneuvers can be freely performed during the arrhythmia because if they cause its termination AFL can be reinduced with the same stimulation protocol.

In addition, easy reinducibility of the AFL offers a clear endpoint for catheter ablation, such as the absence of induction with programmed stimulation, once the isthmus linear lesion has been created.

Activation Mapping: Intracardiac Recording

TAFL has a constant cycle length (200–250 ms) and amplitude, morphology, and sequence of endocardial electrograms (EGMs) are stable.

The tricuspid annulus, the crista terminalis, the inferior vena cava, the Eustachian ridge, and the CS ostium are the anatomic boundaries of the circuit; the simultaneous registration of the EGMs at these sites allows the characterization of the largest portion of the macro re-entrant circuit.

The activation map of the RA is usually done by placing a 20-pole circular catheter along the tricuspid annulus (distal poles just lateral to the isthmus and proximal poles at the high septal region) and a decapolar catheter inside the CS (proximal poles at the CS ostium and distal poles inside CS). Optionally, two additional multipolar catheters can be positioned at the bundle of His region and at the crista terminalis.

During counterclockwise AFL the wavefront from the proximal CS proceeds up to the antero-septum with the activation of the proximal poles of the 20-pole catheter. Then it travels along the anterior tricuspid annulus to descend cranio-caudally along the lateral wall, which results in a proximal-to-distal sequence on the 20-pole catheter. From the distal 20-pole, the next EGM is recorded at the proximal CS with a delay, which is accumulated while traveling from the lateral to the septal portion of the isthmus.

During clockwise AFL the pathway is reversed and the 20-pole catheter sequence is distal-to-proximal followed by the proximal CS. The isthmus is crossed from the septal to the lateral edge and the resulting delay is recorded between the proximal CS and the distal poles of the 20-pole catheter.

The left atrium is passively activated and the catheter inside the CS records a proximal-to-distal activation. Exceptionally, when the catheter tip is deep into the CS at the level of the great cardiac vein, distal-to-proximal or fusion type CS activation can be recorded because of the conduction from the RA to the roof of the left atrium across the Bachmann's bundle.

Activation Mapping: Resetting and Entrainment

TAFL is a macro re-entrant arrhythmia whose entire cycle length can be mapped in the RA. It has a wide, fully excitable gap accounting for the 15%–30% of the tachycardia cycle length and this characteristic allows for delivering atrial extra stimuli at different coupling intervals and from different sites. An atrial extra stimulus is usually able to reset (advancement of the next activation with a pause less than compensatory) the tachycardia. When the site of pacing is close to the pathway even a late coupled extra stimulus can enter the circuit and produce a pause that is less than compensatory. In this case, manifest fusion or intracardiac fusion is found on the surface ECG or EGMs, respectively.

Pacing from the isthmus between the TV and the inferior vena cava produces a concealed fusion with both surface ECG and intracardiac EGM identical to the tachycardia.

When the pacing site is outside the re-entrant path the return cycle is longer than the tachycardia cycle length and there is usually manifest fusion on the surface ECG.

The resetting response is flat in the majority of patients with TAFL but almost 50% demonstrated a trend of progressive conduction delay as the coupling interval becomes shorter.[13] Callans and coworkers[13] demonstrated that the isthmus was the site of conduction delay because the premature impulse encroached this region during its relative refractory period.

Entrainment is the continuous resetting of the tachycardia with fixed fusion, at a given cycle length, and progressive fusion when the pacing rate increases. Tachycardia resumes with the same cycle after pacing is stopped and the interval between the last paced beat and the first tachycardia EGM recorded at the same site defines the post-pacing interval. A post-pacing interval minus tachycardia cycle length less than 20 ms and a difference between the stimulus-F wave onset and local EGM-F wave onset during tachycardia less than 20 ms suggests that the pacing site is on the re-entrant pathway. When the above-mentioned characteristics are associated with concealed fusion (F-wave identical to the tachycardia) the pacing site is in a circuit of the arrhythmia (**Fig. 1**). Entrainment can be performed at different sites and the circuit can be precisely characterized. Olgin and coworkers created an entrainment map of the RA enriched by the anatomic information provided by the intracardiac echo.

The region posterior to the crista terminalis, the fossa ovalis, and the region posterior to the Eustachian ridge were outside of the arrhythmia circuit (**Fig. 2**).

The critical isthmus was identified as the anatomic region between the inferior vena cava and the tricuspid annulus anterior to the Eustachian ridge. Similar findings have been reported by Kalman and coworkers[14] who confirmed that fossa ovalis, right atrial appendage, and the left atrium were not part of the circuit, whereas the tricuspid annulus served as the anterior barrier.

Pacing during AF can cause the termination of the arrhythmia and it usually occurs when the pacing rate is faster than the heart rate required to entrain the arrhythmia. Termination is achieved more easily if the pacing site is within the circuit and if a long-lasting burst is applied.

Pacing from outside the circuit or with a high heart rate may increase the chance to convert AF to atrial fibrillation.

The restoration of the sinus rhythm occurs when the isthmus becomes refractory and the orthodromic-paced wavefront is blocked at this level. The RA is now activated by two wavefronts traveling in the opposite directions, orthodromic and antidromic, and the last paced impulse cannot perpetuate the re-entry with AF termination.

Tri-dimensional Electroanatomic Mapping

The registration of intracardiac signals through the catheters placed inside the CS and around the

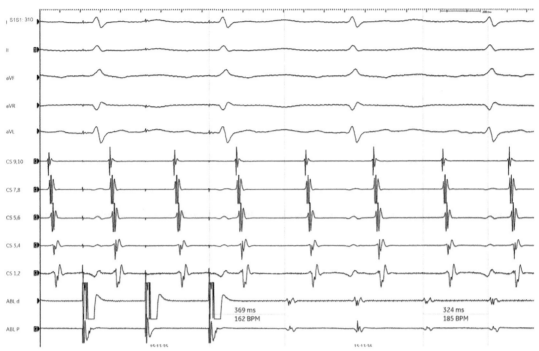

Fig. 1. Intracardiac recording from CS and ablation catheter (Abl d). Pacing at cl shorter than AFL is delivered from distal pole of the ablation catheter (ABL d) during AF. The first return cycle shows a post-pacing interval of 369 millisecond, 45 millisecond longer than AFL cycle length. This delay suggests that the pacing location was outside of the circuit. Abl, recording ablation catheter with distal (d) and proximal (p) poles shown; SVC, superior vena cava; IVC, inferior vena cava.

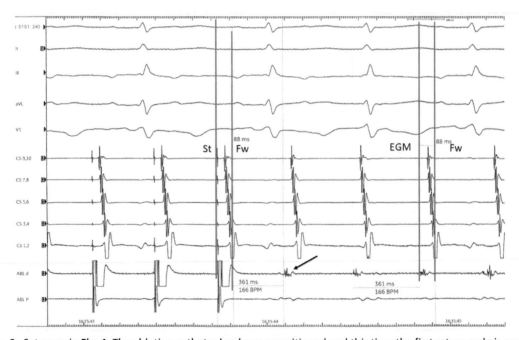

Fig. 2. Set up as in **Fig. 1**. The ablation catheter has been repositioned and this time the first return cycle is equal to the AFL cycle length. Furthermore, the stimulus (St) to F-wave onset was equal to local EGM to F-wave onset during tachycardia. Entrainment showed concealed fusion on the surface ECG and the local EGM (*black arrow*) was fragmented suggesting an area of slow conduction. This location appears to be an ideal ablation site (see text for further explanations).

tricuspid annulus under fluoroscopy is usually able to delineate the circuit of TAFL and to guide ablation.

However, tri-dimensional (3D) electroanatomic mapping systems can provide additional useful information to precisely characterize the re-entrant pathway, to evaluate the voltage of the right atrial myocardium, and reduce X-ray exposure.

Mapping systems reconstruct the 3D anatomy of the cardiac chambers and they are able to display, through a color code, the endocardial activation. Moreover, they allow real-time visualization of mapping and ablating catheters while being positioned inside the cardiac chambers.

A reference catheter is placed in a stable position inside the CS and the clearest atrial EGM is used as a reference. A time interval, called the window of interest, will define the period during which an arbitrary relationship (before or after) is established between local EGMs recorded at different locations and the one at the reference catheter.

The window of interest usually covers 90% of the cycle length and it allows classifying and color display of the bipolar signal recorded by the mapping catheter at different sites as early or late.[15]

The mapping catheter as well as recording the local bipolar EGMs can reconstruct or annotate anatomic landmarks, such as the inferior vena cava, the bundle of His, and the tricuspid annulus, completing the anatomic map.

For TAFL, as for all macro re-entrant arrhythmias, the final result is a map with an ordered succession of colors and the one representing the earliest activation meets the latest **Fig. 3**.

In the common type, the activation spreads from the CTI around the tricuspid annulus and double potentials are recorded along two lines of a block at the level of the crista terminalis and the Eustachian ridge.

The high-resolution and high-density mapping can reveal double potentials at the crista terminalis and at the Eustachian ridge. The activation wavefront travels in opposite directions along with these two barriers. The line of the block is encountered when mapping is performed during AF, during pacing below a critical cycle length and it is usually absent during sinus rhythm. These data suggest that the conduction block is functional in the majority of patients and that the conduction properties across these sites are crucial for the arrhythmia initiation and perpetuation.[16,17]

In addition to the activation map, additional maps can be created to provide complementary information.

The post-pacing intervals at different sites can be displayed to highlight the re-entrant pathway and the isochronal maps can clearly show the re-entrant pathway.

Interesting data to guide the ablation can be retrieved from the acquisition of the voltage map, which is based on the amplitude of the EGM. Pre-existing spontaneous scars can be embedded in the ablation line as well as the thinner region of the isthmus to make the ablation more effective and straightforward.

TYPICAL ATRIAL FLUTTER ABLATION

As detailed in the section titled, "Typical Atrial Flutter Re-entrant Circuit Identification and Ablation", the target of TAFL ablation is the isthmus between the tricuspid annulus and the inferior vena. The middle portion of the isthmus is the preferred site for ablation because it is shorter and thinner than both the septal (from the tricuspid annulus to the CS ostium and from the CS ostium to the inferior vena cava) and the lateral sides. The ablation line in this region is away from the right coronary artery and from both the AV node slow pathway and the AV node supplying artery thus reducing the risk of complications potentially seen in a more lateral or septal lesion set (**Fig. 4**).

Technique

A steerable ablation catheter advance to the RA through a fixed shape or steerable sheath is used for CTI ablation.[18] On the right anterior oblique projection, the catheter is advanced inside the right ventricle and it is bent to reach the right ventricle inferior wall. The catheter is then withdrawn at the level of the tricuspid annulus where the ratio between atrial and ventricular EGM is around 1:4. On the left anterior oblique projection, the tip is positioned at 6 o'clock midway between the septum and the lateral wall. Radiofrequency is nowadays the preferred source of energy for CTI ablation delivered through a 4 mm irrigated tip catheter. Ablation is usually started at the level of the tricuspid annulus and it is continued until the catheter has reached the inferior vena cava where no further atrial EGMs are recorded. Between the tricuspid annulus and the inferior vena cava, the relationship between atrial and ventricular EGMs is 1:1 or 1:2, whereas before falling inside the inferior vena cava it becomes 2:1 or 4:1. Ablation can be carried out by withdrawing the catheter during continuous radiofrequency delivery or with a point-by-point technique.

The local atrial EGM during effective ablation becomes smaller. It may fragment and disappear. A complete conduction block across the isthmus is characterized by the presence of a continuous

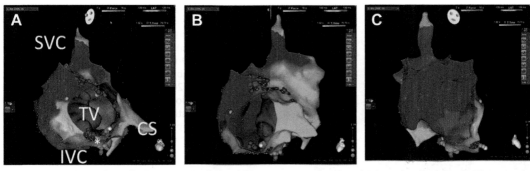

Fig. 3. 3D mapping of RA during TAFL in three different nonconventional RA projections (*A–C*). The mapping shows very clearly all the relevant anatomic land marking and identifies the CTI isthmus (*asterisk*). Furthermore, the entire re-entrant circuit is represented with the (relative) early activation wavefront in red and the latest in purple color. IVC, inferior vena cava; SVC, superior vena cava.

sequence of widely spaced double potentials (**Fig. 5**), whereas a gap in the ablation line is identified by closely spaced double potentials or by fragmented signals between two EGMs (**Fig. 6**).

When gaps are identified, a second attempt is made delivering radiofrequency either over the same line to consolidate it or, more often, medially or laterally to achieve a permanent block.

The standard power setting for irrigated tip catheters is between 50 W and 70 W with a temperature limit of 55° to 60° but recently very high power short duration (90 W for 4 s) has been shown to be effective and safe.[19]

Despite the fact that CTI block can be achieved in the majority of patients, different strategies have been developed to increase the likelihood of

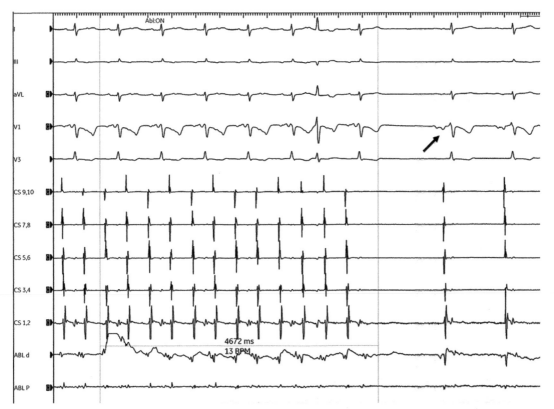

Fig. 4. Set up as in **Figs. 1** and **2**. Ablation is shown during the same arrhythmia at the CTI site shown in **Fig. 2**. During ablation, the AF was terminated. The black arrow highlights the first sinus P-wave morphology.

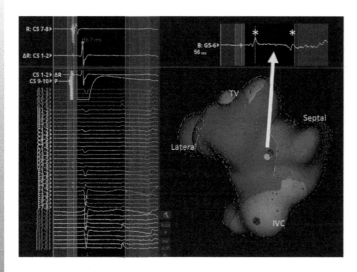

Fig. 5. Limited 3D mapping of the CTI isthmus in a steep caudo-cranial projection. The catheter is shown over the line of ablation during CS ostium pacing. Double potentials are recorded over the ablation line separated by more than 120 millisecond delay. The earliest activation (*red*) in the proximal end of the isthmus meets the latest (*purple*) on the opposite side of the CTI line. IVC, inferior vena cava; RV, right ventricle.

creating transmural and irreversible lesions and to reduce procedural and fluoroscopy duration.

The precise anatomy of the isthmus can be reconstructed with the electroanatomic mapping system and the most important landmarks to be acquired are the inferior portion of the tricuspid annulus and the ostium of the inferior vena cava. The ablation points can be tracked with the mapping system to avoid repeated radiofrequency application on the same spot and to identify more easily the presence of gaps.

The mapping system allows the operators to create a voltage map of the isthmus and this information has been used to plan the course of the ablation line.

The use of 3D mapping systems during TAFL ablation reduces the fluoroscopy time compared with the conventional technique but the former was more expensive and it did not reduce recurrences or total procedure time.[20]

A voltage-guided approach for CTI ablation has been proposed as an alternative to the traditional anatomic approach although it lacks standardization.

Some groups have suggested selectively identifying and ablating areas of high EGM amplitude within the isthmus as these may represent bands of myocardium essential for AFL maintenance.[21] On the contrary, other groups have proposed to avoid these high-amplitude regions as they

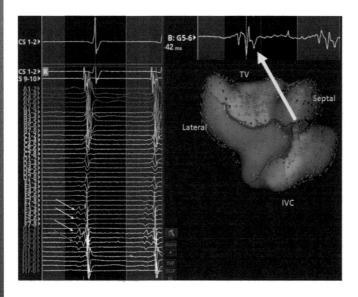

Fig. 6. Similar set up as in **Fig. 5**. During CS pacing the mapping catheter situated over the ablation line records a fragmented EGM. Some electrodes of the multipolar mapping catheter close to the gap displayed single (*white arrows*) or closely spaced potentials (*red arrows*). IVC, inferior vena cava; RV, right ventricle.

represent thicker myocardium rendering transmural ablation more difficult.[22]

Lesion size indicators, such as the ablation index or the local impedance drop, demonstrated even in this setting to increase the effectiveness and safety of the ablation.[19,23]

Endpoints of Ablation

The endpoint of the ablation is the achievement of bidirectional block across the CTI.

The validation of the bidirectional block across the CTI can be obtained by evaluating the atrial activation sequence during pacing medially (proximal CS) and laterally (low lateral wall) to the isthmus.

Before ablation, pacing from the proximal CS results in a clockwise activation across the CTI, which collides with the counterclockwise activation of the lateral wall. After the isthmus line has been created the activation proceeds counterclockwise to activate cranio-caudally the entire lateral wall and subsequently all the points adjacent to the lateral border of the isthmus.

Similarly, pacing from the low lateral wall before the ablation results in an upward clockwise activation of the lateral wall. The activation collides at the high lateral right atrium with the counterclockwise wavefront coming from the CTI and septum. The latter activates the proximal CS before the bundle of His region. After the isthmus has been blocked, the wavefront propagates only in a clockwise direction and the bundle of His region is activated before the proximal CS. Accordingly, the CS activation changes from distal to proximal because the left atrium is activated through the Bachman's bundle.

However, atrial activation sequence recorded with the 20-pole catheter can miss some gaps with very slow conduction especially if they are localized posteriorly.

A simplified approach suggests that a successful long-term ablation is likely to be predicted by a minimum conduction time (measured from the pacing artifact to the EGM recorded on the opposite side of the line) across the isthmus of 150 ms (or an increase of 50% compared with the baseline).

The likelihood of complete CTI block is increased by the observation of a change of morphology of the unipolar signal recorded just medial to the ablation line from an RS pattern to monophasic R during pacing from the CS ostium.

Differential pacing can also add important clues about CTI block. When pacing is performed sequentially from the low lateral RA and from the mid-lateral RA the activation of the CS ostium will be recorded earlier because the wavefront travels clockwise as a result of the isthmus block.[24] On the contrary, if the activation passes across the isthmus because the block is incomplete, the EGM at the CS is delayed and the delay will increase by shortening pacing cycle length, which causes a rate-dependent slower conduction.

The gold standard of bidirectional block demonstration remains the presence of double potentials along the ablation line. Double potentials with an isoelectric interval longer than 110 ms are consistent with bidirectional block, whereas an interval less than 90 ms suggests the presence of possible gaps[25] (see **Fig. 5**).

Electroanatomic mapping, especially when performed with multielectrode catheters, can prove the presence of blocks or help to identify gaps (see **Fig. 6**). During pacing from the proximal CS the activation map can be made by acquiring points on both sides of the line and the result, in the case of complete conduction block, is an "early meets late" appearance.

Signals recorded only at the distal side of the ablation line will demonstrate a continuous progression of colors from the earliest activation (red) recorded at the caval end of the isthmus to the latest (purple) at the tricuspid valve (TV) end.

This is because of the progression of the wavefront from the pacing site in the CS ostium along with the IVC from posterior to anterior meeting the lateral caval site of the line as the earliest site. According to some authors, this approach can increase the chance to identify gaps.[26]

Pitfalls in Typical Atrial Flutter Ablation

TAFL ablation has a high success rate but sometimes procedural difficulties can prevent the achievement of bidirectional block, which in turn increase the probability of arrhythmia recurrences.

When the Eustachian ridge is very thick the catheter maneuverability is limited and the septal aspect of the isthmus cannot be targeted with proper contact unless steerable sheaths are employed.

Deep pouches are often encountered in the isthmus and they cause an impedance and temperature rise during radiofrequency delivery. Ablation at these sites increases the risk of excessive tissue heating with tissue boiling, gas vaporization, and "steam pops" with possible perforation. The solution to this problem is to move the catheters' tip laterally or medially.

Pectinate muscles may extend from the lateral wall to the isthmus and they typically cause high voltage EGM on the ablation catheter. The

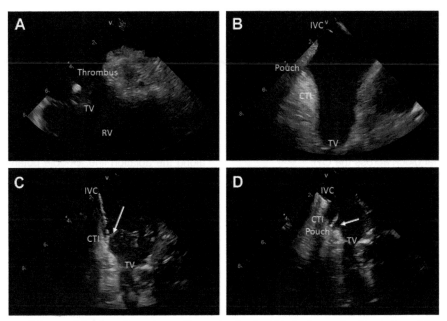

Fig. 7. The usefulness of intracardiac echocardiography in the RA is shown in this series of imagines. (*A*): Thrombus on the TV leaflet. (*B*): Very long CTI in a patient with repaired atrial septal defect and a pouch close to the IVC. (*C*): The tip of the ablation catheter (*white arrow*) is well positioned for ablation being parallel to a straight and smooth CTI. (*D*): The tip of the ablation catheter is inside a deep pouch in the middle of CTI. IVC, inferior vena cava; RV, right ventricle.

presence of these muscular structures may prevent the possibility of creating transmural lesions.

As discussed earlier, steerable sheaths can overcome some anatomic difficulties but an important contribution can be provided by the intracardiac echo.[27] It can guide the ablation by allowing a detailed and real-time visualization of the anatomy and it can also detect some early complications, such as cardiac tamponade (**Fig. 7**).

CLINICS CARE POINTS

- Typical atrial flutter is the prototype of the macro-reentrant tachycardia.

- The macro-reentrant circuit can be precisely characterized with electrophysiological maneuvers and with tri-dimensional mapping systems.

- The target of ablation is the cavo-tricuspid isthmus.

- Typical atrial flutter ablation is the gold standart to manage symptoms and to reverse tachycardia-induced cardiomyopathy.

- CTI ablation has a high success rate but not infrequently some anatomical variants can reduce the efficacy and can increase the risk of complications.

REFERENCES

1. Scherf D, Schaffer AI, Blumenfeld S. Mechanism of flutter and fibrillation. AMA Arch Intern Med 1953; 91:333–52.
2. Boineau JP, Schuessler RB, Mooney CR, et al. Natural and evoked atrial flutter due to circus movement in dogs. Role of abnormal atrial pathways, slow conduction, nonuniform refractory period distribution and premature beats. Am J Cardiol 1980;45: 1167–81.
3. Allessie MA, Bonke FI, Schopman FJ. Circus movement in rabbit atrial muscle as a mechanism of tachycardia. III. The "leading circle" concept: a new model of circus movement in cardiac tissue without the involvement of an anatomical obstacle. Circ Res 1977;41:9–18.
4. Disertori M, Inama G, Vergara G, et al. Evidence of a reentry circuit in the common type of atrial flutter in man. Circulation 1983;67:434–40.
5. Klein GJ, Guiraudon GM, Sharma AD, et al. Demonstration of macroreentry and feasibility of operative therapy in the common type of atrial flutter. Am J Cardiol 1986;57:587–91.
6. Saoudi N, Atallah G, Kirkorian G, et al. Catheter ablation of the atrial myocardium in human type I atrial flutter. Circulation 1990;81:762–71.
7. Feld GK, Fleck RP, Chen PS, et al. Radiofrequency catheter ablation for the treatment of human type 1 atrial flutter. Identification of a critical zone in the

reentrant circuit by endocardial mapping techniques. Circulation 1992;86:1233–40.

8. Cosio FG, Goicolea A, Lopez-Gil M, et al. Catheter ablation of atrial flutter circuits. Pacing Clin Electrophysiol 1993;16:637–42.

9. Fischer B, Jais P, Shah D, et al. Radiofrequency catheter ablation of common atrial flutter in 200 patients. J Cardiovasc Electrophysiol 1996;7:1225–33.

10. Josephson M. Clinical cardiac electrophysiology. 2008285-2008338.

11. Olgin JE, Kalman JM, Saxon LA, et al. Mechanism of initiation of atrial flutter in humans: site of unidirectional block and direction of rotation. J Am Coll Cardiol 1997;29:376–84.

12. Watson RM, Josephson ME. Atrial flutter. I. Electrophysiologic substrates and modes of initiation and termination. Am J Cardiol 1980;45:732–41.

13. Callans DJ, Schwartzman D, Gottlieb CD, et al. Characterization of the excitable gap in human type I atrial flutter. J Am Coll Cardiol 1997;30:1793–801.

14. Kalman JM, Olgin JE, Saxon LA, et al. Activation and entrainment mapping defines the tricuspid annulus as the anterior barrier in typical atrial flutter. Circulation 1996;94:398–406.

15. De Ponti R, Verlato R, Bertaglia E, et al. Treatment of macro-re-entrant atrial tachycardia based on electroanatomic mapping: identification and ablation of the mid-diastolic isthmus. Europace 2007;9:449–57.

16. Arenal A, Almendral J, Alday JM, et al. Rate-dependent conduction block of the crista terminalis in patients with typical atrial flutter: influence on evaluation of cavotricuspid isthmus conduction block. Circulation 1999;99:2771–8.

17. Tai CT, Chen SA, Chen YJ, et al. Conduction properties of the crista terminalis in patients with typical atrial flutter: basis for a line of block in the reentrant circuit. J Cardiovasc Electrophysiol 1998;9:811–9.

18. Marrouche NF, Schweikert R, Saliba W, et al. Use of different catheter ablation technologies for treatment of typical atrial flutter: acute results and long-term follow-up. Pacing Clin Electrophysiol 2003;26:743–6.

19. Schillaci V, Strisciuglio T, Stabile G, et al. Cavotricuspid isthmus ablation by means of very high power, short-duration, temperature-controlled lesions. J Interv Card Electrophysiol 2022. https://doi.org/10.1007/s10840-022-01197-x.

20. Hindricks G, Willems S, Kautzner J, et al. Effect of electroanatomically guided versus conventional catheter ablation of typical atrial flutter on the fluoroscopy time and resource use: a prospective randomized multicenter study. J Cardiovasc Electrophysiol 2009;20:734–40.

21. Posan E, Redfearn DP, Gula LJ, et al. Elimination of cavotricuspid isthmus conduction by a single ablation lesion: observations from a maximum voltage-guided ablation technique. Europace 2007;9:208–11.

22. Hall B, Veerareddy S, Cheung P, et al. Randomized comparison of anatomical versus voltage guided ablation of the cavotricuspid isthmus for atrial flutter. Heart Rhythm 2004;1:43–8.

23. Sakama S, Yagishita A, Sakai T, et al. Ablation index-guided cavotricuspid isthmus ablation with contiguous lesions using fluoroscopy integrated 3D mapping in atrial flutter. J Interv Card Electrophysiol 2022. https://doi.org/10.1007/s10840-022-01182-4.

24. Katritsis DG, Chokesuwattanaskul R, Zografos T, et al. A simplified differential pacing technique for the evaluation of bidirectional cavo-tricuspid isthmus block during ablation of typical atrial flutter. J Interv Card Electrophysiol 2022;63:109–14.

25. Tada H, Oral H, Sticherling C, et al. Double potentials along the ablation line as a guide to radiofrequency ablation of typical atrial flutter. J Am Coll Cardiol 2001;38:750–5.

26. Nakagawa H, Jackman WM. Use of a three-dimensional, nonfluoroscopic mapping system for catheter ablation of typical atrial flutter. Pacing Clin Electrophysiol 1998;21:1279–86.

27. Bencsik G. Novel strategies in the ablation of typical atrial flutter: role of intracardiac echocardiography. Curr Cardiol Rev 2015;11:127–33.

Mapping and Ablation of Atypical Atrial Flutters

Jacopo Marazzato, MD[a,b], Raffaella Marazzi, MD[a], Lorenzo A. Doni, MD[a],
Fabio Angeli, MD[b,c], Giuseppe Bagliani, MD[d], Fabio M. Leonelli, MD[e],
Roberto De Ponti, MD, FHRS[a,b,*]

KEYWORDS

- Atypical atrial flutter • 3-dimensional electroanatomic mapping • Cardiac mapping
- Catheter ablation • Supraventricular arrhythmia

KEY POINTS

- Atypical atrial flutters are regarded as complex atrial arrhythmias leading to clinically relevant events.
- With little role played by antiarrhythmic medications, catheter ablation has emerged as a feasible treatment option in this setting. Moreover, the use of irrigated catheters and 3D electroanatomic mapping has brought far better results over the last decade.
- The ablation results may be still suboptimal due to the progressive atrial remodeling occurring in these patients, which might lead to new arrhythmogenic circuits and atrial fibrillation.
- To improve the overall success, a patient-tailored approach is required. In addition to arrhythmia termination and validation of the ablation lines, any other potential arrhythmogenic source should be identified and treated, especially in patients with clinical history of atrial fibrillation.

INTRODUCTION

Atypical atrial flutters (AAFLs) are complex atrial arrhythmias arising from either atrium,[1] not involving the cavotricuspid isthmus,[2] and generally stemming from a spectrum of different pathophysiological substrates. Surgical correction of acquired[3] and congenital[4] heart disorders, pulmonary vein isolation procedures,[5] and structural heart diseases[6] may all lead to an electroanatomic remodeling of the atrial substrate, which does represent the pathophysiological cornerstone of these macroreentrant circuits. However, AAFLs may also be encountered in patients with structurally normal hearts where atrial myopathy[7] or mechanisms of nonuniform anisotropy might be responsible for the onset and maintenance of these atrial arrhythmias.[8,9]

As for the limited role of antiarrhythmic medication in this complex clinical scenario,[10] catheter ablation has progressively attracted increasing attention as the potentially definitive treatment option for these arrhythmias. Therefore, a general overview regarding the development of different mapping and ablation strategies for AAFLs, their overall feasibility and results, as well as the

Conflicts of interest disclosure: Dr R. De Ponti has received fees for lectures and scientific collaboration from Biosense Webster. None for the other authors.
No funding sources to be acknowledged.
[a] Department of Heart and Vessels, Ospedale di Circolo - University of Insubria, Viale Borri, 57, Varese 21100, Italy; [b] Department of Medicine and Surgery, University of Insubria, Viale Guicciardini, 9, Varese 21100, Italy; [c] Department of Medicine and Cardiopulmonary Rehabilitation, Maugeri Care and Research Institutes, IRCCS, Via Crotto Roncacci, 16, Tradate, Varese 21049, Italy; [d] Cardiology and Arrhythmology Clinic, Marche Polytechnic University, University Hospital "Ospedali Riuniti Umberto I-Lancisi-Salesi", Via Conca 71, Ancona 60126, Italy; [e] Cardiology Department, James A. Haley Veterans' Hospital, University of South Florida, 13000 Bruce B Down Boulevard, Tampa, FL 33612, USA
* Corresponding author. Department of Heart and Vessels, Ospedale di Circolo and Macchi Foundation, University of Insubria - Varese, Viale Borri, 57. Varese 21100, Italy.
E-mail address: roberto.deponti@uninsubria.it

Card Electrophysiol Clin 14 (2022) 471–481
https://doi.org/10.1016/j.ccep.2022.03.003
1877-9182/22/© 2022 Elsevier Inc. All rights reserved.

authors' experience in this field are given herein.[11,12]

DIFFERENT MAPPING AND ABLATION STRATEGIES FOR ATYPICAL ATRIAL FLUTTERS

Accurate mapping and specific pacing maneuvers have been regarded as essential cornerstones for the identification of appropriate ablation targets of AAFLs. Although conventional mapping with the systematic use of entrainment and assessment of postpacing interval have been seminal in the study of complex reentrant arrhythmias in different surgical[4] and nonsurgical settings,[13] the progressive implementation of 3-dimensional electroanatomic mapping proved very helpful in the straightforward assessment of macroreentrant circuits in the right[6,14] and left atrial chambers.[15,16] Indeed, as reported by studies investigating the use of these mapping systems for the evaluation of AAFLs,[6,14–16] tachycardia termination is usually achieved by radiofrequency delivery to narrow anatomic channels or isthmi with remarkably slow conductive properties and well identified on activation and bipolar voltage maps. However, complex circuits may pose significant challenges for ablation,[17] and, in some cases, electroanatomic activation mapping may provide ambiguous data.[18] Although the integration of these systems with more traditional mapping strategies proved useful,[19,20] the feasibility of entrainment, when systematically attempted, can be limited in this setting. Arrhythmia termination or degeneration into atrial fibrillation or failure to capture the tested sites due to increased pacing thresholds are all well-acknowledged shortcomings associated with these complex pacing maneuvers.[11,15,21,22] Moreover, antiarrhythmic medications may alter the assessment of postpacing intervals[23] in a clinical setting where standard criteria for entrainment have not been experimentally validated so far[24] and the results highly depend on the pacing rate and site where these maneuverers are performed.[25]

To further complicate this scenario, not all anatomic isthmi are equally associated with successful results when targeted for ablation. Some anatomic areas are difficult to ablate due to high voltages as the result of remarkable myocardial thickness[12] and, in case of double loop reentry, which could be as high as 60% of all macroreentrant atrial arrhythmias,[11,12,26] more anatomic areas or isthmi are to be approached to achieve tachycardia interruption, thus leading to time-consuming and potentially unsuccessful procedures.[27]

To overcome these issues, a mapping and ablation strategy based on a specific setting of the window of interest on 3-dimensional electroanatomic mapping systems to properly identify and ablate the mid-diastolic isthmus of the investigated macroreentrant circuits was validated in a multicenter study.[11] Indeed, the mid-diastolic isthmus should be regarded as the weakest part of the tachycardia circuit, very frequently associated with low-amplitude potentials and area of slow conduction, and the ideal site for ablation.[11] In our experience,[11,12] the mid-diastolic isthmus can be easily identified based on electroanatomic mapping alone and successfully ablated with tachycardia termination in most cases, regardless of entrainment mapping validation,[11] especially when radiofrequency applications are delivered to areas with remarkably slow conduction velocity and low bipolar voltages.[12]

In the following paragraphs, an overview of this specific mapping and ablation strategy is provided together with a literature review on catheter ablation feasibility, postablation arrhythmia recurrence, and related issues occurring in this complex clinical scenario.

MAPPING AND ABLATION BASED ON 3-DIMENSIONAL ELECTROANATOMIC MAPPING
Specific Setting of the Window of Interest

The window of interest is the part of the tachycardia cycle length analyzed by the mapping system to identify electrical signals that are annotated for both activation and voltage mapping. All bipolar signals that precede and follow a prespecified reference signal are included in the window of interest. In case they precede the reference signal they have a negative value, whereas in the opposite case, they have a positive value. A diagnostic catheter is commonly placed in the coronary sinus to provide a stable atrial reference signal throughout the procedure. As already described elsewhere,[11] the onset of the window is set exactly at mid-diastole and its duration spans from 90% to 95% of the tachycardia cycle length so to consider minimal variations of tachycardia cycle and to avoid ambiguous mapping results. To correctly identify the diastole, that is, the isoelectric line between P waves, and consequently the mid-diastole, clear identification of the P wave is crucial. To this purpose, carotid sinus massage or adenosine bolus injection may be required to induce a transient modification of the atrioventricular conduction ratio, which can help identify the surface P wave during the ongoing tachycardia. As already discussed,[11] a

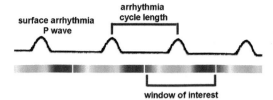

Fig. 1. Schematic representation of the specific setting of the window of interest for 3-dimensional electroanatomic mapping of atypical atrial flutter. The onset of the window of interest is set in the mid-diastole, and it lasts for 90% to 95% of the arrhythmia cycle length, so that the surface P wave, corresponding to systolic activation, is central. By doing this, each color represents a specific chronology in the reentry circuit. If the reentry circuit is fully reconstructed, the rainbow of colors identifies the reentrant activation sequence, and the mid-diastolic isthmus is where the red-colored area meets the purple-colored area.

distinct surface P wave can be properly identified in AAFLs by increasing the sweep speed on the recording system to 100 mm/s, because the continuously waving pattern of the surface P wave with no isoelectric line is observed at the

speed of standard electrocardiogram of 25 mm/ s. Once the reentry circuit is fully reconstructed in the atrial chamber of origin, the color code used for activation identifies the activation sequence from what has been arbitrarily defined early (red) to late (purple), and each color represents a specific activation time during the arrhythmia cycle (**Fig. 1**). Therefore, the mid-diastolic isthmus can be clearly identified in the site where the red-colored area meets the purple-colored area, as shown in **Fig. 1**. When activation spanning at least 90% of the arrhythmia cycle length cannot be reconstructed in an atrial chamber, this strongly favors the hypothesis that atrial flutter originates in the opposite atrial chamber, provided a focal tachycardia has been already excluded.

Activation Mapping

Mapping is usually commenced in the right atrium to be continued in the left atrial chamber when a right-sided circuit has been thoroughly ruled out. The acquired mapping points should be homogeneously distributed to cover greater than or equal

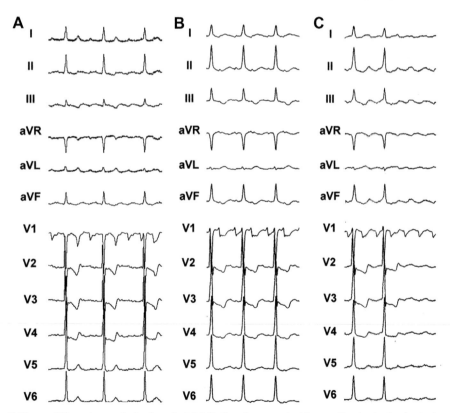

Fig. 2. (A–C) Three different morphologies of atrial flutter documented in a patient who had priorly undergone Fontan operation for pulmonary valve atresia and tricuspid valve dysplasia. Morphology displayed in (A and B) are consistent with atypical atrial flutter, whereas the one shown in (C) seems to match a typical reverse isthmus-dependent atrial flutter. In the 3 different morphologies, cycle length varies from 290 (A) to 220 ms (C).

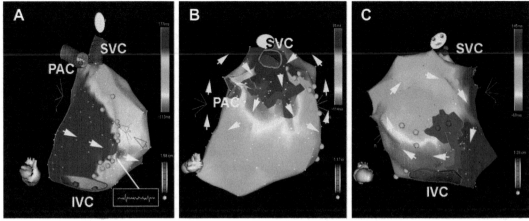

Fig. 3. (A–C) Three-dimensional activation mapping of the right atrium, each corresponding to the 3 morphologies shown in the previous figure. According to the previous Fontan operation, the tricuspid orifice was closed with a patch and a conduit connects the pulmonary artery with the right atrium. The right atrium is shown in lateral projection in (A), posteroanterior in (B), and left anterior oblique in (C). In (A), a single loop clockwise reentry (*arrows*) sustains the atypical atrial flutter, and the mid-diastolic isthmus is identified by the red area where red encounters the purple, corresponding to a gap in a line of double potentials (*blue dots*), a prior right lateral atriotomy; in the inset, a long-lasting, fragmented, low-amplitude bipolar electrogram recorded in this small isthmus identifies a very slow conduction area. In (B), a double loop reentry with one loop around the conduit orifice and the second in the lateral right atrium (*arrows*) is identified, with both loops sharing the mid-diastolic isthmus in the posterosuperior right atrium. In (C), a single clockwise loop around the tricuspid patch is identified with the critical isthmus between the patch (*gray area*) and the inferior vena cava os; this would depict a peculiar form of typical reverse atrial flutter, which explains the morphology shown in **Fig. 2C**. IVC, inferior vena cava os; PAC, pulmonary atrial conduit; SVC, superior vena cava os.

to 90% of the tachycardia cycle length in the investigated atrial chamber.[11] Whether acquired manually[11] or automatically[28] by ablation or multipolar catheters, the importance of proper analysis of the acquired mapping points is paramount. Bipolar signals in sites with minimal but still discernible amplitude should be carefully considered not to miss out critical target areas for ablation. If fractionated and prolonged electrograms pose a challenge, the first sharp deflection is usually annotated.[11] Moreover, the available cutting-edge technologies can detect regions with a bipolar signal amplitude as low as 0.03 mV, at the limit of the definition of noise using conventional ablation catheters (0.05 mV), which may, nonetheless, be critical for the maintenance of the reentrant circuit.[28] Therefore, every effort should be made to precisely define the border between an electrically silent area and the surrounding still viable myocardial tissue.[29,30]

Cycle length stability and proper catheter manipulation during the mapping phase are greatly important to prevent ambiguous mapping results. Therefore, arrhythmia variations, surface P wave morphology, tachycardia cycle, and the intracavitary activation sequence should all be properly monitored throughout the procedure to avert these issues. In addition to careful

monitoring, mechanical arrhythmia termination or modification should be avoided to prevent creation of incomplete or misleading activation maps.

Once the activation mapping has been completed, the reentry course of AAFL can be identified following the sequence of colors of the color-coded scale. In this analysis, single loop or double loop reentry circuits can be identified so that the arrhythmia can be better characterized. **Figs. 2** and **3** show a case of 3 different atrial flutters morphologies sustained by single or double loop reentry circuit in a post-Fontan patient. Independently from entrainment pacing maneuvers and provided that the entire reentry circuit has been reconstructed, the mid-diastolic isthmus is identified at the interface between the red and the purple areas, marked by red band, as shown in **Fig. 3**. In this site, when applied, entrainment maneuvers confirm the presence of a protected isthmus of slow conduction, critical for the reentry circuit and, therefore, representing the ablation target.[11] Higher-density mapping may be required at this site to accurately define its boundaries and better clarify the arrhythmogenic substrate. In fact, the boundaries of the critical isthmus can be anatomic structures, scar areas with no electrical signal, or lines of double potentials possibly related to prior atriotomy.

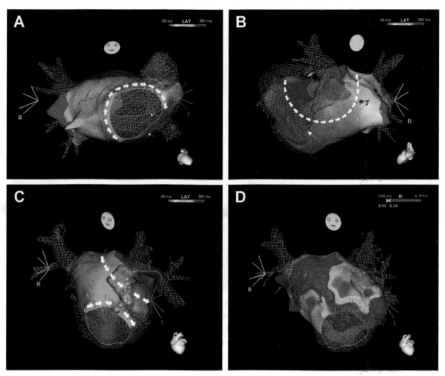

Fig. 4. (*A–D*) In (*A–C*), left atrial activation electroanatomic mapping superimposed to the 3-dimensional computed tomography rendering is shown, whereas bipolar voltage mapping is shown in (*D*). In this patient, who underwent pulmonary vein isolation in a previous procedure, a double-loop left atrial flutter is now identified, with one clockwise loop around the mitral annulus (*arrows in A*) and a second counterclockwise loop around the left pulmonary veins (*arrows in B*). Both loops share the mid-diastolic isthmus, identified by the red band in B (*dotted arrow*), in the posterolateral isthmus between the inferior pulmonary vein and the postero-lateral mitral annulus. In consideration of the extension, high voltages displayed in this area, and the issues related to ablation of posterior mitral isthmus, an alternative ablation strategy was carried out, transecting a more anterior isthmus where both loops passed through (*white arrows in C*). Radiofrequency energy delivery to this site of low atrial voltages, as assessed by the red color in the bipolar voltage map in (*D*), led to progressive cycle length prolongation and successful tachycardia interruption (*pink and red dots in C*). Validation of the ablation line was then performed during left atrial appendage pacing, and sinus rhythm was persistently observed during follow-up.

Choice of the Ablation Strategy

If ablation of the mid-diastolic isthmus is generally the first-line strategy to treat AAFLs, this is even more true in case of more complex atrial substrates. In fact, up to 60% all AAFLs are made up of double reentrant loops[11,17] where each observed loop emerges from the common mid-diastolic isthmus and spans more than 90% of tachycardia cycle length as observed on propagation maps.[11] In most of these cases, catheter ablation based on electroanatomic mapping findings proves an invaluable strategy, because a single ablation line at mid-diastolic isthmus commonly leads to arrhythmia suppression, thus sparing ablation and mapping time compared with separate targeting of each loop.[11,27] However, under certain circumstances,[31] ablation of the mid-diastolic isthmus might be challenging. In these cases, an alternative ablation strategy should be thoroughly chosen, deploying radiofrequency energy applications to more practical isthmi, which could be more easily and effectively ablated.[11,31] **Fig. 4** shows an example of this alternative strategy in a patient with a left-sided double loop AAFL. Instead of targeting the posterolateral left isthmus, ablation is performed in the anterior isthmus between the left superior pulmonary vein os and the anterior mitral annulus, shorter and with low-amplitude potentials.

Finally, complex atrial substrates with different low-voltage channels commingled with areas of dense scar may underpin the development of different arrhythmias with varying atrial P wave morphologies and cycle lengths.[32] Therefore, as an alternative to activation mapping and ablation during the AAFL, high-density mapping in sinus rhythm for detection and ablation of protected

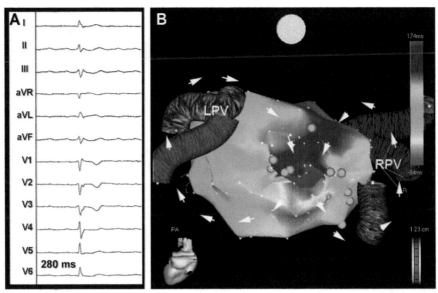

Fig. 5. (*A, B*). Atypical atrial flutter after mitral valve surgery. (*A*) The surface morphology of the flutter is shown with positive P-waves in the inferior and precordial leads and a cycle length of 280 ms. (*B*) Electroanatomic activation mapping of the left atrium is shown in a posteroanterior view. A double loop reentry, with each loop rotating around the left and right pulmonary veins, respectively (*arrows*), and the critical isthmus (*red band*) in a gap of the line of double potentials (*blue dots*) related to prior atriotomy are identified. LPV, left pulmonary veins; RPV, right pulmonary veins.

isthmi has proved a helpful strategy to obtain scar homogenization and arrhythmia suppression.[32]

Ablation Settings

Over the years, different ablation catheters have been used for ablation of AAFLs. Initially, 4-mm-[4,15] and 8-mm-tip[33] catheters for radiofrequency ablation were used with a temperature threshold set to 55°C to 65°C and energy delivery set to 65 W and up to 80 W in case of 8-mm-tip ones.[11] However, over the years, open-irrigation catheters have been more extensively used to become the first adopted option[11,28] with a preset temperature generally set to 43°C, power output between 30 and 50 W, and maximum application duration preset at 60 seconds.[11,34] The irrigation flow rate is generally set at 20 mL/min for power settings less than 30 W and 30 mL/min for power settings between 30 and 50 W.[11] Finally, implementation of contact force sensing technologies is generally recommended because, in recent years, it has been associated with a greater procedure success.[34]

Procedure End Points

Whatever the strategy used, in case of mappable arrhythmia, the ablation end point of macroreentrant AAFLs is conduction block across the targeted isthmus. During pacing from one side of the line, similarly to typical atrial flutter ablation, conduction block is confirmed by evidence of double potentials along the ablation line and by demonstration of wavefront detour around the ablation line resulting in late activation at the opposite site.[35] **Figs. 5** and **6** show the ablation target of a double loop left atrial flutter and demonstration of conduction block in the target isthmus by electroanatomic propagation mapping. Differential pacing maneuvers may also prove helpful in the validation of the targeted line.[35] However, outside the cavotricuspid isthmus, demonstration of bidirectional conduction block over the ablation line may be difficult. For this reason, complete disappearance of electrical activity at the site of ablation can be considered a surrogate for conduction block.[11,12] In this setting, as well as in case of substrate ablation and scar homogenization performed in sinus rhythm, tachycardia noninducibility by aggressive atrial pacing also should be regarded as major procedure end point,[11,34] and, in the event of any tachycardia induction, remapping and ablation should be performed to minimize recurrences.

EFFICACY AND SAFETY USING DIFFERENT MAPPING AND ABLATION STRATEGIES

A variable procedure efficacy is generally reported in literature, spanning from limited success rate

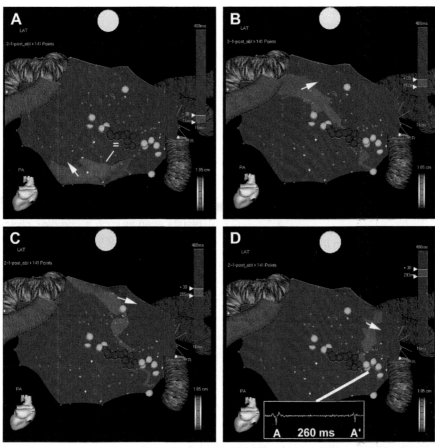

Fig. 6. Display of 4 frames (*A-D*) of postablation electroanatomic propagation map in the case presented in the previous figure. During coronary sinus pacing, the red band of propagation clearly shows the presence of a line of continuous block along the line of ablation (*red dots*) and double potentials (*blue dots*) with wavefront detour (*arrows*). Conduction block is confirmed also by double potentials separated by an isoelectric line of 260 ms in the posteromedial left atrium (*inset in D*).

recorded in seminal studies[36] to the far greater efficacy shown in a recently published experience using the available cutting-edge technologies in the field.[28] Different reasons may explain these findings. It stands to reason that a suboptimal result is generally expected in remarkably complex atrial substrates, such as in case of congenital heart disease[37] where longer procedure and fluoroscopy times[26] are generally expected. On the other hand, regardless of the underlying substrate to ablate, a trend showing a progressive improvement in catheter ablation results has been clearly observed over the past years with reported success rate ranging from 65% to greater than 90%.[11,15,28,38] Similar findings have been recently reported in a meta-analysis assessing the feasibility of catheter ablation of macroreentrant atrial circuits after mitral valve surgery.[39] If the systematic use of conventional mapping[16,38] is not generally associated with better results when compared with ablation strategies based on 3-dimensional

mapping systems alone,[11,12,26] proper handling of these systems is crucial with the aid of newer technologies, which over the past decade proved extremely helpful to achieve better results and lower procedure and fluoroscopy times.[28,40,41] In addition to the progressive implementation of these mapping systems, the use of radiofrequency, open-irrigated-tip catheters has also played a pivotal role in achieving a better procedure-related efficacy[42] due to larger and deeper myocardial lesions yielded by homogeneous catheter cooling.[43]

However, the acute success rate might still be suboptimal in a few cases.[34,40] The anatomic extension and thickness of the targeted isthmus can be an important variable, because the greater the anatomic extension and the conduction velocity of the mid-diastolic isthmus, the lower the procedural success.[12,26] Moreover, peculiar anatomic locations are incredibly difficult to ablate, such as arrhythmias stemming from the mitral isthmus[31] or other atrial septal circuits. In this latter case, catheter ablation might be interrupted for safety issues to avoid modification of the atrioventricular conduction properties.[11]

Regarding the procedural safety, catheter ablation of AALFs is generally deemed safe, although associated with a non-negligible prevalence of major and minor complications. If groin hematoma accounts for up to 7%,[16] arteriovenous fistula for up to 4%,[11,12] and femoral pseudoaneurysm for 1.4%, more severe complications, such as cerebral[15,44] and peripheral[38] embolism, could be reported in 4% to 6% of the cases, whereas major bleedings are only sparingly reported.[45] These data suggest that antithrombotic therapy should be carefully managed in these patients, especially when ablation is performed in the presence of mechanical prostheses.[39]

Finally, particular attention should be devoted to catheter ablation and handling in specific anatomic sites, to avoid right hemidiaphragm palsy[38] or damage to the sinus node, both potentially associated with lack of localization of these structures in potentially complex postsurgical anatomies.

ARRHYTHMIA RECURRENCE AND ISSUES RELATED TO LONG-TERM FOLLOW-UP

After an initially successful ablation procedure, a recurrence rate ranging from 7%[11] to 62%[44,46] can be generally expected after catheter ablation of AAFLs. Although a different follow-up duration might partly explain these variable findings,[39] the progressive implementation of electroanatomic systems,[11,12] high-density mapping technologies,[28] and irrigated-tip catheters[42] has been associated with better ablation results over a mid- and long-term follow-up.[11] However, in patients undergoing repeat catheter ablation for recurrent arrhythmias, most of these circuits do not represent true tachycardia recurrence, but different arrhythmias located in different sites compared with first ablation procedures.[47] In fact, despite a huge number of procedures over time,[39] the overall maintenance of sinus rhythm on/off antiarrhythmic medications is generally suboptimal in these patients.[16,48] These findings are well explained by the progressive atrial substrate evolution occurring in these patients,[39,47] with occurrence of clinical atrial fibrillation, which could be as high as 20% in these patients.[39] To improve the overall success rate, in addition to arrhythmia termination and validation of the ablation lines, any other potential arrhythmogenic source should be identified and treated, especially in patients with clinical history of atrial fibrillation or any prior surgical/nonsurgical treatment of this cardiac arrhythmia.[49]

SUMMARY

AAFLs are complex arrhythmias leading to significant symptoms in the affected patients with little role played by antiarrhythmic medications. With the aim to overcome these issues, catheter ablation has progressively emerged as the potentially definitive treatment option in this setting, and, despite a non-negligible number of complications and the remarkable complexity of some cases, the procedure is deemed useful and associated with an improved mid-term clinical impact. Of note, the use of irrigated catheters and 3-dimensional electroanatomic mapping with cutting-edge mapping technologies warranted far better results even in such a complex clinical scenario. The higher recurrence rate despite repeat procedures should be regarded in the light of atrial substrate evolution leading to new arrhythmia circuits and to atrial fibrillation. Hence, to improve the overall success, a patient-tailored approach is required, aiming at detecting any potential arrhythmogenic substrate especially in complex cases.

CLINICS CARE POINTS

Preprocedure

- Collect and analyze the 12-lead electrocardiogram recorded during the clinical episodes to evaluate the presence of multiple morphologies, including assessment of atrial fibrillation.

- In case of prior surgical cardiac operations, obtain a detailed report including the surgical approach used and anatomic location of surgical lesions.

- In case of peculiar anatomy, obtain a 3-dimensional imaging by computed tomography or cardiac magnetic resonance scan.

During mapping

- Verification of arrhythmia stability in terms of P-wave morphology and cycle length.

- Setting of the electroanatomic mapping system to obtain a meaningful activation map.

- Identification on activation and propagation maps the reentry course and critical isthmus to set out a proper ablation strategy.

- Defining of the boundaries of the critical isthmus and of sensitive structures, such as sinus node, atrioventricular node, and phrenic nerve, to avoid potentially dreadful complications.

During ablation

- Optimize parameters for durable lesion formation, including appropriate radiofrequency energy settings, catheter stability, and contact force.
- In case of significant arrhythmia modification, evaluate the need for remapping.
- Upon arrhythmia termination, assess achievement of conduction block over the ablation line by dedicated pacing maneuvers, propagation mapping, and/or electrical signal disappearance.
- Evaluate the suppression of atrial flutter inducibility by programmed electrical stimulation.

Follow-up

- Define the need for antiarrhythmic drug therapy continuation based on the severity of atrial myopathy.
- Define the frequency and strategy for future outpatient evaluation to assess long-term sinus rhythm maintenance/arrhythmia recurrence.

REFERENCES

1. Bun SS, Latcu DG, Marchlinski F, et al. Atrial flutter: more than just one of a kind. Eur Heart J 2015;36: 2356–63.
2. Saoudi N, Chairman MD, Cosio F, et al. Classification of atrial flutter and regular atrial tachycardia according to electrophysiologic mechanism and anatomic bases: a statement from a joint expert Group from the Working Group of arrhythmias of the European Society of Cardiology and the North A. J Cardiovasc Electrophysiol 2001;12:852–66.
3. Markowitz SM, Brodman RF, Stein KM, et al. Lesional tachycardias related to mitral valve surgery. J Am Coll Cardiol 2002;39:1973–83.
4. Kalman JM, VanHare GF, Olgin JE, et al. Ablation of 'Incisional' reentrant atrial tachycardia complicating surgery for congenital heart disease. Circulation 1996;93:502–12.
5. Morady F, Oral H, Chugh A. Diagnosis and ablation of atypical atrial tachycardia and flutter complicating atrial fibrillation ablation. Heart Rhythm 2009;6(8 SUPPL):S29–32.
6. Kall JG, Rubenstein DS, Kopp DE, et al. Atypical atrial flutter originating in the right atrial free wall. Circulation 2000;101:270–9.
7. Fiala M, Chovančík J, Neuwirth R, et al. Atrial macroreentry tachycardia in patients without obvious structural heart disease or previous cardiac surgical or catheter intervention: characterization of arrhythmogenic substrates, reentry circuits, and results of catheter ablation. J Cardiovasc Electrophysiol 2007;18:824–32.
8. Tai CT, Huang JL, Lin YK, et al. Noncontact three-dimensional mapping and ablation of upper loop re-entry originating in the right atrium. J Am Coll Cardiol 2002;40:746–53.
9. Marrouche NF, Natale A, Wazni OM, et al. Left septal atrial flutter: electrophysiology, anatomy, and results of ablation. Circulation 2004;109:2440–7.
10. Natale A, Newby KH, Pisanó E, et al. Prospective randomized comparison of antiarrhythmic therapy versus first- line radiofrequency ablation in patients with atrial flutter. J Am Coll Cardiol 2000;35: 1898–904.
11. De Ponti R, Verlato R, Bertaglia E, et al. Treatment of macro-re-entrant atrial tachycardia based on electroanatomic mapping: identification and ablation of the mid-diastolic isthmus. Europace 2007;9:449–57.
12. De Ponti R, Marazzi R, Zoli L, et al. Electroanatomic mapping and ablation of macroreentrant atrial tachycardia: comparison between successfully and unsuccessfully treated cases. J Cardiovasc Electrophysiol 2010;21:155–62.
13. Bogun F, Bender B, Li YG, et al. Ablation of atypical atrial flutter guided by the use of concealed entrainment in patients without prior cardiac surgery. J Cardiovasc Electrophysiol 2000;11:136–45.
14. Nakagawa H, Shah N, Matsudaira K, et al. Characterization of reentrant circuit in macroreentrant right atrial tachycardia after surgical repair of congenital heart disease: isolated channels between scars allow "focal" ablation. Circulation 2001;103:699–709.
15. Jaïs P, Shah DC, Haïssaguerre M, et al. Mapping and ablation of left atrial flutters. Circulation 2000; 101:2928–34.
16. Ouyang F, Ernst S, Vogtmann T, et al. Characterization of reentrant circuits in left atrial macroreentrant tachycardia: critical isthmus block can prevent atrial tachycardia recurrence. Circulation 2002;105: 1934–42.
17. Shah D, Jaïs P, Takahashi A, et al. Dual-loop intra-atrial reentry in humans. Circulation 2000;101:631–9.
18. Irtel TA, Delacrétaz E. Intra-atrial reentrant tachycardia with ambiguous data from activation mapping: what to do next? Heart Rhythm 2005;2: 780–1.
19. Jaïs P, Matsuo S, Knecht S, et al. A deductive mapping strategy for atrial tachycardia following atrial fibrillation ablation: importance of localized reentry. J Cardiovasc Electrophysiol 2009;20:480–91.
20. Esato M, Hindricks G, Sommer P, et al. Color-coded three-dimensional entrainment mapping for analysis and treatment of atrial macroreentrant tachycardia. Heart Rhythm 2009;6:349–58.
21. Stevenson IH, Kistler PM, Spence SJ, et al. Scar-related right atrial macroreentrant tachycardia in

patients without prior atrial surgery: electroanatomic characterization and ablation outcome. Heart Rhythm 2005;2:594–601.

22. Magnin-Poull I, De Chillou C, Miljoen H, et al. Mechanisms of right atrial tachycardia occurring late after surgical closure of atrial septal defects. J Cardiovasc Electrophysiol 2005;16:681–7.

23. Fatemi M, Mansourati J, Rosu R, et al. Value of entrainment mapping in determining the isthmus-dependent nature of atrial flutter in the presence of amiodarone. J Cardiovasc Electrophysiol 2004;15:1409–15.

24. Triedman JK, Alexander ME, Berul CI, et al. Electroanatomic mapping of entrained and exit zones in patients with repaired congenital heart disease and intra-atrial reentrant tachycardia. Circulation 2001;103:2060–5.

25. Morton JB, Sanders P, Deen V, et al. Sensitivity and specificity of concealed entrainment for the identification of a critical isthmus in the atrium: relationship to rate, anatomic location and antidromic penetration. J Am Coll Cardiol 2002;39:896–906.

26. Drago F, Russo MS, Marazzi R, et al. Atrial tachycardias in patients with congenital heart disease: a minimally invasive simplified approach in the use of three-dimensional electroanatomic mapping. Europace 2011;13:689–95.

27. Seiler J, Schmid DK, Irtel TA, et al. Dual-loop circuits in postoperative atrial macro re-entrant tachycardias. Heart 2007;93:325–30.

28. Vlachos K, Efremidis M, Derval N, et al. Use of high-density activation and voltage mapping in combination with entrainment to delineate gap-related atrial tachycardias post atrial fibrillation ablation. Europace 2021;23:1052–62.

29. Sanders P, Morton JB, Kistler PM, et al. Electrophysiological and electroanatomic characterization of the atria in sinus node disease: evidence of diffuse atrial remodeling. Circulation 2004;109:1514–22.

30. Marcus GM, Yang Y, Varosy PD, et al. Regional left atrial voltage in patients with atrial fibrillation. Heart Rhythm 2007;4:138–44.

31. Maheshwari A, Shirai Y, Hyman MC, et al. Septal versus lateral mitral isthmus ablation for treatment of mitral annular flutter. JACC Clin Electrophysiol 2019;5:1292–9.

32. Methachittiphan N, Akoum N, Gopinathannair R, et al. Dynamic voltage threshold adjusted substrate modification technique for complex atypical atrial flutters with varying circuits. Pacing Clin Electrophysiol 2020;43:1273–80.

33. Zrenner B, Dong J, Schreieck J, et al. Delineation of intra-atrial reentrant tachycardia circuits after mustard operation for transposition of the Great arteries using biatrial electroanatomic mapping and entrainment mapping. J Cardiovasc Electrophysiol 2003;14:1302–10.

34. Balt JC, Klaver MN, Mahmoodi BK, et al. High-density versus low-density mapping in ablation of atypical atrial flutter. J Interv Card Electrophysiol 2021;62:587–99.

35. Jaïs P, Hocini M, O'Neill MD, et al. How to perform linear lesions. Heart Rhythm 2007;4:803–9.

36. Delacretaz E, Ganz LI, Soejima K, et al. Multi atrial maco-re-entry circuits in adults with repaired congenital heart disease: entrainment mapping combined with three-dimensional electroanatomic mapping. J Am Coll Cardiol 2001;37:1665–76.

37. Yap SC, Harris L, Silversides CK, et al. Outcome of intra-atrial re-entrant tachycardia catheter ablation in adults with congenital heart disease: negative impact of age and complex atrial surgery. J Am Coll Cardiol 2010;56:1589–96.

38. Triedman JK, Bergau DM, Saul JP, et al. Efficacy of radiofrequency ablation for control of intraatrial reentrant tachycardia in patients with congenital heart disease. J Am Coll Cardiol 1997;30:1032–8.

39. Marazzato J, Cappabianca G, Angeli F, et al. Catheter ablation of atrial tachycardias after mitral valve surgery: a systematic review and meta-analysis. J Cardiovasc Electrophysiol 2020;31:2632–41.

40. Derval N, Takigawa M, Frontera A, et al. Characterization of complex atrial tachycardia in patients with previous atrial Interventions using high-resolution mapping. JACC Clin Electrophysiol 2020;6:815–26.

41. Liu SH, Lin YJ, Lee PT, et al. The isthmus characteristics of scar-related macroreentrant atrial tachycardia in patients with and without cardiac surgery. J Cardiovasc Electrophysiol 2021;32:1921–30.

42. Bai R, Fahmy TS, Patel D, et al. Radiofrequency ablation of atypical atrial flutter after cardiac surgery or atrial fibrillation ablation: a randomized comparison of open-irrigation-tip and 8-mm-tip catheters. Heart Rhythm 2007;4:1489–96.

43. Demazumder D, Mirotznik MS, Schwartzman D. Comparison of irrigated electrode designs for radiofrequency ablation of myocardium. J Interv Card Electrophysiol 2001;5:391–400.

44. Deisenhofer I, Estner H, Zrenner B, et al. Left atrial tachycardia after circumferential pulmonary vein ablation for atrial fibrillation: Incidence, electrophysiological characteristics, and results of radiofrequency ablation. Europace 2006;8:573–82.

45. Enriquez A, Santangeli P, Zado ES, et al. Postoperative atrial tachycardias after mitral valve surgery: mechanisms and outcomes of catheter ablation. Heart Rhythm 2017;14:520–6.

46. Grubb CS, Lewis M, Whang W, et al. Catheter ablation for atrial tachycardia in adults with congenital heart disease: electrophysiological predictors of acute procedural success and post-procedure atrial tachycardia recurrence. JACC Clin Electrophysiol 2019;5:438–47.

47. De Groot NMS, Atary JZ, Blom NA, et al. Long-term outcome after ablative therapy of postoperative atrial tachyarrhythmia in patients with congenital heart disease and characteristics of atrial tachyarrhythmia recurrences. Circ Arrhythmia Electrophysiol 2010;3:148–54.

48. Tanner H, Lukac P, Schwick N, et al. Irrigated-tip catheter ablation of intraatrial reentrant tachycardia in patients late after surgery of congenital heart disease. Heart Rhythm 2004;1:268–75.

49. Marazzato J, Cappabianca G, Angeli F, et al. Ablation of atrial tachycardia in the setting of prior mitral valve surgery. Minerva Cardiol Angiol 2021;69:94–101.

Atypical Cases of Typical Atrial Flutter? A Case Study

Roberto De Ponti, MD, FHRS[a,b,*], Jacopo Marazzato, MD[a,b], Fabio Angeli, MD[b,c], Manola Vilotta, EP Tech[a], Federico Blasi, MD[a,b], Giuseppe Bagliani, MD[d], Fabio M. Leonelli, MD[e], Raffaella Marazzi, MD[a]

KEYWORDS

- Typical atrial flutter • Atypical atrial flutter • Electroanatomic mapping • Catheter ablation
- Electrophysiologic study

KEY POINTS

- A longer cycle length or isoelectric lines between flutter waves can be associated with a different or more complex arrhythmogenic substrate.
- In patients with prior cardiac surgery, hidden pitfalls are present in apparently typical flutter cases.
- The coronary sinus os can be a source of arrhythmias mimicking typical atrial flutter.
- Electroanatomic mapping can be useful in particular cases to identify the reentry course and the ablation target.

INTRODUCTION

Over the years, techniques for typical atrial flutter ablation have been improved, so that ablation of cavotricuspid isthmus (CTI) is currently considered a well-established therapy for the treatment of these patients. In fact, the success rate after a single ablation procedure is reported to be as high as 91.7% and adverse events as low as 0.5%.[1] Nevertheless, difficulties that may be encountered during ablation of these arrhythmias should not be underestimated to avoid alterations of the safety and efficacy profile of this procedure. In some cases, the pitfalls can be anticipated by the presence of a variant of the electrocardiographic pattern, such as a longer cycle length, or by a specific context, such as prior cardiac surgery for a congenital or acquired heart disease. Therefore, these cases should be approached with a sufficient knowledge of the substrate and with all the necessary technologies. In the following paragraphs, a short series of 4 cases encountered during the last decade with a "supposed-to-be" typical atrial flutter with pitfalls during ablation is presented and discussed.

CASE 1
Case Presentation

In 2010, a male patient, aged 78 years, was electively admitted for ablation of a persistent atrial flutter after evaluation for palpitation in the outpatient clinic. He was affected by hypertension and

No funding sources to be acknowledged.

[a] Department of Heart and Vessels, Ospedale di Circolo, Viale Borri, 57, Varese 21100, Italy; [b] Department of Medicine and Surgery, University of Insubria, Viale Guicciardini, 9, Varese 21100, Italy; [c] Department of Medicine and Cardiopulmonary Rehabilitation, Maugeri Care and Research Institutes, IRCCS, Via Crotto Roncaccio, 16, Tradate, Varese 21049, Italy; [d] Cardiology and Arrhythmology Clinic, Marche Polytechnic University, University Hospital "Ospedali Riuniti Umberto I-Lancisi-Salesi", Via Conca 71, Ancona 60126, Italy; [e] Cardiology Department, James A. Haley Veterans' Hospital, University of South Florida, 13000 Bruce B Down Boulevard, Tampa, FL 33612, USA

* Corresponding author. Department of Heart and Vessels, Ospedale di Circolo and Macchi Foundation, University of Insubria-Varese, Viale Borri, 57, Varese 21100, Italy.
E-mail address: roberto.deponti@uninsubria.it

Card Electrophysiol Clin 14 (2022) 483–494
https://doi.org/10.1016/j.ccep.2022.03.004

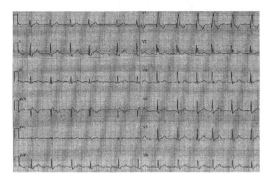

Fig. 1. Case 1. Twelve-lead ECG on hospital admission. ECG, electrocardiogram.

5 years before he underwent surgical revascularization for unstable angina with no complications. At transthoracic echocardiogram, only mild hypertrophy of the left ventricle was reported, whereas the other findings were unremarkable. On admission, the 12-lead electrocardiogram evidenced the persistence of the arrhythmia with right bundle branch block (**Fig. 1**). Although the morphology of the P wave was consistent with typical counterclockwise atrial flutter (negative in the inferior and left precordial leads and positive in V1), an isoelectric line was clearly present between the flutter waves with a longer cycle length of 290 ms. This may not be surprising in an elderly patient with ischemic heart disease, who in the previous months had received amiodarone and withdrawn short before hospital admission. Therefore, typical counterclockwise atrial flutter was considered the most suitable working hypothesis.

Electrophysiologic Procedure

After placing 2 decapolar catheters in the coronary sinus and cresta terminalis and a tetrapolar catheter in the His bundle area while the patient was on arrhythmia, it was clear that the intracavitary activation sequence was not consistent with the preprocedure diagnosis and electroanatomic mapping right atrium was commenced. As shown by the color-coded scale in **Fig. 2**A, the right atrium was activated centrifugally from the infero-medial region and the CTI showed an activation sequence from medial to lateral. Moreover, the right atrial activation lasted 175 ms corresponding to 60% of the tachycardia cycle length, which could be consistent with a focal form. However, as shown in **Fig. 2**B, the earliest activated area showed a wider extension and, although the earliest activated site preceded the reference signal in the proximal coronary sinus by 69 ms and a prepotential was evident, a steep negative intrinsecoid deflection was not present in the unipolar recording from the distal electrode of the mapping catheter. This was not consistent with a focal atrial tachycardia originating from this site

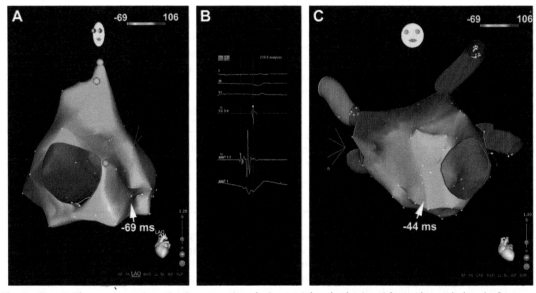

Fig. 2. Case 1. Electroanatomic activation mapping during atrial arrhythmia with a color-coded scale from red (early) to purple (late). In Panel A, electroanatomic mapping of the right atrium in left anterior oblique view showing a centrifugal propagation from the earliest site in the infero-medial region. Panel B shows tracings at the earliest activated site. From top to bottom: surface leads I, III, V1, reference signal in the coronary sinus (CS 3–4), bipolar signal from the mapping catheter (MAP 1–2) and unipolar signal from the distal electrode of the mapping catheter (MAP 1). In Panel C, electroanatomic mapping of the left atrium in antero-poster view. See text for further explanation. MAP, mapping catheter.

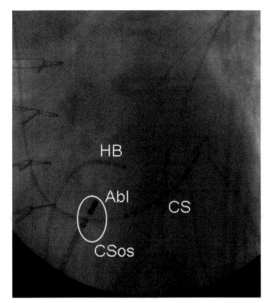

Fig. 3. Case 1. Catheter positioning during coronary sinus mapping in 30° left anterior oblique view. Abl, ablation catheter; CS, coronary sinus catheter; HB, His bundle catheter.

and suggested an origin from the medial left atrium. Therefore, after transseptal catheterization, the left atrium was mapped (**Fig. 2**C). Surprisingly, it was activated later than the right and the left earliest activated site preceded the reference signal only by 44 ms. Therefore, the catheter was pulled back in the right atrium for further mapping. As shown in **Fig. 3**, the coronary sinus os was markedly enlarged, and both the distal and proximal electrode pairs of the mapping catheter could be stably placed in its mouth. Here, as shown in **Fig. 4**A, low-amplitude, long-lasting, fragmented bipolar recordings spanning the whole atrial diastole between the P-waves was recorded by the mapping catheter. Entrainment attempts failed to capture the local electrograms. The activation

recorded in the 2 contiguous electrode pair spanned greater than 90% of the tachycardia cycle length and, hence, localized reentry was hypothesized. Irrigated-tip radiofrequency ablation at 35 W in this area, where diastolic potentials before the surface P-wave were recorded, abruptly prolonged the tachycardia cycle length, and interrupted the arrhythmia (**Fig. 4**B). Subsequently, no arrhythmia was inducted even by aggressive stimulation protocols. Therefore, conduction block of the CTI was considered pointless. The patient was discharged the day after with no antiarrhythmic drug therapy and remained arrhythmia free for the following 5 years, after which he was lost at follow-up.

Commentary

As stated more than 20 years ago,[2] the term flutter refers to a continuously waving pattern on the surface electrocardiogram with no isoelectric line in at least one lead regardless of the cycle length. It was also underlined that the presence or the absence of an isoelectric line between P-waves contributes little to the underlying mechanism. Accordingly, the presence of isoelectric line between the P-waves is considered an exclusion criterion in algorithms used for diagnosis of typical counterclockwise atrial flutter.[3] Based on this consideration, the diagnosis of typical atrial flutter should have been excluded since the first patient evaluation. However, enlarged right atrium, prior surgery, prior catheter ablation, elderly age, use of antiarrhythmic drugs can cause conduction delays resulting in isoelectric lines between P-waves in the inferior leads in typical counterclockwise atrial flutter, as shown in **Fig. 5** and in one of the following cases. The presence of an arrhythmogenic substrate close to the coronary sinus os generating an electrocardiographic pattern very similar to the one of the typical counterclockwise isthmus-dependent atrial flutter has been reported

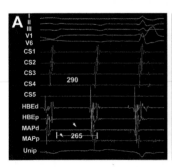
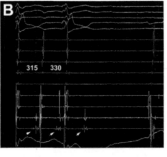

Fig. 4. Case 1. Tracings during coronary sinus mapping (A) and ablation (B). From top to bottom, tracings are displayed as follows: peripheral and precordial leads, coronary sinus bipolar recording (C1–C5) from distal to proximal, bipolar His bundle electrograms (HBEd and HBEp) from distal to proximal, bipolar recordings from the mapping/ablation catheter (MAPd and MAPp) from distal to proximal, and unipolar recordings from the distal electrode of the mapping catheter (Unip). Arrows indicate fragmented diastolic potentials. Notably, in B, radiofrequency energy application progressively and significantly prolongs the arrhythmia cycle length until conduction block is obtained distal to the late diastolic potentials, favoring the hypothesis of a localized reentry against a focal form. HBE, His-bundle catheter.

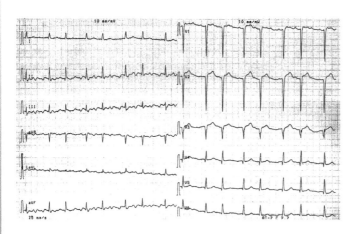

Fig. 5. Twelve-lead ECG showing atrial arrhythmia in an elderly patient with hypertensive cardiomyopathy on amiodarone therapy. The morphology of the P-waves is consistent with typical counterclockwise atrial flutter, but the cycle length is longer (280 ms) and isoelectric lines between P-waves are present. However, a counterclockwise CTI-dependent right atrial reentry was identified at electrophysiologic study and ablation permanently suppressed the arrhythmia.

as the cause of early recurrence after successful CTI ablation, both in patient with and without prior cardiac surgery.[4–6] In the area of the earliest activation, fragmented and long-lasting bipolar electrograms are recorded, which combined with a centrifugal pattern of the right atrial activation favors the hypothesis of a focal arrhythmia based on micro-reentry.[6] In our case, the fragmented bipolar electrogram spanning the whole diastole with a recorded electrical activity in the mouth of the coronary sinus for greater than 90% of the arrhythmia cycle length favors the hypothesis of a localized reentry, possible for an extremely slow conduction and an abnormally dilated coronary sinus os. Based on these experiences, the os and the proximal part of the coronary sinus should be carefully mapped, before considering a left atrial approach, as erroneously done in this case when detailed knowledge of these forms was poor. In this and similar cases, if the ablation procedure had been performed when the patient was on sinus rhythm and CTI block obtained during coronary sinus pacing, the clinical arrhythmia would have recurred postablation. This leads to plan the procedure when the patient is on arrhythmia, especially when surface electrocardiographic pattern does not completely match the one of typical atrial flutter and to perform accurate mapping in all these cases.

CASE 2
Case Presentation

In 2012, a male patient aged 61 years was referred for a persistent atrial arrhythmia detected at Holter monitoring. Six months earlier, he had undergone a surgical intervention for sinus venosus type of atrial septal defect with partial anomalous pulmonary venous return. The atrial septal defect was closed with a pericardial patch and the right superior pulmonary vein redirected to the left atrium. The postoperative course was uneventful until the arrhythmia was detected. At Holter monitoring, the arrhythmia was not easy to interpret because of the fast ventricular response, but in a rest 12-lead electrocardiogram (**Fig. 6**), P-waves consistent with a typical atrial flutter with a cycle of 240 could be observed when the atrioventricular conduction ratio was different from 2:1. Then, an electrophysiologic procedure was planned while the patient was on atrial flutter and oral anticoagulation.

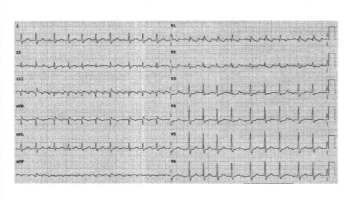

Fig. 6. Case 2. Twelve-lead ECG.

Electrophysiologic Procedure

After placing 2 decapolar catheters in the coronary sinus and cresta terminalis and a mapping/ablation catheter in the CTI, the activation sequence confirmed the presence of a counterclockwise peritricuspid loop in the right atrium (**Fig. 7**). To avoid the risk of arrhythmia modification, no entrainment maneuvers were attempted. Because the patient exhibited a postsurgical arrhythmia, electroanatomic mapping was commenced in the right atrium with a specific setting of the window of interest.[7] It seemed clear that the atrial anatomy was modified by previous surgery. Particularly, in the postero-lateral wall, 2 areas of double potentials were present, one superior and one inferior, separated by a 1.5 cm gap of single fragmented potentials. These 2 areas were likely to correspond to prior atriotomy for the right atrial cannula of the cardiopulmonary by-pass and for the access to the septum, respectively. When right atrial activation mapping was completed with greater than 95% of the activation sequence acquired, it was clear that 2 codominant loops were present in the right atrium: one, as expected, was counterclockwise around the tricuspid annulus (**Fig. 8**A) and the other was clockwise in the upper right atrium around the superior vena cava os (**Fig. 8**B). This pattern was different from the typical form of figure of 8 reentry where both loops share the same slow conduction isthmus. In this case, each loop was sustained by a critical slow conduction isthmus with diastolic activation, which was the CTI for the first loop and the gap between the areas of double potentials for the second. This justified a separate approach for each

loop, targeting the 2 separate diastolic pathways, as no other ablation strategy seemed appropriate. Therefore, the peritricuspid loop was targeted first and achievement of conduction block in this site by irrigated-tip radiofrequency ablation modified the intracavitary sequence of atrial activation with no change in the flutter cycle length, whereas the surface P-wave morphology was not discernible for the 2:1 atrioventricular conduction ratio (**Fig. 9**A). Positioning the ablation catheter in the second gap as shown in distal pole of the ablation catheter (ABLd) in **Fig. 9**A, a fragmented and long-lasting bipolar potential was recorded between P-waves in this site. After assessing that slow rate pacing at 10 mA did not result in phrenic capture, radiofrequency energy was delivered also in this area with early arrhythmia interruption (**Fig. 9**B). This second isthmus was finally blocked by further ablation, after the position of the sinus node was assessed in a more superior position. The patient was discharged with no antiarrhythmic drug the following day and the subsequent follow-up was uneventful.

Commentary

Intra-atrial reentrant tachycardias or flutters are frequently sustained by a double-loop reentry mechanism.[8] Using entrainment mapping, also typical atrial flutter has been reported to involve 2 loops around the tricuspid annulus and the inferior vena cava with a shared isthmus corresponding to the CTI.[9] Using electroanatomic mapping with a specific setting of the window of interest,[7] double loop reentry with a shared mid-diastolic isthmus has been observed frequently in atypical

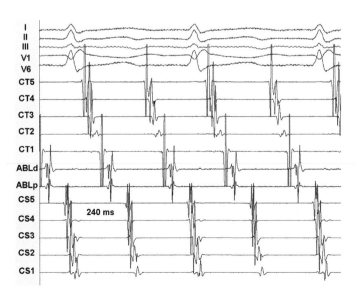

I
II
III
V1
V6
CT5
CT4
CT3
CT2
CT1
ABLd
ABLp
CS5
CS4
CS3
CS2
CS1

240 ms

Fig. 7. Case 2. Tracings during the clinical arrhythmia exhibiting a cycle length of 240 ms. From top to bottom, tracings are displayed as follows: peripheral and precordial leads, crista terminalis bipolar recordings (CT5-CT1 [cavo-tricuspid isthmus]) from proximal to distal, bipolar recordings from the mapping/ablation catheter positioned in the CTI (ABLd and ABLp) from distal to proximal, and coronary sinus bipolar recordings (C5-C1) from proximal to distal. Keeping the negative P-wave in the inferior leads as reference, the crista terminalis shows a cranio-caudal activation inscribed in the terminal part of the P-wave, followed by activation of the CTI and followed by the coronary sinus activation from proximal to distal just before the next P-wave. This intracavitary activation pattern is consistent with a peritricuspid counterclockwise loop.

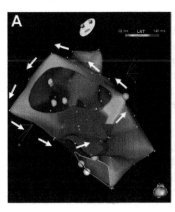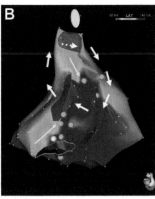

Fig. 8. Case 2. Right atrial electroanatomic mapping during the clinical arrhythmia in left oblique view (*A*) and postero-lateral view (*B*). The right atrial activation was fully reconstructed, and 2 loops are evident: one counterclockwise around the tricuspid annulus (*arrows* in *A*) and the second clockwise in the upper right atrium around the os of the superior vena cava (*arrows* in *B*). The red areas indicate the isthmus of mid-diastolic activation, the yellow arrows indicate the areas of double potentials (*blue dots*), and the orange dot indicates the His bundle area.

atrial flutters. Exceptionally, in atypical atrial flutter/tachycardias, 2 independent loops in the same atrial chamber have been observed after cardiac surgery,[10] as in the present case.

Interestingly, in this case, the upper loop did not grossly affect the P-wave morphology, probably because the atrial mass involved by this second loop was quite limited compared with the amount

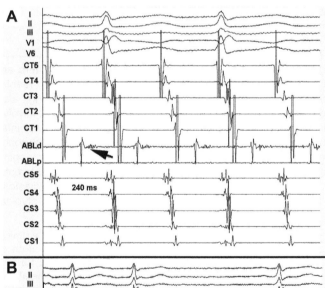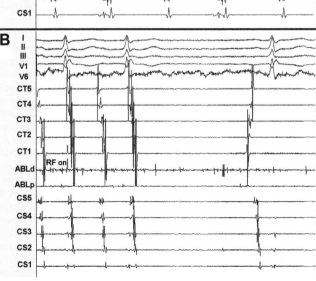

Fig. 9. Case 2. Tracings after ablation of the CTI (*A*) and during ablation of the second isthmus (*B*). Tracings are displayed as in **Fig. 7**. In A, the right atrial activation sequence has changed with an almost simultaneous activation of the crista terminalis and coronary sinus. Interestingly, a fragmented long-lasting potential (*arrow*) suggesting the presence of slow conduction is recorded between the P-waves in the critical isthmus of the second loop. In B, irrigated-tip radiofrequency ablation in this site early interrupted the arrhythmia and subsequently achieved conduction block (see text for further explanation).

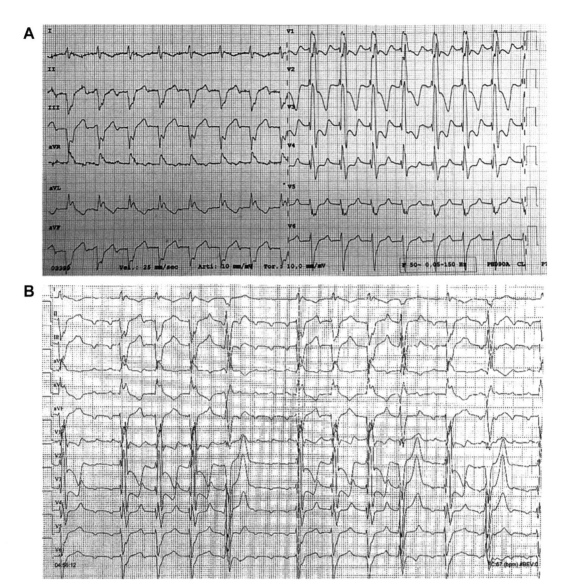

Fig. 10. Case 3. Twelve-lead electrocardiogram at hospital admission (*A*) and the day after (*B*).

of the right and left atrium activated by the peritricuspid loop. Moreover, although the upper loop had also a limited size, it was rendered possible by the slow conduction assessed by fragmented potentials found in the gap between the 2 areas of double potentials. Nevertheless, this second loop could have been the substrate for postablation recurrences if left untreated. Finally, this specific case underlines the importance of extensive mapping even in case of typical atrial flutter diagnosed on surface electrocardiogram, if the patient underwent prior cardiac surgery implying atriotomy. Electroanatomic mapping allows precise localization of sensitive structures, such as the sinus node area or the phrenic nerve.

CASE 3
Case Presentation

In 2019, a 52-year-old female patient presented at the Emergency Department with symptoms and signs of congestive heart failure. In 1973 and 1981, she had undergone surgical interventions for correction of tetralogy of Fallot with right ventricular infundibulectomy and positioning of a transannular pericardial patch, closure of the ventricular septal defect, and positioning of a biological pulmonary valve prosthesis. The intervention had implied also extensive right atrial atriotomy. On admission, the electrocardiogram showed a regular wide QRS complex tachycardia at 100 bpm with no visible P-waves (**Fig. 10**A), which

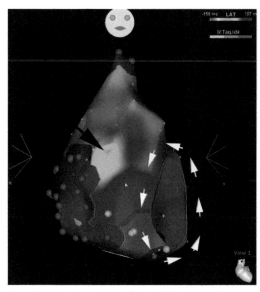

Fig. 11. Case 3. Electroanatomic activation mapping of the right atrium in antero-posterior projection during atrial flutter. Activation during the whole arrhythmia cycle length was reconstructed, and a single counterclockwise peritricuspid reentrant loop is evident (*white arrows*). Notably, an area of earlier activation not consistent with the reentrant loop is observed in the antero-lateral position at 11 o'clock of the tricuspid annulus (*black arrow*). Gray areas identify scar tissue with no electrical activity, blue dot double potential, and pink dots fragmented potentials.

was correctly diagnosed as supraventricular tachycardia for the presence of complete right bundle branch block and anterior hemiblock in sinus rhythm in previous tracings. The patient was then admitted to the Cardiology Department and pharmacologic therapy for heart failure administered. A transthoracic echocardiogram showed a severely depressed left ventricular function with ejection fraction of 30% associated with right ventricular dysfunction associated with initial degeneration of the prosthetic pulmonary valve. Early after admission, improvement of the general conditions was observed, and the electrocardiographic monitoring showed a persistent atrial

arrhythmia with a P-wave morphology consistent with typical atrial flutter but a longer cycle length of 350 ms, with variable atrioventricular conduction ratio (**Fig. 10**B). The arrhythmia persisted for the following days, and electrophysiologic procedure was deemed necessary for arrhythmia ablation and sinus rhythm restoration.

Electrophysiologic Procedure

After insertion of a decapolar catheter in the coronary sinus, used as reference, electroanatomic mapping of the arrhythmia was performed in the right atrium. At first sight, mapping highlighted

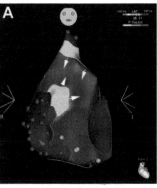
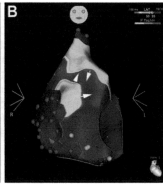

Fig. 12. Case 3. Two subsequent frames of the propagation map of the arrhythmia shown in the previous figure. Two independent and colliding wavefronts, one generated from the peritricuspid loop and the other from the site of origin of the focal atrial tachycardia, are evident. White arrows indicate the direction of the wavefronts. Dots as in the previous figure. See text for further explanation.

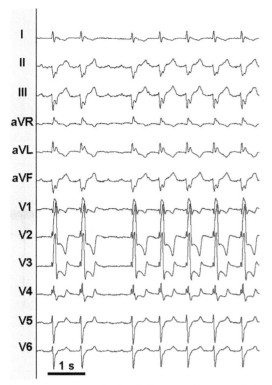

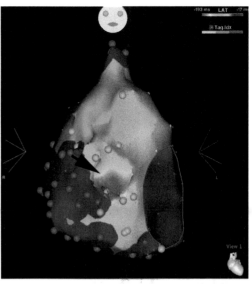

Fig. 14. Case 3. Electroanatomic activation map of the tachycardia shown in the previous figure. The red color identifies the area of early activation (black arrow in the figure), already evident during atrial flutter. The orange dot identifies the earliest activated area and the red dot the site of successful ablation. Other dots as in **Fig. 11**.

Fig. 13. Case 3. Twelve-lead electrocardiogram of the tachycardia appeared after CTI block by ablation. Positive P-waves in the inferior leads and negative in V1 are evident and consistent with the site of origin of the focal atrial tachycardia. The tachycardia cycle length is 360 ms.

the presence of a large area with no electric signal in the postero-lateral region. Spotty areas of scar tissue were also observed in the CTI. After reconstruction of the entire course of the reentry, it was clear that the arrhythmia was sustained by a single counterclockwise reentry around the tricuspid annulus with slow conduction in the CTI for the presence of scar tissue (**Fig. 11**). Interestingly, a relatively early activated area was observed at 11 o'clock of the tricuspid annulus very close to the border of the scar tissue. According to the color-coded scale, the activation of this area was not consistent with the peritricuspid loop and produced a second wavefront of activation, spreading from the border of the scar tissue anteriorly anticipating the propagation from the peritricuspid loop (**Fig. 12**). Peritricuspid loop (**Fig. 12**), thus potentially representing the presence of a second arrhythmia, partially suppressed but the dominant flutter. Therefore, the CTI was targeted first, and when conduction block was achieved in this site, a second arrhythmia appeared with a similar cycle length (**Fig. 13**). The right atrium was then

remapped, and now the electroanatomic map (**Fig. 14**) showed a centrifugal activation from the area of earliest activation located where the region of earlier activation during flutter was identified. The presence of no residual conduction in the CTI and the fact that right atrial activation spanned only roughly 50% of the tachycardia cycle length confirmed the presence of a different arrhythmia of focal origin. Further ablation in this site suppressed the tachycardia and its inducibility by pacing maneuvers. The patients then remained in sinus rhythm and in the following months were referred to surgeons for further evaluation.

Commentary

In addition to macro-reentrant atrial tachycardias or flutters, focal atrial tachycardia can be found in patient with prior cardiac surgery for congenital heart disease, valvuloplasty, or valve replacement, or, eventually, for other acquired heart diseases. In this population, although most of the arrhythmias are macro-reentrant, a focal mechanism can account for 7% to 18% of the arrhythmia morphologies encountered, according to different patient series.[11–15] The site of origin of focal tachycardias can be the same found in the nonsurgical population,[13] but in some cases, as the one presented, can be very close to large areas of scar, where very low-amplitude potentials are found and

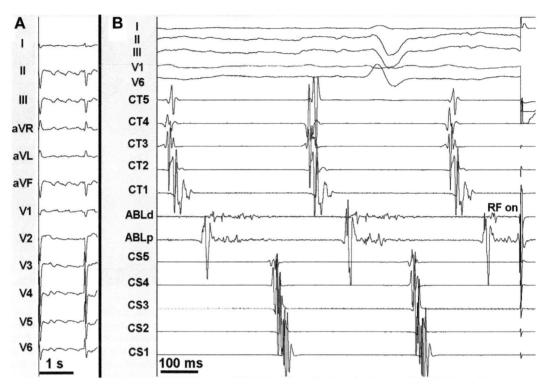

Fig. 15. Case 4. Twelve-lead electrocardiogram (*A*) and intracavitary signals (*B*) of a typical atrial flutter with a longer cycle length. In B, tracings are displayed as in **Fig. 7**. RF on identifies when radiofrequency energy delivery is initiated. See text for further explanation.

micro-reentry can be the putative mechanism. The peculiarity of this case resides in the fact that the focal arrhythmia coexisted with typical counterclockwise atrial flutter as clearly identified by electroanatomic propagation mapping. This was possible only because both arrhythmias had a similar cycle length, as the peritricuspid reentry was delayed by scar tissue in the CTI. Interestingly, the ventricular rate in the first arrhythmia observed (see **Fig. 10**A) does not exactly match any of the possible atrioventricular conduction ratio during the atrial flutter with a cycle length of 350 ms, subsequently observed. Because reentrant arrhythmias usually exhibit a stable cycle length opposite to focal ones, it seems reasonable to hypothesize that the first arrhythmia in **Fig. 10**A could have been the focal atrial tachycardia found during electrophysiology procedure and that the two arrhythmias alternate in this patient.

CASE 4
Case Presentation

In 2020, a 78-year-old male patient on flecainide for paroxysmal atrial fibrillation presented with typical atrial flutter with a longer cycle length (**Fig. 15**A). In the past, the patient had undergone DDDR pacemaker implantation for bradycardia-

tachycardia syndrome. Transthoracic echocardiogram showed only mild left ventricular hypertrophy consistent with hypertension. An ablation procedure was then proposed, and the patient gave informed consent only for right atrial ablation.

Electrophysiologic Procedure

After placing 2 decapolar catheters in the coronary sinus and cresta terminalis and a mapping/ablation catheter in the CTI, the activation sequence confirmed the presence of a counterclockwise peritricuspid loop in the right atrium with a cycle length of 350 ms (**Fig. 15**B). Because both the surface P-wave morphology and the intracavitary activation sequence were consistent with an isthmus-dependent loop entrainment, maneuvers were avoided for the risk of arrhythmia modification and concomitant antiarrhythmic drug therapy. Instead, a detailed mapping of the CTI was performed to search for an area of conduction delay. In the medial region of the CTI, at the os of the coronary sinus, low-amplitude and fragmented bipolar signals were recorded with a duration of 100 ms (see **Fig. 15**B). Radiofrequency energy ablation in this area from the tricuspid annulus to the os of the inferior vena cava, early terminated the arrhythmia and blocked conduction over the

CTI with the disappearance of the delayed potential. The patient was discharged the day after with an uneventful follow-up on flecainide.

Commentary

High-resolution mapping has recently demonstrated that in general in isthmus-dependent right atrial arrhythmias conduction velocity at the CTI is not slower than in other regions of the right atrium, showing values consistent with normal conduction velocity (>100 cm/s).[16,17] However, in some cases, there could be a conduction slowing especially in the medial CTI.[17] In addition, the proximal coronary sinus is involved in the reentry circuit in a substantial subset of patients with typical atrial flutter[18] and, when slow conduction is present in this area, it could represent the substrate for other reentrant arrhythmias if left untreated after typical atrial flutter ablation at the central isthmus.[18,19] Therefore, although it seems reasonable to target the maximum voltage in the CTI in typical atrial flutter in the general population,[20] it could be appropriate to consider for ablation also slow conduction areas around the coronary sinus, especially in cases with a longer flutter cycle length as the one herein presented.

SUMMARY

Ablation of typical atrial flutter is considered an easy procedure with a high safety and efficacy profile, but hidden pitfalls may be encountered, which may alter this profile. A careful preprocedure clinical evaluation may reveal variants of the morphologies of typical atrial flutter, which may suggest a different arrhythmogenic substrate from the CTI. Similarly, prior surgery may have consistently modified the atrial substrate, which, according to the complexity of the case, may sustain multiple arrhythmias, in term of both reentrant circuits and arrhythmia mechanism. Finally, slow conduction in the region of the coronary sinus os even in regular cases may represent a problem. In fact, if not directly involved in the typical atrial flutter circuit and therefore not ablated, it can sustain other arrhythmias during the follow-up, which may mimic typical atrial flutter recurrences.

CLINICS CARE POINTS

- Evaluate carefully typical atrial flutters with longer cycle length and/or isoelectric lines between flutter waves

- Consider routine use of electroanatomic mapping in postsurgical patients with typical atrial flutter
- Be prepared to face multiple arrhythmias in patients with complex heart diseases
- Identify the presence of slow conduction around the coronary sinus os because it can be a potential source of recurrent postablation arrhythmias

CONFLICTS OF INTEREST DISCLOSURE

Dr R. De Ponti has received fees for lectures and scientific cooperation from Biosense Webster.

REFERENCES

1. Spector P, Reynolds MR, Calkins H, et al. Meta-analysis of ablation of atrial flutter and supraventricular tachycardia. Am J Cardiol 2009;104:671–7.
2. Saoudi N, Cosio F, Waldo A, et al. Classification of atrial flutter and regular atrial tachycardia according to electrophysiologic mechanism and anatomic bases: a statement from a joint expert group from the Working Group of Arrhythmias of the European Society of Cardiology and the North American Society of Pacing and Electrophysiology. J Cardiovasc Electrophysiol 2001;12:852–66.
3. Frisch DR, Frankel E, Gill D, et al. Algorithm for cavotricuspid isthmus flutter on surface ECGs: the ACTIONS study. Open Heart 2021;8:e001431.
4. Yoshida N, Yamada T. Pseudo typical atrial flutter occurring after cavotricuspid isthmus ablation in a patient with a prior history of Senning operation. Heart Rhythm Case Rep 2015;1:54–7.
5. Itoh T, Yoshida Y, Morishima I, et al. Focal intracavotricuspid isthmus atrial tachycardias occurring after typical atrial flutter ablation: incidence and electrocardiographic and electrophysiological characteristics. J Interv Card Electrophysiol 2018;52: 237–45.
6. Muresan L, Le Bouar R, Schiau S, et al. What is the mechanism of this post ablation atrial flutter "recurrence. J Electrocardiol 2020;60:110–3.
7. De Ponti R, Verlato R, Bertaglia E, et al. Treatment of macro-re-entrant atrial tachycardia based on electroanatomic mapping: identification and ablation of the mid-diastolic isthmus. Europace 2007;9:449–57.
8. Shah D, Jaïs P, Takahashi A, et al. Dual-loop intra-atrial reentry in humans. Circulation 2000;101:631–9.
9. Fujiki A, Nishida K, Sakabe M, et al. Entrainment mapping of dual-loop macroreentry in common atrial flutter: new insights into the atrial flutter circuit. J Cardiovasc Electrophysiol 2004;15:679–85.
10. De Ponti R. A non-clinical macroreentrant right atrial tachycardia with two independent loops: the

exception to the rule of a shared mid-diastolic isthmus in doble-loop reentry. In: From signals to colours: a case-based atlas of electroanatomic mapping in complex atrial arrhythmias. Milan: Springer-Verlag; 2008. p. 151–6.

11. de Groot NM, Zeppenfeld K, Wijffels MC, et al. Ablation of focal atrial arrhythmia in patients wlth congenital heart defects after surgery: role of circumscribed areas with heterogeneous conduction. Heart Rhythm 2006;3:526–35.

12. Pap R, Kohári M, Makai A, et al. Surgical technique and the mechanism of atrial tachycardia late after open heart surgery. J Interv Card Electrophysiol 2012;35:127–35.

13. Kohári M, Pap R. Atrial tachycardias occurring late after open heart surgery. Curr Cardiol Rev 2015; 11:134–40.

14. Moore JP, Gallotti RG, Chiriac A, et al. Catheter ablation of supraventricular tachycardia after tricuspid valve surgery in patients with congenital heart disease: a multicenter comparative study. Heart Rhythm 2020;17:58–65.

15. Marazzato J, Cappabianca G, Angeli F, et al. Ablation of atrial tachycardia in the setting of prior mitral valve surgery. Minerva Cardiol Angiol 2021;69: 94–101.

16. Sau A, Sikkel MB, Luther V, et al. The sawtooth EKG pattern of typical atrial flutter is not related to slow conduction velocity at the cavotricuspid isthmus. J Cardiovasc Electrophysiol 2017;28:1445–53.

17. Pathik B, Lee G, Sacher F, et al. New Insights into an old arrhythmia: high-resolution mapping demonstrates conduction and substrate variability in right atrial macro-re-entrant tachycardia. JACC Clin Electrophysiol 2017;3:971–86.

18. De Sisti A, Andronache M, Damiano P, et al. Is proximal coronary sinus involved in the circuit in some cases of ECG "typical" atrial flutter? J Cardiovasc Electrophysiol 2018;29:1508-1514.

19. Yang Y, Varma N, Badhwar N, et al. Prospective observations in the clinical and electrophysiological characteristics of intra-isthmus reentry. J Cardiovasc Electrophysiol 2010;21:1099–106.

20. Gula LJ, Redfearn DP, Veenhuyzen GD, et al. Reduction in atrial flutter ablation time by targeting maximum voltage: results of a prospective randomized clinical trial. J Cardiovasc Electrophysiol 2009; 20:1108–12.

Atrial Flutter in Pediatric Patients

Fabrizio Drago, MD, FAIAC*, Pietro Paolo Tamborrino, MD

KEYWORDS

- Atrial flutter • Children • Treatment

KEY POINTS

- Atrial flutter (AFL) in pediatric patients is a rare condition as the physical dimensions of the immature heart are inadequate to support the arrhythmia.
- Even in children, the analysis of the surface electrocardiogram (ECG) allows us to make the diagnosis of AFL which in the typical form.
- AFL represents about 10% to 30% of fetal tachycardias.
- Beyond the neonatal period, AFL primarily occurs in the presence of CHD, in patients with accessory AV pathways, myocarditis, and with various types of cardiomyopathies.
- In children and adolescents, depending on clinical presentation and efficacy of antiarrhythmic medication, electrophysiological study (EPS) and catheter ablation is the treatment of choice allowing for substrate-specific treatment of AFL.

INTRODUCTION

Atrial flutter (AFL) in pediatric patients is a rare condition as the physical dimensions of the immature heart are inadequate to support the arrhythmia. This low incidence makes it difficult for patients in this particular setting to be studied.

Atrial flutter accounts for 30% of fetal tachyarrhythmias, 11% to 18% of neonatal tachyarrhythmias, and 8% of supraventricular tachyarrhythmias in children older than 1 year of age.

The substrate for this tachyarrhythmia consists of a macro-reentrant circuit around fixed or functional barriers with areas of relatively slow conduction and unidirectional block. This circuit is confined principally to the right atrium.

In details, activation moves from the region of the sinus node, along the right anterior free wall toward the atrio-ventricular (AV) rings whereby the delayed conduction, in the region of Koch's triangle or in the cavo-tricuspid isthmus (CTI), allows a subsequent caudo-cranial activation through the inter-atrial septum to complete the circuit.

In a sentinel study from 1985 on AFL in the young, with limited diagnostic methods available at that time, less than 10% of the patients had an "otherwise" normal heart ("lone AFL").[1]

ELECTROCARDIOGRAM FEATURES

Even in children, the analysis of the surface electrocardiogram (ECG) allows us to make the diagnosis of AFL which in the typical form is characterized by a sawtooth pattern in inferior leads which replaces normal P-waves.

The wave front may rotate around the above-mentioned circuit with a counterclockwise (typical common AFL) or clockwise rotation (uncommon AFL).

The cycle length is usually between 190 and 300 msec with QRS complexes normal and mathematically related to the flutter waves. The normal conduction pattern is 2:1 or 3:1, occasionally 1:1 conduction may occur especially in the small children, because the normal AV node imposes much less conduction delay than in adult patients. In this case, when the ventricular response rate is rapid,

Paediatric Cardiology and Cardiac Arrhythmias Complex Unit, Department of Paediatric Cardiology and Cardiac Surgery, Bambino Gesù Children's Hospital and Research Institute, Piazza S. Onofrio 4, Rome 00165, Italy
* Corresponding author.
E-mail address: fabrizio.drago@opbg.net

Card Electrophysiol Clin 14 (2022) 495–500
https://doi.org/10.1016/j.ccep.2022.05.005

ECG can show a wide QRS with bundle branch block.

The definition of atypical AFL includes a broad spectrum of other macro-reentrant tachycardia for which the wave front does not travel around the tricuspid annulus and can occur especially in children with congenital heart disease (CHD). The mean cycle length is usually from 170 to 250 msec.

ATRIAL FLUTTER IN THE FETAL AND PERINATAL PERIOD

AFL represents about 10% to 30% of fetal tachycardias.[2]

Fetal AFL generally occurs in the third trimester probably in relation to the atrial size which is large and highly vulnerable to atrial extrasystoles.

This fetal tachyarrhythmia may be associated with an accessory AV pathway (in about 25% of the cases), myocarditis, positive SSA/SSB autoantibody, or CHD such as Ebstein anomaly.

Moreover, fetuses and neonates with AFL are more likely to be macrosomic or to be born to diabetic mothers than the general population.[3]

Fetal AFL can cause hydrops fetalis or heart failure especially if AV nodal conduction is fast and 1:1 AV conduction occurs with a ventricular rate of more than 300 bpm which inevitably leads to circulatory compromise. Without treatment, hydrops is found in 7% to 43% of fetuses with AFL.[4]

Fetal hydrops is the most important prognostic factor in terms of mortality.[5,6] Consequently, in case of hydrops, elective preterm delivery and other life-saving interventions are often attempted.

Generally, the treatment goal is to suppress the arrhythmia or to slow down the ventricular rate.

For fetuses with no signs of fetal hydrops, maternal digoxin is a routinely used therapy. Unfortunately, digoxin alone is not so effective in fetuses with hydrops due to poor trans-placental transfer. In these cases, flecainide, sotalol, or amiodarone can be used, though flecainide should not be used alone because it does not decrease AV nodal conduction.

Considering that no single agent is universally effective, it is important to administer the most effective drug at the lowest effective dose to avoid the risk of maternal and fetal morbidity.

In a recent multicenter prospective study, transplacental treatment with digoxin alone showed a resolution rate of 59% and an overall resolution rate of 93% in 28 patients with fetal AFL.[7]

In neonates, AFL mostly occurs within the first 2 days after birth. Sex distribution is known to be equal.

The ECG appearance is similar to that seen in the adult, with continuous regular atrial sawtooth waves, which are best seen in leads II, III, and aVF, suggesting either clockwise or counterclockwise rotation around the tricuspid annulus. The atrial rate ranges from 400 to 700 bpm and AV conduction is generally 2:1 with ventricular rates ranging between 150 and 250 bpm but, as mentioned above, 1:1 conduction can occur. Normal or near-normal ventricular rates are observed in AFL with slower 3:1 or 4:1 AV conduction.[8–10]

Despite the often high atrial and ventricular rates, AFL is generally tolerated and heart failure or death is rare. In neonates with good hemodynamic tolerance, treatment can be postponed, as almost always the arrhythmia spontaneously ends within 24 to 48h.

In case of poor hemodynamic tolerance of the neonate affected, synchronized electrical cardioversion (2 J/kg) is the most straightforward treatment to establish sinus rhythm with a success rate of about 85% to 90%. Transesophageal overdrive pacing, instead, has a lower success rate (60%–70%), probably because the atrial cycle is too short to be penetrated by the overdrive pacing. In a stable hemodynamic condition, pharmacologic treatment may be initiated. The recommended drugs are digoxin which can decrease the ventricular rate until the spontaneous interruption of the AFL. Digoxin can be combined with flecainide or amiodarone in case of failure.

During infancy, AFL cycle lengths can range from 125 to 200 ms with 2:1 or 3:1 conduction (heart rates between 150 and 300 bpm). These patients are often asymptomatic but may present with tachypnea, poor feeding, and diaphoresis. The development of symptoms does not correlate with rapid atrial or ventricular rates or conduction ratio, but appears to be related to the duration of the tachycardia.[11] In an infant with AFL and a structurally normal heart, once sinus rhythm is achieved, recurrences are unlikely to occur in the absence of concomitant arrhythmias, and long-term prophylactic antiarrhythmic drug therapy is unnecessary as recurrences are very rare.[8–10]

ATRIAL FLUTTER IN CHILDREN AND ADOLESCENTS

Beyond the neonatal period, AFL primarily occurs in the presence of CHD,[1,8,12] in patients with accessory AV pathways,[9] myocarditis,[5,10] and with various types of cardiomyopathies[13] (see case report later in discussion).

In a very recent study about 8 children who underwent transcatheter ablation of the CTI for an apparently lone AFL, the endomyocardial biopsy (EMB), was performed in 6 patients showing myocarditis in 2 and minor fibro-fatty changes, consistent with an early state of arrhythmogenic right ventricular cardiomyopathy, in another one. One patient with recurrent AFL had a negative EMB but Brugada syndrome was diagnosed during further follow-up confirming the possibility that a channelopathy can be the cause of an apparently idiopathic AFL at any age.[14] Consequently, detailed noninvasive and invasive diagnostic work-up including EMB is recommended in young patients with presumed "lone AFL" allowing disease-specific treatment. The role of cardiac magnetic resonance and genetic testing in this setting remained undetermined but its use can be recommended to obtain relevant data in the future.

In older children, AFL cycle lengths range from 125 to 300 ms (atrial rates 200–450 bpm). In these patients, the arrhythmia can be asymptomatic particularly if AV conduction ratios preclude an elevated ventricular rate. However, symptomatic patients can have palpitations, shortness of breath, and asthenia.

Once again, the diagnosis can be made from the surface ECG, which most frequently demonstrates 2:1 or variable AV conduction. If the classic AFL pattern is difficult to discern, as for other pediatric age groups, adenosine administration can help by inducing AV block to unmask classic "flutter" P waves. Moreover, transesophageal atrial recordings can also aid in delineating the P-QRS relationship.

Conversion to sinus rhythm could be spontaneous or by the intervention of direct current cardioversion, transesophageal pacing, and/or antiarrhythmic drugs. Although conversion to sinus rhythm by antiarrhythmic drugs has been observed, available studies concluded that synchronized electrical cardioversion was the most straightforward procedure to rapidly establish sinus rhythm with a response rate of 87%. Patients with hemodynamically unstable AFL should undergo immediate direct current cardioversion.

In children and adolescents, depending on clinical presentation and efficacy of antiarrhythmic medication, electrophysiological study (EPS) and catheter ablation is the treatment of choice allowing for substrate-specific treatment of AFL.[15] As reported in the guidelines,[16] ablation is recommended for complex supraventricular tachycardia, recurrent or persistent, associated with ventricular dysfunction or when medical therapy is either not effective or is associated with intolerable adverse effects or in case the family wishes to avoid chronic antiarrhythmic medications.

The success rate of radiofrequency catheter ablation is near 90%, as reported for adults, and it is similar between patients with and without CHD.

ATRIAL FLUTTER AFTER SURGICAL REPAIRS OF CHILDREN WITH CONGENITAL HEART DISEASE

Atrial arrhythmias represent a major source of long-term morbidity and are a significant contributor to mortality after CHD repairs.

AFL or intra-atrial reentry-tachycardia (IART) can be firstly observed or in the immediate postsurgical period or months or years after cardiac surgery for CHD, especially in patients younger than 4 years of age. The development of the AFL/IART is associated with several variables including the complexity of CHD, number of surgical procedures, hemodynamic status, and the time after cardiac surgery. Moreover, the reentry can be more frequently observed around surgical scars. Precipitating factors for the development of AFL are the presence of prosthetic material and electro-pathological alterations of the atrial architecture.

This arrhythmia may develop in patients with ventricular septal defect, as a result of atrial enlargement, but it is most often observed after repair or palliation of complex CHD.

In Fontan circulation, risk factors related to the development of AFL and IART are: right atrial enlargement, elevated atrial pressure, dispersion of atrial refractoriness, sinus node dysfunction, cardiac surgery at older age, elevated pulmonary pressure, low oxygen saturation, preoperative arrhythmias, a longer time after cardiac surgery, long sutures lines or scar tissue.[17,18]

In patients with the transposition of the great arteries, the arterial switch operation (Jatene procedure) is associated with a lower incidence of atrial tachyarrhythmias (about 5%) in comparison to Mustard or Senning procedures,[19] because it does not require an atrial septectomy and, consequently, atrial sutures.

After a surgical repair for tetralogy of Fallot, performed through a trans-atrial approach, atrial tachyarrhythmias could be observed. Their incidence is associated with pulmonary regurgitation, atrial volume overload, and older age at the time of surgical correction.[20]

In patients with an atrial septal defect (ASD), early surgery may prevent the development of AFL because it is associated in particular with the presence and severity of pulmonary hypertension causing right atrial stretch for the right-sided volume overload[21] (see case report later in discussion).

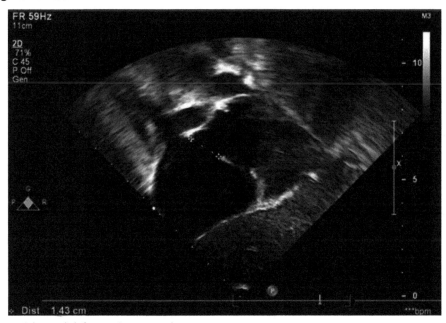

Fig. 1. The atrial septal defect ostium secundum type.

In a large series of patient with CHD, CTI-dependent AFL was the most common arrhythmia, while in non–CTI-dependent AFL become progressively more common with the more extensive atrial incision. Moreover, in patients operated on for CHD, the reentrant circuits were highly variable because of individual differences in original anatomy and surgical modifications.[22]

CASE REPORT

In a one-year-old child, a first-degree AV block, junctional premature complexes, and idioventricular escape rhythm were detected during a routine ECG. For this reason, the child underwent a 24-h ECG Holter monitoring and an echocardiogram.

Sinus node dysfunction and an atrial septal defect (ASD, ostium secundum type), associated with a moderate bi-atrial enlargement (particularly the right atrial) in absence of ventricular dysfunction, were diagnosed (**Fig. 1**).

After 1 year a CTI-dependent AFL with a mean ventricular rate of 180 bpm with 2:1 AV occurred (**Fig. 2**) and was successfully treated by transesophageal pacing. Then an oral treatment with sotalol was started.

As Sotalol was only partially effective, the child underwent radiofrequency transcatheter ablation (RFTA) of CTI. The procedure was acutely effective, but at its end, the ECG showed a Brugada pattern (**Fig. 3**). Two days after the RFTA, AFL recurred and the child underwent surgical correction of ASD, epicardial dual-chamber pace-maker implantation (DDD), and surgical ablation of CTI.

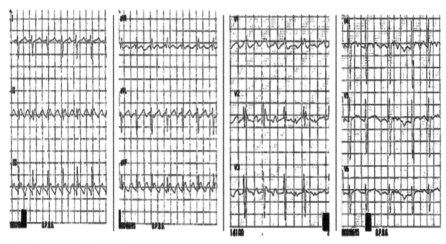

Fig. 2. AFL with a 2:1 AV conduction.

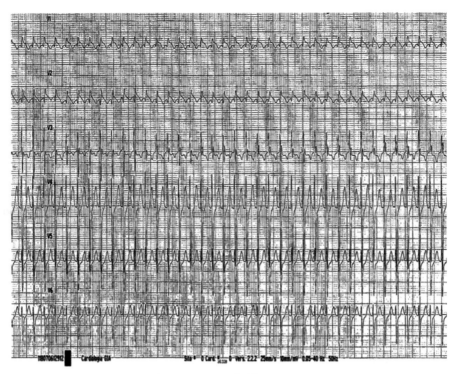

Fig. 3. AFL with a 2:1 AV conduction and pattern Brugada-like.

In the first 2 months after the procedure, the patient experienced 2 episodes of AFL/IART treated with antitachycardia pacing. So that, a therapy with hydroquinidine and propranolol was started.

Subsequently, due to the detection of various episodes of AFL/IART and junctional tachycardia on the Holter monitoring and remote monitoring system, Nadolol was started and successfully replaced propranolol.

Genetic testing showed c.1202 G > A mutation in the gene TBX5 associated with Holt-Oram syndrome and c.2441 G > A mutation in the gene SCN5A.

CLINICS CARE POINTS

- Atrial flutter in neonates can disappear in the first 2 days of life. Therefore, if it is not hemodinamically relevant, it may not be treated.

- The occurrence of atrial flutter during infancy can indicate the presence of a channellopaty.

- The occurrence of atrial flutter in children and adolescents is generally due to the presence of structural heart diseases.

- Complex congenital heart disease can experience atrial flutter during post-operative follow-up.

DISCLOSURE

The authors have nothing to disclose.

REFERENCES

1. Garson A, Bink-Boelkens M, Hesslein PS, et al. Atrial flutter in the young: a collaborative study of 380 cases. J Am Coll Cardiol 1985;6(4):871–8.
2. Frohn-Mulder IM, Stewart PA, Witsenburg M, et al. The efficacy of flecainide versus digoxin in the management of fetal supraventricular tachycardia. Prenat Diagn 1995;15(13):1297–302.
3. Pike JI, Krishnan A, Kaltman J, et al. Fetal and neonatal atrial arrhythmias: an association with maternal diabetes and neonatal macrosomia. Prenat Diagn 2013;33(12):1152–7.
4. Krapp M, Kohl T, Simpson JM, et al. Review of diagnosis, treatment, and outcome of fetal atrial flutter compared with supraventricular tachycardia. Heart 2003;89(8):913–7.
5. Skinner JR, Sharland G. Detection and management of life threatening arrhythmias in the perinatal period. Early Hum Dev 2008;84(3):161–72.
6. Oudijk MA, Visser GHA, Meijboom EJ. Fetal tachyarrhythmia - Part II: treatment. Indian Pacing Electrophysiol J 2004;4(4):185–94.
7. Miyoshi T, Maeno Y, Hamasaki T, et al. Antenatal therapy for fetal supraventricular tachyarrhythmias: multicenter trial. J Am Coll Cardiol 2019;74(7):874–85.

8. Texter KM, Kertesz NJ, Friedman RA, et al. Atrial flutter in infants. J Am Coll Cardiol 2006;48(5):1040–6.

9. Casey FA, McCrindle BW, Hamilton RM, et al. Neonatal atrial flutter: significant early morbidity and excellent long-term prognosis. Am Heart J 1997;133(3):302–6.

10. Mendelsohn A, Dick M, Serwer GA. Natural history of isolated atrial flutter in infancy. J Pediatr 1991;119(3):386–91.

11. Martin TC, Hernandez A. Atrial flutter in infancy. J Pediatr 1982;100(2):239–42.

12. Brugada J, Blom N, Sarquella-Brugada G, et al. Pharmacological and non-pharmacological therapy for arrhythmias in the pediatric population: EHRA and AEPC-Arrhythmia Working Group joint consensus statement. Europace 2013;15(9):1337–82.

13. Jaeggi ET, Carvalho JS, De Groot E, et al. Comparison of transplacental treatment of fetal supraventricular tachyarrhythmias with digoxin, flecainide, and sotalol: results of a nonrandomized multicenter study. Circulation 2011;124(16):1747–54.

14. Dieks JK, Backhoff D, Schneider HE, et al. Lone atrial flutter in children and adolescents: is it really "lone". Pediatr Cardiol 2021;42(2):361–9.

15. Roberts JD, Hsu JC, Aouizerat BE, et al. Impact of a 4q25 genetic variant in atrial flutter and on the risk of atrial fibrillation after cavotricuspid isthmus ablation. J Cardiovasc Electrophysiol 2014;25(3):271–7.

16. Philip Saul J, Kanter RJ, Abrams D, et al. PACES/HRS expert consensus statement on the use of catheter ablation in children and patients with congenital heart disease: developed in partnership with the pediatric and congenital Electrophysiology Society (PACES) and the Heart Rhythm Society (HRS) Endorsed by the governing bodies of PACES, HRS, the American Academy of Pediatrics (AAP), the American Heart Association (AHA), and the Association for European Pediatric and Congenital Cardiology (AEPC). Hear Rhythm 2016;13(6):e251–89.

17. Driscoll DJ, Offord KP, Feldt RH, et al. Five- to fifteen-year follow-up after Fontan operation. Circulation 1992;85(2):469–96.

18. Balaji S, Johnson TB, Sade RM, et al. Management of atrial flutter after the Fontan procedure. J Am Coll Cardiol 1994;23(5):1209–15.

19. Van Hare GF, Lesh MD, Ross BA, et al. Mapping and radiofrequency ablation of intraatrial reentrant tachycardia after the Senning or Mustard procedure for transposition ofthe great arteries. Am J Cardiol 1996;77(11):985 91.

20. Folino AF, Daliento L. Arrhythmias after tetralogy of fallot repair. Indian Pacing Electrophysiol J 2005;5(4):312–24.

21. Gatzoulis MA, Freeman MA, Siu SC, et al. Atrial arrhythmia after surgical closure of atrial septal defects in adults. N Engl J Med 1999;340(11):839–46.

22. Anguera I, Dallaglio P, Macías R, et al. Long-term outcome after ablation of right atrial tachyarrhythmias after the surgical repair of congenital and Acquired heart disease. Am J Cardiol 2015;115(12):1705–13.

Atrial Flutters in Adults with Congenital Heart Disease

Alessandro Capestro, MD[a],*, Elli Soura, MD[a], Paolo Compagnucci, MD[b,c],
Michela Casella, MD, PhD[b,d], Raffaella Marzullo, MD[e],
Antonio Dello Russo, MD, PhD[b,c]

KEYWORDS

- Macroreentrant atrial tachycardia • Atrial flutter • Congenital heart disease

KEY POINTS

- The adult with congenital heart disease frequently have macroreentrant atrial tachycardia.
- The correct ECG interpretation is the key to understand the mechanism of the arrhythmias and the more appropriate treatment.
- The following congenital heart disease are mainly involved: atrial septal defect and atrioventricular septal defect, Ebstein's anomaly, tetralogy of Fallot, transposition of great arteries after atrial switch operation and post-Fontan palliation.

INTRODUCTION

Congenital heart disease (CHD) affects about 8/1000 of live births.[1] The improvement of interventional and medical management of CHD over the past decades has caused a dramatic change in the panorama of patients with CHD in adulthood so that there are more adults with CHD (ACHD) than children.[2,3]

The arrhythmias are the most common complication during the follow-up of ACHD and represent an important cause of morbidity, mortality, and hospitalization.[4–7] Up to 25% of ACHD die suddenly for cardiac arrhythmia.[8]

The risk of death of atrial arrhythmias in adults with CHD is significant: Yap and colleagues identified an overall mortality of 2.0% per patient-year. Independent predictors of mortality resulted in poor functional class, single-ventricle physiology, pulmonary hypertension, and valvular heart disease.[9]

The last guideline for management of ACHD classified disease according to anatomic or physiologic features. *In particular, the anatomic and physiologic classification divides patients* into three following anatomic groups:

- *Simple* (native disease or repaired conditions) like small atrial septal defect (ASD) or ventricular septal defect (VSD), repaired secundum ASD, sinus venosus (SV) defect, or VSD without significant residual shunt or chamber enlargement
- *Moderate complexity* (repaired or unrepaired conditions) like partial or complete atrioventricular septal defect (AVSD), Ebstein anomaly

[a] Department of Paediatric and Congenital Cardiac Surgery and Cardiology, University Hospital "Ospedali Riuniti", via Conca 71, Ancona 60100, Italy; [b] Cardiology And Arrhythmology Clinic, University Hospital "Ospedali Riuniti", via Conca 71, Ancona 60100, Italy; [c] Department of Biomedical Sciences and Public Health, Marche Polytechnic University, via Conca 71, Ancona 60100, Italy; [d] Department of Clinical, Special and Dental Sciences, Marche Polytechnic University, via Conca 71, Ancona 60100, Italy; [e] Department of Pediatric Cardiology, University of Campania "Luigi Vanvitelli", Former Second University of Naples, "Monaldi Hospital-AORN Ospedale dei Colli", piazzale E Ruggieri, Naples 80131, Italy
* Corresponding author. via Monte Venanzio 8, Ancona 60129, Italy.
E-mail address: alcapest@gmail.com

Card Electrophysiol Clin 14 (2022) 501–515
https://doi.org/10.1016/j.ccep.2022.05.008

(EA) of tricuspid valve (TV), or repaired tetral-ogy of Fallot (TOF)

- *Great complexity* like cyanotic CHD, double-outlet ventricle, Fontan procedure, single ventricle (including double inlet left ventricle, tricuspid atresia, hypoplastic left heart, all abnormality with a functionally single ventricle), transposition of great arteries (TGA), and other abnormalities of atrioventricular (AV) and ventriculoarterial connections (heterotaxy syndromes, isomerism).

The second 4 physiologic stages from A to D based on functional status or symptoms and presence or absence of some conditions such as cyanosis, hypoxemia, ventricular dysfunction, haemodynamic sequelae, valvular disease, shunt, arrhythmias, aortic disease, pulmonary hypertension, and end-organ dysfunction.[10]

The Adult with Congenital Heart Disease and Supraventricular Tachycardia

In 2001, the European Society of Cardiology and the North American Society of Pacing and Electrophysiology proposed a new classification where macroreentrant atrial tachycardia (MAT) was defined as "atrial tachycardia due to a reentry circuit of large size with fixed and/or functional barriers." MAT includes atrial flutter (typical, reverse typical, lower loop flutter) and other macroreentrant tachycardia (lesion-related, left atrial, right atrial free wall without atriotomy). Intra-atrial reentry tachycardia (IART) was comprehended among the MAT.[11] In 2015, the joint American College of Cardiology/American Heart Association/Heart Rhythm Society guidelines specified that MAT in ACHD use the cavotricuspid isthmus (CTI) as a critical pathway for the reentry to perpetuate in greater than 60% of atrial reentry circuits. One of the more represented settings of IART is postsurgical repair of CHD.[12]

Table 1 illustrates the main sites of intra-atrial reentry tachycardia reentry circuit and respective anatomic issues.

IARTs are the most common arrhythmias in the ACHD population and are also known as incisional tachycardia to differentiate them from the typical atrial flutter of "structurally normal heart." The main mechanism of the IART is a macroreentry circuit within atrial muscle revolving around a nonconductive or highly anisotropic barrier, identifiable in the natural anatomic barriers such as AV valve, crista terminalis, and inferior and superior vena cava orifices and acquired post-interventional substrates such as scar areas, atriotomy, ASD patch, intra-atrial baffle, on which chronic pressure and volume overload,

hypoxemia, and other factors act generating fibrosis and remodeling atrium.[7,13]

Most of the MAT present a cavo-tricuspid isthmus-dependent circuit (or cavomitral in L-looped transposition) resembling typical atrial flutter. The differentiating characteristics of IART with respect to atrial flutter are slower atrial rates in the range of 150 to 250 per minute with variable grade of AV block depending on the function of AV node and the relationship with history of heart surgery or interventional treatment.[14] In the presence of normal AV conduction, rapid ventricular rate could cause hemodynamic decompensation. Conversely, when a 2:1 or 3:1 AV conduction is present, the diagnosis of IART could be missed for hidden P waves. Sometimes atypical P wave of different morphology may suggest the existence of multiple circuits. The return to isoelectric baseline in all leads is not a discriminating feature between atrial flutter and IART, although the identification of a reentrant arrhythmia is based on electrophysiological characteristics.

The flutter waves are easily recognizable in less complex CHD (**Fig. 1**), whereas at times recognition of IART is challenging (**Fig. 2**).

The grade of atrial dilatation or thickening, the manipulation and scarring of the atrium, the older age at time of heart surgery, and hemodynamic sequelae are known risk factors for IART.[15–17]

In a large population of 3311 young adults (median age of 22.6 years at entry) with CHD during a median follow-up of 5 years 4.6% had atrial tachycardia with highest burden in complex CHD like single ventricle (22.8%) and d-TGA (22.1%) and TOF (9.2%). The independent risk factors for developing atrial tachycardia were univentricular physiology, previous intracardiac repair, systemic right ventricle (SRV), pulmonary hypertension, pulmonary regurgitation, right-sided AV valve regurgitation, and ventricular dysfunction.[18]

Roca-Luque and colleagues defined a voltage cut off value of 0.5 mV for the identification of unhealthy tissue in the atria of adult patients with CHD and MAT. An important aspect of this study is that more than one-third of patients with CTI-related IART had a concomitant bystander circuit around the scar tissue, deserving electrophysiological maneuvers for determining an ablation strategy.[19]

As expected, electroanatomic mapping of patients with CHD and postoperative atrial tachyarrhythmias detects larger low-voltage areas of the right atrium, especially in the posterior wall, in comparison to patients without CHD.[20]

A priori knowledge of the specific congenital anatomy, all available surgical and interventional procedures, hemodynamic issues, and state of

Table 1
Synthesis of the main electrophysiological substrates and anatomic issues in CHD described

Congenital Heart Disease	Main Sites of IART Reentry Circuit	Anatomic Issue
ASD and AVSD	• Right AFl • Reentry on free right atrial wall (atriotomy)	• Difficulty of trans-catheter ablation in presence of interatrial septal closure device • The opening of CS in left atrium (post-repair of AVSD) • Posterior displacement of AV node (AVSD)
Ebstein anomaly	• CTI-dependent AFl	• TR is often severe • Thin ventricular and atrial wall • Limited access to arrhythmic substrate after tricuspid repair/replacement
Tetralogy of Fallot	• CTI-dependent AFl • Reentry at lateral wall of RA	• High incidence of anomalies of superior caval veins and brachiocephalic vein • RA enlargement and tricuspid regurgitation (catheter instability)
TGA post-atrial switch	• CTI-dependent AFl • Non-CTI-dependent: superior baffle line, peri-inferior vena cava and near pulmonary veins	• Anatomic information from EAM 3D merge CT, CMR, or ICE is useful • Access to PVA and SVA is very often necessary • PVA is reachable through retrograde aortic approach or trans-baffle puncture • Localization of CS could be challenging
Post-Fontan repair	• CTI-dependent AFl • Area close to intra-atrial baffle and lateral native RA	• Knowledge of CHD and surgical procedure is crucial • Anatomic information from EAM 3D merge CT, CMR, or ICE is useful • Vascular access could be challenging (multiple and previous procedures) • Access to RA through fenestration or trans-baffle puncture

Abbreviations: AFl, atrial flutter; ASD, atrial septal defect; AV, atrioventricular; AVSD, atrioventricular septal defect; CMR, cardiovascular magnetic resonance; CS, coronary sinus; CT, cardiovascular tomography; CTI, cavo-tricuspid isthmus; ICE, intracardiac echocardiography; PVA, pulmonary vein atrium; RA, right atriomegaly; SVA, systemic vein atrium; TGA, transposition of great arteries; TR, tricuspide regurgitation.

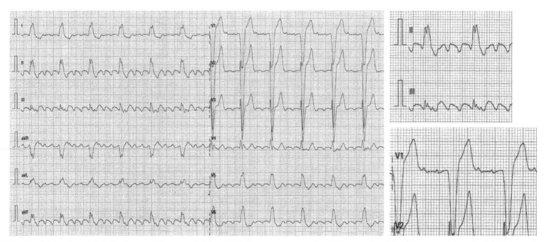

Fig. 1. A typical atrial flutter with cavo-tricuspid isthmus in a patient 32 years old with a postsurgical left bundle branch block. At the age of 11 years, a resection of subaortic membrane was performed and 13 years later a new surgery with septal myectomy was carried out for a recurrence. The P waves appear negative in the inferior leads and positive in V1.

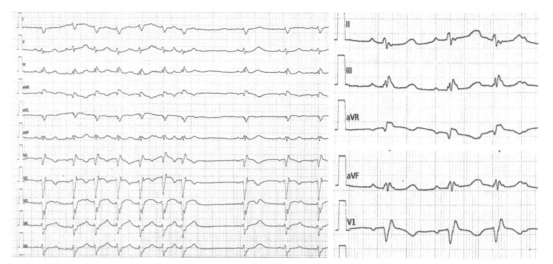

Fig. 2. IART in a 57-year-old patient with severe pulmonary regurgitation and postoperative tetralogy of Fallot repair. The patient had a concomitant left ventricular dysfunction and mild palpitations. It represented the conversion of supraventricular tachycardia to sinus rhythm, demonstrating the challenge of recognizing the IART mostly when present at not high heart rate.

vascular access is necessary for an optimal management of IART.

The therapeutic options for IART must be tailored to the single patient, according to age, clinical and hemodynamic status, and complexity of electrophysiological procedure. The choice of antiarrhythmic drugs is often limited by the coexistence of sinus node dysfunction, AV block, delay of intraventricular conduction, the risk of adverse effects (eg, pulmonary fibrosis in Fontan repair) and ventricular dysfunction/heart failure and by ineffectiveness of long-term prophylaxis.[21] For this reason and for the improvement of ablative technique, currently ablation of symptomatic MAT is recommended as an alternative to antiarrhythmic drugs and/or electrical cardioversion at experienced centers depending on complexity of CHD. Overall, the acute success rate varies between 76% and 96% with best results for CTI-dependent tachycardia than other forms of IART.[22] The use of new technologies such as three-dimensional (3D) electroanatomical mapping (EAM), irrigated radiofrequency catheter, intracardiac echocardiography, and remote magnetic navigation has improved the results of ablative therapy.[23,24] In a cohort of 144 patients (mean age of 32 ± 15 years) with atrial tachyarrhythmias (>80% IART) undergoing radiofrequency catheter ablation and CHD, no difference was observed in term of acute success regard of complexity of CHD.[25] Atrial tachycardia recurrence was associated with complex surgical anatomy (Fontan, atrial switch procedure). In another study, predictors of recurrence were non-CTI IART, long pulmonary regurgitation (PR) interval (>200 msec), previous or induced atrial fibrillation, and indicators of advanced atrial disease.[26]

The rate of recurrence after catheter ablation of atrial tachycardia remains very high. Grubb and colleagues highlighted 44% cases of recidive at a median follow-up of 49.9 months in a population with median age of 45 years where the 93% of patients had a MAT. Interestingly, they noted that 52% of patients had a second catheter ablation procedure and the mechanism of arrhythmia was different than the previous.[27]

Recent data show high risk of intracardiac thrombus in the CHD population with first presentation of atrial fibrillation or atrial flutter/IART (prevalence of thrombus in the entire cohort 9.5% without difference between atrial fibrillation (AF) and AFl/IART) irrespective of CHADS2/CHA2DS-VASc score, suggesting the importance of preventive transesophageal echocardiography (TEE).[28]

Finally, a valid option for managing adults with CHD and tachy-arrhythmias is the surgical treatment that seems to have good results in selected cases with freedom from arrhythmia recurrence at 1 and 10 years of 94% and 85% for atrial arrhythmias.[29]

Remains to be evaluated the long-term efficacy of surgical technique to prevent MAT in patients undergoing surgery for CHD like suturing the intact right atrial free wall in a manner to construct a transmural suture line from the inferior vena cava (IVC) to right atrial incision.[30]

The Macroreentrant Atrial Tachycardia in Specific Settings

Atrial septal defect and atrioventricular septal defect

ASD is one of the most common CHDs and is characterized by absence of atrial tissue at the interatrial septum and by varying degree of interatrial shunt.[31] The four major types of ASD are

- Ostium secundum (OS): communication at the level of fossa ovalis
- Sinus venosus: defect at the orifice of the superior or IVC; the superior SV defect is sometimes associated with sinoatrial node dysfunction and partial anomalous pulmonary venous return
- Ostium primum (or partial AVSD): characterized by the presence of a common AV junction without a ventricular component to the defect
- Coronary sinus (CS): communication between the atria through the mouth of the sinus.

When all components of the atrial septum are absent, it is a common atrium.

The surgical closure of ASD is performed by using a direct suture or a patch of pericardium. The OS type is also suitable for percutaneous closure with different devices.

The magnitude of interatrial shunt is determined by compliance of the right ventricle and size of defect. The result of left to right atrial shunt is the progressive enlargement of the right atrium and stretching and electrical remodeling of its walls together with right ventricular dilatation and dysfunction, elevation in pulmonary arterial pressure, and tricuspid and mitral regurgitation. The presence of an ASD alone has been shown to be associated with the development of atrial tachycardia, especially atrial fibrillation, in 10% of patients by the age of 40 years.[32] The surgical or percutaneous closure of ASD is demonstrated efficacious for the reduction of arrhythmic events.[32,33]

The risk of atrial flutter or atrial fibrillation is not canceled by surgical closure and is related to age and pulmonary arterial pressure, although a meta-analysis of 2020 has not demonstrated a significant reduction of atrial arrhythmias after percutaneous ASD closure.[33]

Different mechanisms of MATs are involved after surgical closure of ASD:

- Common right atrial flutter circuit around TV as leading one
- Reentry around the atriotomy on free lateral wall
- Reentry with a double loop[34–36]

The AVSDs, alias AV canal, or endocardial cushion defects are classified in the following:

- Partial: sometimes associated with mitral cleft
- Complete: large septal defect with an atrial component (ostium primum defect) and a ventricular component (inlet septal defect), common AV valve ring, and common AV valve
- Intermediate: two separate AV valves with primum ASD and small restrictive inlet VSD.

Important variables over the size of the defects in the pathophysiology are the regurgitation of portions of AV valves and the balance of the ventricles. The surgical correction of the defect implies closure of intracardiac communications and reconstruction of two separate and functional AV valves. An important point of the surgery regards the ostium of the CS that usually is placed to the left side to avoid AV block.[37,38] The anatomy of the electric conduction system presents peculiar aspect[39]:

1) Posterior displacement of the AV node related to deficiency of AV septum
2) Altered relation between AV node and ostium of the CS with AV node close to the mouth of CS when AV septum is very deficient
3) Long non-branching bundle
4) Intra-atrial and AV-nodal conduction delay

The predominant circuits of IART are dependent on the right-sided cavo-annular isthmus. An example of typical atrial flutter in a repaired AV canal is reported in **Fig. 3**.

Ebstein anomaly

EA is a rare CHD, accounting for less than 1% of all CHD, characterized by adherence of the septal and posterior leaflets to the underlying myocardium, apical displacement of the functional annulus (septal > posterior > anterior), and dilation of the "atrialized" portion of the right ventricle, with various degrees of hypertrophy and thinning of the wall, anomaly of the anterior leaflet (fenestration, tethering), and dilatation of the anatomic annulus.[40]

The grade of displacement of septal and posterior leaflets generates different clinical spectra with variable reduction of functional right ventricle for the atrialization of ventricular inflow and degrees of tricuspid regurgitation.[40]

The additional cardiac malformations are in most cases interatrial communication but also bicuspid or atretic aortic valves, pulmonary atresia or hypoplastic pulmonary artery, subaortic stenosis, coarctation, mitral valve prolapse, accessory

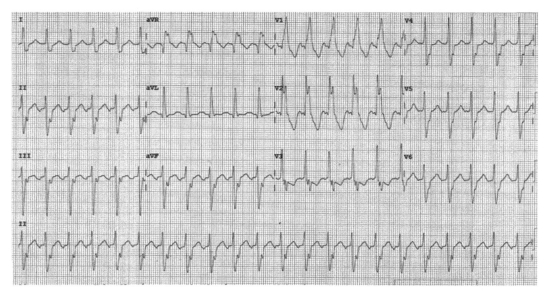

Fig. 3. An atypical atrial flutter with cavo-tricuspid critical isthmus in a 44-year-old man with repaired partial atrioventricular canal at 2 years. Note the bifascicular block (anterior hemiblock related to an elongation and displacement of left anterior fascicle and right bundle branch block related to surgical lesion).

mitral valve tissue or muscle bands of the left ventricle, VSDs, and pulmonary stenosis.[40]

The physiopathology is determined by the TV insufficiency, right ventricular dysfunction, and associated lesions.

The surgical repair of the TV is preferred to valve replacement. Various surgical techniques have been proposed and include valvuloplasty, right ventriculorrhaphy, subtotal ASD closure, and reduction of atrialized right ventricle.

A 1.5-ventricular repair (bidirectional Glenn shunt) is indicated for patients with poor RV function.[41,42]

There are various conduction anomalies: first AV block for the effect of right atrial dilatation, a de-. gree of right branch bundle block, and preexcitation syndrome. The ECG baseline is characterized by tall and broad P waves, short—when preexcitation is present—or prolonged PR interval and polyphasic and fragmented QRS complexes with similar right bundle branch block (RBBB) morphology.[43]

Accessory conduction pathways are present up to 30% and are often multiple and right sided. Interestingly, when a right-sided AV pathway is present, the right branch bundle block could be not evident.[44,45]

The patients with EA have an elevated risk of supraventricular and ventricular arrhythmias.

MAT is one of the most frequent arrhythmias in EA. The dominant mechanism is CTI-dependent

atrial flutter, favored by chronic hemodynamic stress of the right atrium for tricuspid insufficiency and sequelae of surgical intervention. Non-CTI-dependent atrial flutters are present particularly in patients with prior cardiac surgery.[44,45]

It is important to remember that any surgery involving annuloplasty ring or valve replacement could limit the catheter's access to atrial tissue that is part of the critical isthmus. A multicenter retrospective study showed how after surgery for CHD catheter ablation success was lower and tachycardia recurrence was higher after TV ring/replacement surgery. Acute success rate for annular substrate in CTI-IART was achieved in 71% of TV ring/replacement, 91% of TV repair, and 94% of no TV surgery group procedures.[46]

The risk of recurrence in patients undergoing catheter ablation for MAT and EA is high, 26% at 10 years.[47]

The use of reduced power is suggested in areas of potentially thinned atrial or atrialized ventricular myocardium to reduce the risk of cardiac perforation.

Some authors point out a cohort of 143 young patients with a median age of 10 years who underwent cone reconstruction with preoperative arrhythmias in 31% of patients.[48] This finding supports the chance for surgical ablation of preoperative atrial arrhythmias in patients with EA.[49]

In **Fig. 4**, a singular case of EA is described.

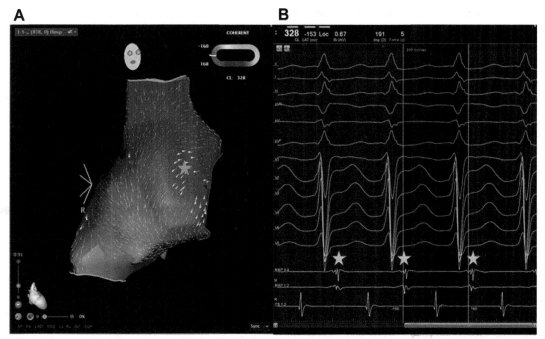

Fig. 4. Intra-atrial reentrant tachycardia in a 20-year-old male patient with congenitally corrected transposition of the great arteries—a combination of atrioventricular and ventricular-arterial discordance—and status post-pulmonary artery banding, post-closure of perimembranous interventricular septal defect, and post-tricuspid valve replacement with a mechanical valve prosthesis for Ebstein anomaly. The patient received an endocardial pacemaker at the age of 2 years for a postsurgical complete atrioventricular block. The tachycardia has a cycle length of 328 msec, and a proximal-to-distal activation pattern is recorded on the coronary sinus catheter. (A) Activation mapping with the Coherent Mapping module (Biosense Webster, Diamond Bar, CA) in the right anterior oblique view, showing an area of early activation (*red*) meeting late activation (*purple*) in the lateral wall of the right atrium (*blue star*). Note that conduction velocity in that region is markedly slowed, as represented by thick white propagation vectors. (B) 12 lead electrocardiogram and intracavitary signals. The ablation catheter records fragmented mid-diastolic electrograms (*white stars*) in the region of maximum conduction velocity slowing (*blue star* in panel A). The arrhythmia was terminated with radiofrequency energy delivery at this point.

Tetralogy of Fallot

TOF is the most common cyanotic CHD characterized by four anatomic features: subpulmonary infundibular stenosis, VSD, aortic overriding, and right ventricular hypertrophy. The anatomic hallmark is antero-cephalad deviation of the outlet septum.

The VSD may be perimembranous or muscular. When the postero-inferior border of VSD is muscular, the AV node is more distant from the margin of VSD. Usually, the conduction branches run to the left, off the septal crest.[50]

The cyanosis depends on the right to left interventricular shunt by effect of the degree of right ventricle outflow tract (RVOT) obstruction. The stenosis or hypoplasia of pulmonary valve and pulmonary trunk is often associated.

The surgical treatment of TOF consists of the following:

- Systemic-pulmonary shunt (usually a Blalock–Taussig shunt with anastomosis of the subclavian artery and pulmonary artery [PA]) as palliation
- Closure of VSD with a patch of pericardium or prosthetic material and disobstruction of RVOT through resection of muscular bundles in the infundibulum and a placement of a transannular patch between the infundibulum and the pulmonary valve in case of a restrictive pulmonary valve annulus. Initially, large ventriculotomy with wide resection of infundibular musculature was performed. Actually, a patch is placed to enlarge RVOT without resection of muscle preferring transatrial and transpulmonary artery approaches.[51]

The main late complications after repair of TOF are pulmonary regurgitation[52] leading to right ventricular dilatation and dysfunction,[53] aortic root enlargement (about 30% of all patients) with moderate/severe aortic valve regurgitation (3.5% of cases),[54] atrial arrhythmias,[55] and ventricular tachycardias with risk of sudden death.[56]

An important issue in postoperative TOF is the left ventricular dysfunction that is present in 20% to 25% of the patients.[57,58] Many factors could take part in its development: the interventricular interaction with the role of right ventricle dysfunction, the interventricular dyssynchrony for the right bundle branch block, the degree of fibrosis of left ventricle, the presence of concomitant aortic regurgitation, the chronic hypoxemia before corrective surgery, and the previous palliative shunt.[58,59]

In a multicenter study, Ait Ali and colleagues observed that at follow-up of 24.1 years from correction left ventricle ejection fraction and left ventricle end-diastolic volume, evaluated by cardiac magnetic resonance, were associated with atrial arrhythmias. However, at the multivariate analysis only tricuspid regurgitation and lower right ventricle ejection fraction were associated with atrial arrhythmias.[60]

A large cross-sectional study found an elevated arrhythmic (43.3%) burden in 556 patients (mean age 36.8 ± 12 years) with repaired TOF. IART (11.5%) was the most common tachyarrhythmias after ventricular tachycardia (14.2%), especially for patients under 45 years (above 45 years the atrial fibrillation was dominant). The factors associated with IART were right atrial enlargement and prior cardiac surgeries.[61]

Wu and colleagues confirmed these dates, arguing that after a quiescent period of 10 to 15 years after corrective surgery a steady increase of the atrial and ventricular arrhythmias starts.[62]

The MAT occurs in the right atrium, often involving the cavo-tricuspid isthmus. It is reasonable that the chronic pressure overload in the right atrium facilitates the development of areas of slow conduction between IVC and tricuspid annulus.[63]

The other prevalent reentry circuit is on the lateral wall of the right atrium corresponding to the area of prior atriotomy or past incisions used for bicaval venous or atrial cannulation.[64]

The acute success rate for ablation was over 90% in particular for patients with critical CTI. Most recurrences occur in different locations with respect to the initial ablation site.[65] Some attentions must be considered as follows:

- The altered anatomy of right atrium and concomitant tricuspid regurgitation may create problems for the stability of catheter and tip pressure.

- The variability of atriotomy does not provide well-defined landmark of CTI.
- The careful identification of phrenic nerve before applying radiofrequency through pacing the lateral wall of right atrium prevents the risk of palsy.
- The use of bidirectional block after CTI ablation could be a useful endpoint for a successful atrial flutter ablation.

Transposition of great arteries after atrial switch operation (Mustard/Senning)

The TGA is the most common cyanotic CHD in the newborn period and is characterized by the pulmonary trunk originating from the left ventricle and by the aorta originating from the right ventricle.[66] Before the introduction of arterial switch operation by Jatene, until the mid-1980s, TGA was corrected at atrial level by Mustard[67] or Senning procedure.[68] The atrial switch is made through the use of atrial baffles, derived from autologous atrial tissue (Senning) or pericardial patch (Mustard), to direct systemic venous blood into the left ventricle and the pulmonary venous blood into the right ventricle, constituting an a systemic venous atrium (SVA) and pulmonary venous atrium (PVA). The location of coronary sinus ostium (CSO) after surgery usually drains in the PVA.

The patients after atrial switch operation are particularly vulnerable to atrial tachyarrhythmias for the risk of myocardial ischemia and consequent sudden death[69] related to:

- Dysfunction of SRV
- Baffle obstruction
- Systemic AV valve regurgitation
- Postcapillary hypertension
- Abnormal coronary perfusion (monocoronary circulation of SRV)
- Failure to control ventricular preload (intra-atrial passive conduits)
- CS congestion resulting in a reduced coronary perfusion pressure

The patients with TGA following atrial-level repair (Mustard or Senning) have a risk of 30% and of more than 40% to develop atrial tachyarrhythmias, respectively, within 10 years and 35 years after surgery.[70]

An important complication of atrial surgery regards the loss of sinus rhythm.[71] Gewillig and colleagues demonstrated that only 47% of patients maintain a normal sinus rhythm after 20 years from Senning/Mustard operation, resulting in an annual risk of 2.4%. An early sinus node dysfunction appeared associated with the development of atrial flutter.[72]

The study of Gelatt and colleagues better defined previous observations: the prevalence of atrial flutter was 24% at 20 years and bradycardia during the operative period, permanente heart block, need for reoperation and loss of sinus rhythm during follow-up were recognized as independent risk factors for the occurrence of atrial flutter.[73]

An important question concerns the seat of the AV node, CTI, and the CSO after atrial surgery.

The intra-atrial baffle is generally sutured posterior to the AV node, placing the AV node in PVA, whereas the CSO may drain into the PVA or SVA depending on baffle suture lines, respectively, posterior and anterior to the CSO. In addition, the CSO is opened in SVA when the CS is surgically incised and incorporated in the baffle. Furthermore, the CTI often overrides the two atria.[74–77]

The main MATs reported are CTI-dependent tachycardia where both portions of the isthmus, sectioned by baffle, are involved in the atrial reentry circuit, needing access to both atria for the ablation.[74–77] For the demonstration of bidirectional block through CTI, Balaji and colleagues[78] proposed a simple method in Mustard patients, using three catheters: one high in SVA, a second in the low SVA, and a third placed in the low PVA; when a bidirectional block is present pacing in the lower SVA determines an earlier activation of the high SVA respect of the lower PVA, likewise pacing in the lower PVA showed lower SVA activation preceding high SVA preablation with reversal after ablation.

Other MATs are IART without CTI-dependent tachycardia where the critical isthmuses may be the region between the orifice of SVC and the superoposterior remnant of the atrial septum (superior baffle line), peri-IVC, and near pulmonary veins.[15]

The PVA is reachable from the catheter through retrograde transaortic-transtricuspid valve approach or transbaffle puncture. The transbaffle puncture is burdened by the theoretical risk of pericardial effusion/cardiac tamponade or damage of intra-atrial baffle and should be guided by intracardiac or TEE.[15]

Catheter ablation of IART in Senning/Mustard patients has a high acute success rate (83.3%); however, the risk of recurrence at an average follow-up of 7 months is not negligible (33%). The remote magnetic navigation ablation seems to have better results with a significant reduction of fluoroscopy time and procedure duration.[79]

Functional single ventricle and post-Fontan palliation

For over 50 years, the Fontan operation has represented the final palliation for patients with complex CHD who have a functional single ventricle or the surgical impossibility to perform a biventricular circulation.[80]

The systemic venous blood returns to the PA bypassing the ventricle, determining a passive and laminar blood flow in the PA. The final palliation is reached through a stepwise approach connecting the superior vena cava to the PA at the age of 3 to 9 months (bidirectional Glenn) and completing the total cavopulmonary circulation at the age of 2 to 5 years anastomosing also the IVC to right pulmonary artery.

The main surgical variations of Fontan circulation are the following (**Fig. 5**):

1) The atriopulmonary Fontan where the right atrium is directly connected to right pulmonary artery.[80]
2) The lateral tunnel technique connects the IVC to the PA via an intra-atrial patch created inside of right atrium.[81]
3) The extracardiac conduit connects the IVC with the PA via a rigid Gore-Tex conduit outside the heart.[82]

The lateral tunnel and the extracardiac conduit can be fenestrated to produce a right-to-left shunt and therefore to allow the maintenance of cardiac output and to limit the increase of right atriomegaly pressure especially in patients with elevated risk as like valvular regurgitation or pulmonary vascular resistance >2 Woods' units.

The long-term effects of this circulation and its complications are the marked elevation of systemic venous pressure and the reduction of cardiac output.[83] Furthermore, the limited preload impairs the diastolic function and possible increases of the pulmonary vascular resistances, induced by dynamic (eg, pain, pleural effusion, and so forth) and fixed (eg, pulmonary anomalies) factors could have dramatic impact on the functioning of the circulation itself.[84,85]

In this context, it is understandable how the atrial arrhythmias produce significant hemodynamic effects. Loss of AV synchronization and tachycardia are poorly tolerated by Fontan patients because they could produce an increase of the pulmonary venous atrial pressure and a diminished ventricular preload resulting in cardiac output reduction.[85]

Atrial surgical scars, chamber dilatation, atrial hypertrophy, neonatal hypoxia, and atrial effect of cardiopulmonary bypass will determine

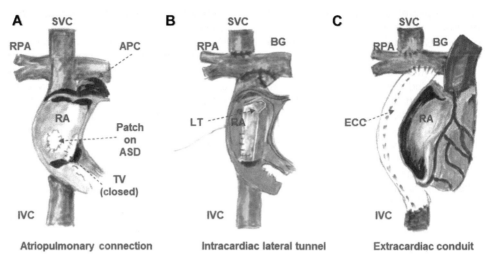

Fig. 5. Types of Fontan palliation. The main mechanisms for the development of IART in Fontan patients are the presence of atrial incision and suture lines, the elevation of atrial pressure producing stretch of atrial wall and atrial fibrosis with constitution of both anatomic conduction barriers and area of functional block. (*A*) Classic Fontan: ASD and TV are sutured and the right auricle is anastomosed with the RPA. Patients with APC are more likely to have IART because of progressive and severe dilation of RA. (*B*) Lateral (intracardiac) tunnel: placement of an intra-atrial Gore-Tex or pericardial baffle directing the blood from IVC through RA to RPA. The area closes the baffle act for the main arrhythmic substrate. (*C*) ECC, the extracardiac total cavo-pulmonary connection, uses an extracardiac conduit between IVC and RPA, determining a lower risk of late atrial arrhythmias. In ECC, the isthmus is often between the atrioventricular valve annulus and the oversewn IVC. APC, atriopulmonary connection; ASD, atrial septal defect; BG, bidirectional Glenn connection (between SVC and RPA); ECC, extracardiac conduit; IVC, inferior vein cava; LT, lateral tunnel; RA, right atrium; RPA, right pulmonary artery; SVC, superior caval vein; TV, tricuspid valve.

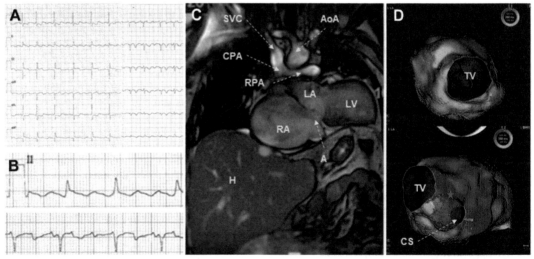

Fig. 6. (*A*) IART with critical isthmus on antero-septal wall of right atrium between tricuspid valve and coronary sinus ostium in 24 patients with bidirectional Glenn anastomosis S/P surgical correction of double outlet right ventricle, pulmonary atresia, and hypoplastic right ventricle. (*B*) Magnification of leads II and V1: the flutter waves are negative in lead II and positive in V1 like counterclockwise reentry. (*C*) CMR frontal image with evidence of marked right atriomegaly and other anatomic and surgical details (bidirectional cavo-pulmonary anastomosis between superior vena cava and right pulmonary artery; atrial septostomy (A); left ventricle; aortic arch; hepatomegaly [H]). (*D*) Activation pattern of IART in the LAO (*top*) and LL (*bottom*) view. Note that the region of early activation (red) encounters a region of late activation (*purple*) in the zone (*red star*) between the tricuspid valve and the coronary sinus ostium. The arrhythmia was terminated with radiofrequency energy delivery in the septal cavotricuspid isthmus. CS, coronary sinus; LAO, left anterior oblique view; LL, left lateral view; S/P, status post; TV, tricuspid valve.

predisposition to IART and sinus node dysfunction, trough formation of fibrosis, and alteration of electrical propagation.[86]

The burden of atrial tachyarrhythmias in patients with Fontan repair is very high: MAT or atrial fibrillation will occur in 50% of all patients within 10 years, reaching 100% after 26 years.[87]

Egbe and colleagues[88] found that the risk of thromboembolism in Fontan patients (age 26 ± 7 years) with atrial arrhythmias was very high with incidence of 0.6% per year and a cumulative incidence of 4% and 7% at 5 and 10 years, respectively, from the time of first atrial arrhythmia diagnosis (mean age at diagnosis age 13 ± 5 years).

Previous studies have shown that IART is the most common arrhythmia in Fontan patients, varying from 7% to 60%, although the current surgical techniques may reduce this burden. The incidence of IART appeared correlated with[87,89,90]:

- Aging, probably for a mechanism atrial fibrosis related
- Type of Fontan operation with an atriopulmonary connection more likely to have IART and no significant difference between lateral tunnel and extracardiac conduit
- The time since surgery with more incidence in patient undertaken to Fontan late

Correa and colleagues,[91] using activation mapping alone or in combination with entrainment mapping, noted that the CTI was critical in over 50% of cases. Successful ablation was performed via trans-baffle puncture into PVA creating a line between IVC and tricuspid annulus. In patients without CTI-dependent circuit, the reentry was located within the intracardiac baffle as the effect of small area remodeling of right atrium including crista terminalis or confined in the intra-atrial lateral tunnel in patients where the native lateral atrium wall is part of the tunnel.[15]

The site where pace the atria and record atrial signals are:

- Directly into intra-atrial tunnel or in the extracardiac conduit via retrograde aortic or the transtube approach
- In left pulmonary artery above the atrium
- Transesophageal
- Through fenestration between the tube and the atrium if possible (usually small).

The risk of mid-term recurrence after ablation of MAT is relatively high up to 50% especially in atriopulmonary Fontan.[92]

A case of right IART in a patient with pulmonary atresia with hypoplastic right ventricle and cavopulmonary anastomosis is described in **Fig. 6**.

CLINICS CARE POINTS

- The knowledge of the anatomy of the congenital heart disease through acquisition of the surgical and past medical history and the use of multimodal cardiac imaging are fundamental for planning and guiding study and ablation of MAT in this population.
- The use of 3D mapping system for the treatment of supraventricular arrhythmias in CHD is reccomended not only to reduce the procedure time and radiation exposure but also for the reconstruction of complex anatomy in CHD.
- The intracardiac echocardiography (ICE) is very useful for real time visualization of anatomy and catheter positioning, identification of suture lines, patch and conduit from repaired CHD and assistance during trans-baffle or interatrial septal puncture.
- The role of expert anesthesiologist is fundamental to support the procedures especially for moderate or severe patients with moderate-severe CHD patients. For example most anesthetic agents produce some vasodilation, which could cause detrimental effects in patients with intracardiac shunts or single-ventricle physiology as well as the modality of ventilation used.
- Pitfalls: The evaluation of systemic venous system before the procedure is an important point because in moderate-complex CHD the venous anomalies are not infrequent like the persistent left superior cava vein draining into coronary sinus or are specific to some conditions like interruption of inferior caval vein in left atrial isomerism. SImilarly the study of vascular access in patients who have already undergone to previous surgical or interventional procedures is required for the identification of the central vein or arterial occlusions and the consequent choice of catheter and materials (ICE.)

DISCLOSURE

Nil.

REFERENCES

1. Liu Y, Chen S, Zühlke L, et al. Global birth prevalence of congenital heart defects 1970-2017:

updated systematic review and meta-analysis of 260 studies. Int J Epidemiol 2019;48(2):455–63.

2. van der Bom T, Zomer AC, Zwinderman AH, et al. The changing epidemiology of congenital heart disease. Nat Rev Cardiol 2011;8(1):50–60.

3. Bouma BJ, Mulder BJ. Changing landscape of congenital heart disease. Circ Res 2017;120(6): 908–22.

4. Kaemmerer H, Bauer U, Pensl U, et al. Management of emergencies in adults with congenital cardiac disease. Am J Cardiol 2008;101(4):521–5.

5. Verheugt CL, Uiterwaal CS, van der Velde ET, et al. Mortality in adult congenital heart disease. Eur Heart J 2010;31(10):1220–9.

6. Silka MJ, Hardy BG, Menashe VD, et al. A population-based prospective evaluation of risk of sudden cardiac death after operation for common congenital heart defects. J Am Coll Cardiol 1998; 32(1):245–51.

7. Walsh EP, Cecchin F. Arrhythmias in adult patients with congenital heart disease. Circulation 2007; 115(4):534–45.

8. Koyak Z, Harris L, de Groot JR, et al. Sudden cardiac death in adult congenital heart disease. Circulation 2012;126(16):1944–54.

9. Stout KK, Daniels CJ, Aboulhosn JA, et al. 2018 AHA/ACC guideline for the management of adults with congenital heart disease: executive summary: a report of the american college of cardiology/american heart association task force on clinical practice guidelines. J Am Coll Cardiol 2019;73(12): 1494–563. Erratum in: J Am Coll Cardiol. 2019; 73(18):2361.

10. Yap SC, Harris L, Chauhan VS, et al. Identifying high risk in adults with congenital heart disease and atrial arrhythmias. Am J Cardiol 2011;108(5):723–38.

11. Saoudi N, Cosío F, Waldo A, et al. Working group of arrhythmias of the european of cardiology and the north american society of pacing and electrophysiology. a classification of atrial flutter and regular atrial tachycardia according to electrophysiological mechanisms and anatomical bases; a Statement from a Joint Expert Group from the Working Group of Arrhythmias of the European Society of Cardiology and the North American Society of Pacing and Electrophysiology. Eur Heart J 2001;22(14): 1162–82.

12. Page RL, Joglar JA, Caldwell MA, et al. 2015 ACC/AHA/HRS guideline for the management of adult patients with supraventricular tachycardia: a report of the American college of cardiology/American heart association task force on clinical practice guidelines and the heart rhythm society. Heart Rhythm 2016; 13(4):e136–221.

13. Kumar S, Tedrow UB, Triedman JK. Arrhythmias in adult congenital heart disease. diagnosis and management. Cardiol Clin 2015;33(4):571–88.

14. Uhm JS, Mun HS, Wi J, et al. Importance of tachycardia cycle length for differentiating typical atrial flutter from scar-related in adult congenital heart disease. Pacing Clin Electrophysiol 2012;35(11): 1338–47.

15. Waldmann V, Bessière F, Raimondo C, et al. Atrial flutter catheter ablation in adult congenital heart diseases. Indian Pacing Electrophysiol J 2021;21(5): 291–302.

16. Hernández-Madrid A, Paul T, Abrams D, et al. ESC scientific document group. arrhythmias in congenital heart disease: a position paper of the european heart rhythm association (EHRA), association for european paediatric and congenital cardiology (aepc), and the European society of cardiology (esc) working group on grown-up congenital heart disease, endorsed by HRS, PACES, APHRS, and SOLAECE. Europace 2018;20(11):1719–53.

17. Ávila P, Oliver JM, Gallego P, et al. Natural history and clinical predictors of atrial tachycardia in adults with congenital heart disease. Circ Arrhythm Electrophysiol 2017;10(9):e005396.

18. Combes N, Derval N, Hascoët S, et al. Ablation of supraventricular arrhythmias in adult congenital heart disease: a contemporary review. Arch Cardiovasc Dis 2017;110(5):334–45.

19. Roca-Luque I, Rivas Gándara N, Dos Subirà L, et al. Intra-atrial re-entrant tachycardia in congenital heart disease: types and relation of isthmus to atrial voltage. Europace 2018;20(2):353–61.

20. Kondo M, Fukuda K, Wakayama Y, et al. Different characteristics of postoperative atrial tachyarrhythmias between congenital and non-congenital heart disease. J Interv Card Electrophysiol 2020;58(1): 1–8.

21. Kawada S, Chakraborty P, Roche L, et al. Role of amiodarone in the management of atrial arrhythmias in adult Fontan patients. Heart 2020;28:317378. Epub ahead of print.

22. Kim YH, Chen SA, Ernst S, et al. 2019 APHRS expert consensus statement on three-dimensional mapping systems for tachycardia developed in collaboration with HRS, EHRA, and LAHRS. J Arrhythm 2020;36(2):215–70.

23. Triedman JK, DeLucca JM, Alexander ME, et al. Prospective trial of electroanatomically guided, irrigated catheter ablation of atrial tachycardia in patients with congenital heart disease. Heart Rhythm 2005;2(7): 700–5.

24. Akca F, Bauernfeind T, Witsenburg M, et al. Acute and long-term outcomes of catheter ablation using remote magnetic navigation in patients with congenital heart disease. Am J Cardiol 2012; 110(3):409–14.

25. Klehs S, Schneider HE, Backhoff D, et al. Radiofrequency catheter ablation of atrial tachycardias in congenital heart disease: results with special

reference to complexity of underlying anatomy. Circ Arrhythm Electrophysiol 2017;10(12):e005451.

26. Roca-Luque I, Rivas-Gándara N, Dos Subirà L, et al. Long-term follow-up after ablation of intra-atrial re-entrant tachycardia in patients with congenital heart disease: types and predictors of recurrence. JACC Clin Electrophysiol 2018;4(6):771–80.

27. Grubb CS, Lewis M, Whang W, et al. Catheter ablation for atrial tachycardia in adults with congenital heart disease: electrophysiological predictors of acute procedural success and post-procedure atrial tachycardia recurrence. JACC Clin Electrophysiol 2019;5(4):438–47.

28. Meziab O, Marcondes L, Friedman KG, et al. Difference in the prevalence of intracardiac thrombus on the first presentation of atrial fibrillation versus flutter in the pediatric and congenital heart disease population. J Cardiovasc Electrophysiol 2020;31(12): 3243–50.

29. Mavroudis C, Deal BJ, Backer CL, et al. Arrhythmia surgery in patients with and without congenital heart disease. Ann Thorac Surg 2008;86(3):857–68. discussion 857–868.

30. Hosseinpour AR, Adsuar-Gómez A, González-Calle A, et al. A simple surgical technique to prevent atrial reentrant tachycardia in surgery for congenital heart disease†. Interact Cardiovasc Thorac Surg 2016;22(1):47–52.

31. Geva T, Martins JD, Wald RM. Atrial septal defects. Lancet 2014;383(9932):1921–32.

32. Vecht JA, Saso S, Rao C, et al. Atrial septal defect closure is associated with a reduced prevalence of atrial tachyarrhythmia in the short to medium term: a systematic review and meta-analysis. Heart 2010;96(22):1789–97.

33. O'Neill L, Floyd CN, Sim I, et al. Percutaneous secundum atrial septal defect closure for the treatment of atrial arrhythmia in the adult: a meta-analysis. Int J Cardiol 2020;321:104–12.

34. Wasmer K, Köbe J, Dechering DG, et al. Isthmus-dependent right atrial flutter as the leading cause of atrial tachycardias after surgical atrial septal defect repair. Int J Cardiol 2013;168(3):2447–52.

35. Magnin-Poull I, De Chillou C, Miljoen H, et al. Mechanisms of right atrial tachycardia occurring late after surgical closure of atrial septal defects. J Cardiovasc Electrophysiol 2005;16(7):681–7.

36. Lukac P, Pedersen AK, Mortensen PT, et al. Ablation of atrial tachycardia after surgery for congenital and acquired heart disease using an electroanatomic mapping system: which circuits to expect in which substrate? Heart Rhythm 2005; 2(1):64–72.

37. Backer CL, Mavroudis C, Alboliras ET, et al. Repair of complete atrioventricular canal defects: results with the two-patch technique. Ann Thorac Surg 1995;60(3):530–7.

38. Nicholson IA, Nunn GR, Sholler GF, et al. Simplified single patch technique for the repair of atrioventricular septal defect. J Thorac Cardiovasc Surg 1999; 118(4):642–6.

39. Thiene G, Wenink AC, Frescura C, et al. Surgical anatomy and pathology of the conduction tissues in atrioventricular defects. J Thorac Cardiovasc Surg 1981;82(6):928–37.

40. Attenhofer Jost CH, Connolly HM, Dearani JA, et al. Ebstein's anomaly. Circulation 2007;115(2):277–85.

41. Burri M, Lange R. Surgical treatment of Ebstein's anomaly. Thorac Cardiovasc Surg 2017;65(8): 639–48.

42. Sainathan S, da Fonseca da Silva L, da Silva JP. Ebstein's anomaly: contemporary management strategies. J Thorac Dis 2020;12(3):1161–73.

43. Waldmann V, Combes N, Ladouceur M, et al. Understanding electrocardiography in adult patients with congenital heart disease: a review. JAMA Cardiol 2020;5(12):1435–44.

44. He BJ, Merriman AF, Cakulev I, et al. Ebstein's anomaly: review of arrhythmia types and morphogenesis of the anomaly. JACC Clin Electrophysiol 2021;7(9):1198–206.

45. Sherwin ED, Abrams DJ. Ebstein anomaly. Card Electrophysiol Clin 2017;9(2):245–54.

46. Moore JP, Gallotti RG, Chiriac A, et al. Catheter ablation of supraventricular tachycardia after tricuspid valve surgery in patients with congenital heart disease: a multicenter comparative study. Heart Rhythm 2020;17(1):58–65.

47. Hassan A, Tan NY, Aung H, et al. Outcomes of atrial arrhythmia radiofrequency catheter ablation in patients with Ebstein's anomaly. Europace 2018;20(3): 534–40.

48. Wackel P, Cannon B, Dearani J, et al. Arrhythmia after cone repair for Ebstein anomaly: the mayo clinic experience in 143 young patients. Congenit Heart Dis 2018;13(1):26–30.

49. Stulak JM, Sharma V, Cannon BC, et al. Optimal surgical ablation of atrial tachyarrhythmias during correction of Ebstein anomaly. Ann Thorac Surg 2015;99(5):1700–5. discussion 1705.

50. Anderson RH, Allwork SP, Ho SY, et al. Surgical anatomy of tetralogy of Fallot. J Thorac Cardiovasc Surg 1981;81(6):887–96.

51. McKenzie ED, Maskatia SA, Mery C. Surgical management of tetralogy of Fallot: in defense of the infundibulum. Semin Thorac Cardiovasc Surg 2013;25(3):206–12. Autumn.

52. Krieger EV, Valente AM. Tetralogy of fallot. Cardiol Clin 2020;38(3):365–77.

53. Redington AN. Physiopathology of right ventricular failure. Semin Thorac Cardiovasc Surg Pediatr Card Surg Annu 2006;9(1):3–10.

54. Mongeon FP, Gurvitz MZ, Broberg CS, et al. Alliance for adult research in congenital cardiology

(AARCC). aortic root dilatation in adults with surgically repaired tetralogy of Fallot: a multicenter cross-sectional study. Circulation 2013;127(2): 172–9.

55. Egbe AC, Najam M, Banala K, et al. Impact of atrial arrhythmia on survival in adults with tetralogy of Fallot. Am Heart J 2019;218:1–7.

56. Cohen MI, Khairy P, Zeppenfeld K, et al. Preventing arrhythmic death in patients with tetralogy of fallot: JACC review topic of the week. J Am Coll Cardiol 2021;77(6):761–71.

57. Broberg CS, Aboulhosn J, Mongeon FP, et al. Alliance for adult research in congenital cardiology (AARCC). prevalence of left ventricular systolic dysfunction in adults with repaired tetralogy of Fallot. Am J Cardiol 2011;107(8):1215–20.

58. Egbe AC, Adigun R, Anand V, et al. Left ventricular systolic dysfunction and cardiovascular outcomes in tetralogy of fallot: systematic review and meta-analysis. Can J Cardiol 2019;35(12):1784–90. Erratum in: Can J Cardiol. 2020;36(11):1830.

59. Tretter JT, Redington AN. The forgotten ventricle? the left ventricle in right-sided congenital heart disease. Circ Cardiovasc Imaging 2018;11(3): e007410.

60. Ait Ali L, Trocchio G, Crepaz R, et al. Left ventricular dysfunction in repaired tetralogy of Fallot: incidence and impact on atrial arrhythmias at long term-follow up. Int J Cardiovasc Imaging 2016;32(9):1441–9.

61. Khairy P, Aboulhosn J, Gurvitz MZ, et al. Alliance for adult research in congenital cardiology (AARCC). arrhythmia burden in adults with surgically repaired tetralogy of Fallot: a multi-institutional study. Circulation 2010;122(9):868–75.

62. Wu MH, Lu CW, Chen HC, et al. Arrhythmic burdens in patients with tetralogy of Fallot: a national database study. Heart Rhythm 2015;12(3):604–9.

63. Mah DY, Alexander ME, Cecchin F, et al. The electro-anatomic mechanisms of atrial tachycardia in patients with tetralogy of Fallot and double outlet right ventricle. J Cardiovasc Electrophysiol 2011;22(9): 1013–7.

64. Karamlou T, McCrindle BW, Williams WG. Surgery insight: late complications following repair of tetralogy of Fallot and related surgical strategies for management. Nat Clin Pract Cardiovasc Med 2006; 3(11):611–22.

65. de Groot NM, Lukac P, Schalij MJ, et al. Long-term outcome of ablative therapy of post-operative atrial tachyarrhythmias in patients with tetralogy of Fallot: a European multi-centre study. Europace 2012; 14(4):522–7.

66. van der Linde D, Konings EE, Slager MA, et al. Birth prevalence of congenital heart disease worldwide: a systematic review and meta-analysis. J Am Coll Cardiol 2011;58(21):2241–7.

67. Mustard WT. Successful two-stage correction of transposition of the great vessels. Surgery 1964; 55:469–72.

68. Senning A. Correction of the transposition of the great arteries. Ann Surg 1975;182(3):287–92.

69. Khairy P. Sudden cardiac death in transposition of the great arteries with a Mustard or Senning baffle: the myocardial ischemia hypothesis. Curr Opin Cardiol 2017;32(1):101–7.

70. Wheeler M, Grigg L, Zentner D. Can we predict sudden cardiac death in long-term survivors of atrial switch surgery for transposition of the great arteries? Congenit Heart Dis 2014;9(4):326–32.

71. Flinn CJ, Wolff GS, Dick M 2nd, et al. Cardiac rhythm after the Mustard operation for complete transposition of the great arteries. N Engl J Med 1984; 310(25):1635–8.

72. Gewillig M, Cullen S, Mertens B, et al. Risk factors for arrhythmia and death after Mustard operation for simple transposition of the great arteries. Circulation 1991;84(5 Suppl):III187–92.

73. Gelatt M, Hamilton RM, McCrindle BW, et al. Arrhythmia and mortality after the Mustard procedure: a 30-year single-center experience. J Am Coll Cardiol 1997;29(1):194–201.

74. Houck CA, Teuwen CP, Bogers AJ, et al. Atrial tachyarrhythmias after atrial switch operation for transposition of the great arteries: treating old surgery with new catheters. Heart Rhythm 2016;13(8):1731–8.

75. Kanter RJ, Papagiannis J, Carboni MP, et al. Radiofrequency catheter ablation of supraventricular tachycardia substrates after mustard and senning operations for d-transposition of the great arteries. J Am Coll Cardiol 2000;35(2):428–41.

76. Wu J, Pflaumer A, Deisenhofer I, et al. Mapping of intraatrial reentrant tachycardias by remote magnetic navigation in patients with d-transposition of the great arteries after mustard or senning procedure. J Cardiovasc Electrophysiol 2008;19(11): 1153–9.

77. Baysa SJ, Olen M, Kanter RJ. Arrhythmias following the mustard and senning operations for dextro-transposition of the great arteries: clinical aspects and catheter ablation. Card Electrophysiol Clin 2017;9(2):255–71.

78. Balaji S, Stajduhar KC, Zarraga IG, et al. Simplified demonstration of cavotricuspid isthmus block after catheter ablation in patients after Mustard's operation. Pacing Clin Electrophysiol 2009;32(10):1294–8.

79. Wu J, Deisenhofer I, Ammar S, et al. Acute and long-term outcome after catheter ablation of supraventricular tachycardia in patients after the Mustard or Senning operation for D-transposition of the great arteries. Europace 2013;15(6):886–91.

80. Fontan F, Baudet E. Surgical repair of tricuspid atresia. Thorax 1971;26(3):240–8.

81. de Leval MR, Kilner P, Gewillig M, et al. Total cavo-pulmonary connection: a logical alternative to atrio-pulmonary connection for complex Fontan operations. experimental studies and early clinical experience. J Thorac Cardiovasc Surg 1988;96(5): 682–95.

82. Marcelletti C, Corno A, Giannico S, et al. Inferior vena cava-pulmonary artery extracardiac conduit. a new form of right heart bypass. J Thorac Cardiovasc Surg 1990;100(2):228–32.

83. Gewillig M, Brown SC, van de Bruaene A, et al. Providing a framework of principles for conceptualising the Fontan circulation. Acta Paediatr 2020; 109(4):651–8.

84. Gewillig M, Brown SC, Eyskens B, et al. The Fontan circulation: who controls cardiac output? Interact Cardiovasc Thorac Surg 2010;10(3):428–33.

85. Gewillig M, Brown SC. The Fontan circulation after 45 years: update in physiology. Heart 2016; 102(14):1081–6.

86. Durongpisitkul K, Porter CJ, Cetta F, et al. Predictors of early- and late-onset supraventricular tachyar-rhythmias after Fontan operation. Circulation 1998; 98(11):1099–107.

87. Quinton E, Nightingale P, Hudsmith L, et al. Preva-lence of atrial tachyarrhythmia in adults after Fontan operation. Heart 2015;101(20):1672–7.

88. Egbe AC, Miranda WR, Devara J, et al. Alliance for Adult Research in Congenital Cardiology (AARCC) investigators. Recurrent sustained atrial arrhythmias and thromboembolism in Fontan patients with total cavopulmonary connection. Int J Cardiol Heart Vasc 2021;33:100754.

89. Stephenson EA, Lu M, Berul CI, et al. Pediatric Heart Network Investigators. Arrhythmias in a contempo-rary fontan cohort: prevalence and clinical associa-tions in a multicenter cross-sectional study. J Am Coll Cardiol 2010;56(11):890–6.

90. Giannakoulas G, Dimopoulos K, Yuksel S, et al. Atrial tachyarrhythmias late after Fontan operation are related to increase in mortality and hospitaliza-tion. Int J Cardiol 2012;157(2):221–6.

91. Correa R, Sherwin ED, Kovach J, et al. Mechanism and ablation of arrhythmia following total cavopul-monary connection. Circ Arrhythm Electrophysiol 2015;8(2):318–25.

92. Rychik J, Atz AM, Celermajer DS, et al. American heart association council on cardiovascular disease in the young and council on cardiovascular and stroke nursing. Evaluation and management of the child and adult with fontan circulation: a scientific statement from the American heart association. Cir-culation 2019. CIR0000000000000696. [Epub ahead of print].

Atrial Flutter in Particular Patient Populations

Paolo Compagnucci, MD[a,b,1,]*, Michela Casella, MD, PhD[a,c,1], Giuseppe Bagliani, MD[a,b], Alessandro Capestro, MD[d], Giovanni Volpato, MD[a,b], Yari Valeri, MD[a,b], Laura Cipolletta, MD, PhD[a], Quintino Parisi, MD, PhD[a], Silvano Molini, MD[a], Agostino Misiani, MD[a], Antonio Dello Russo, MD, PhD[a,c]

KEYWORDS

- Atrial flutter • Catheter ablation • Cardiomyopathy • Neuromuscular diseases • Heart transplant
- COVID-19 • Athletes • Preexcitation

KEY POINTS

- The clinical meaning and the prognostic impact of atrial flutter (AFl) is particularly relevant in some groups of patients.
- The therapeutic approach to AFl may change according to the underlying substrate and associated extracardiac comorbidities.
- Catheter ablation of the cavotricuspid isthmus is the first-line therapy in typical AFl, due to the difficulty in adequate pharmacologic rate and/or rhythm control.
- Patients with heart failure (especially if tachycardia-induced cardiomyopathy is suspected), cardiomyopathies, after heart transplantation, and athletes may particularly benefit from catheter ablation.
- Athletes with AFl may return to competitive sports after catheter ablation.

INTRODUCTION

The initial electrocardiographic documentation of atrial flutter (AFl) dates to 1906, when Willem Einthoven published the first tracings depicting AFl and atrial fibrillation (AF).[1,2] In the ensuing 116 years, multiple clinical studies have elucidated in depth the clinical significance, the prognostic weight, and the medical-interventional approaches for the treatment of AF in several contexts,[3,4] but less work has been done concerning AFl.

AFl is a not an uncommon disease in the general population, with a reported overall incidence of 88 cases/100000 person-years, increasing by 2.5 times in men, 3.5 times among patients with heart failure (HF), and 1.9 times in subjects with chronic obstructive pulmonary disease (COPD).[5] Of note, patients with AFl commonly develop AF, and the 2 arrhythmias are often associated, confounding a precise assessment of the clinical-prognostic meaning of AFl.[6]

In this article, the authors first present an updated review of the differences between AFl's and AF's electrophysiological substrates, then provide a concise summary of the available evidence on AFl in specific patient populations, including patients

[a] Cardiology and Arrhythmology Clinic, University Hospital "Ospedali Riuniti", Via Conca 71, Ancona 60126, Italy; [b] Department of Biomedical Sciences and Public Health, Marche Polytechnic University, Ancona, Italy; [c] Department of Clinical, Special and Dental Sciences, Marche Polytechnic University, Ancona, Italy; [d] Department of Pediatric and Congenital Cardiology and Cardiac Surgery, University Hospital "Ospedali Riuniti", Via Conca 71, Ancona 60126, Italy

[1] Drs. Compagnucci and Casella contributed equally to this work.

* Corresponding author. Department of Biomedical Sciences and Public Health and Cardiology and Arrhythmology Clinic, Marche Polytechnic University and University Hospital "Ospedali Riuniti", Via Conca 71, Ancona, 60126 Italy.

E-mail address: paolocompagnucci1@gmail.com

Card Electrophysiol Clin 14 (2022) 517–532
https://doi.org/10.1016/j.ccep.2022.05.002

cardiacEP.theclinics.com

with HF, cardiomyopathies, or neuromuscular diseases; posttransplant patients; athletes; subjects with preexcitation; and subjects with pulmonary diseases, underlining the clinical-prognostic significance of AFl and reviewing the available specific therapeutic opportunities, aiming to stimulate further research on this often-neglected field. Information on AFl epidemiology in these special subsets and selected hints for optimal patient management are provided in **Table 1**.

ATRIAL FLUTTER AND ATRIAL CARDIOMYOPATHY—IS THERE A DIFFERENCE BETWEEN THE ELECTROPHYSIOLOGICAL SUBSTRATES OF ATRIAL FLUTTER AND FIBRILLATION?

AF is known to trigger a vicious cycle of electrophysiological and structural changes, including action potential duration shortening, conduction velocity slowing, as well as atrial wall fibrous replacement, which in turn facilitate AF recurrences and stabilization, following the well-known motto "AF begets AF."[7] Over the past few years, much attention has been devoted to the study of the complex of structural and functional changes associated with AF, which have been labeled under the term "atrial cardiomyopathy,"[8] and a growing body of literature is now supporting the concept that it is this abnormal atrial substrate that independently mediates the most feared AF complications, that is, thromboembolic events.[9,10]

Because of the common association with AF, whether isolated AFl is associated with a specific electrophysiological and structural substrate, distinct from that of AF, is currently unclear. The anatomy of the cavotricuspid isthmus in normal atria sets the stage for slow conduction: the 3-dimensionally irregular disposition of myocardial strands and the interspersed fibrous tissue content of this region favor typical AFl's reentrant circuit.[11,12] According to recent acquisitions in this field, AFl-induced atrial remodeling may differ from that mediated by AF. In fact, in an animal study involving dogs,[13] both sustained AFl and AF were found to be associated with a shortening of the atrial effective refractory period and increased AF vulnerability, but only dogs with sustained AF were found to develop left atrial dilation, conduction slowing, and, at the histologic level, fibrotic and inflammatory changes.[13] These findings suggest that structural left atrial changes do not usually occur in isolated AFl and motivate greater efforts to control AFl at an early stage, before AF develops, and also to detect AF as early as possible among patients with AFl, in order to intervene (with antiarrhythmic drugs,

cardioversion, and catheter ablation) before irreversible and unfavorable left atrial remodeling.[13–15]

ATRIAL FLUTTER AND HEART FAILURE

The relationship between AFl and HF is complex and reciprocating: AFl may complicate the clinical course of patients with HF of various causes, and, on the other hand, AFl may induce a form of HF known as "tachycardia-induced cardiomyopathy," which resolves on restoration of sinus rhythm.[16] As of today, no study has reported on the incidence or prevalence of AFl among unselected patients with HF. However, HF is common in subjects with AFl, with a reported prevalence ranging between 8% and 56%.[16]

The main mechanism linking AFl and tachycardia-induced cardiomyopathy is the elevated ventricular response during AFl, which is notoriously more difficult to rate control than AF. In a Canadian study, 75% of patients with a ventricular rate of 100/min or higher during persistent AFl and left ventricular dysfunction had significant improvement of left ventricular ejection fraction after catheter ablation, as compared with 25% with a ventricular rate of less than 100/min[17]; furthermore, heart rate was the only independent predictor of recovery from left ventricular dysfunction.[17] The recovery of atrial contribution to ventricular filling may explain the improvement in left ventricular systolic function seldomly seen with restoration of sinus rhythm among patients with AFl, HF, and a well-controlled ventricular rate.[17]

Because of its high acute (87%–100%) and long-term success rate (70%–95%),[16] catheter ablation is a preferrable therapeutic option for patients with typical AFl and HF, especially when tachycardia-induced cardiomyopathy is suspected.[18] Furthermore, left ventricular systolic function improvement or normalization is reported in 57% to 100% and 33% to 88% of patients with HF undergoing catheter ablation of AFl, respectively, mandating a judicious and patient approach to defibrillator implantation for the primary prevention of sudden cardiac death.[16,18] Electrical cardioversion is a reasonable alternative in the short term (acute effectiveness, 89%–96%), but its long-term effectiveness is suboptimal, ranging between 42% and 90%,[16] often requiring multiple shocks and antiarrhythmic drug treatment, with a theoretic risk of drug-induced proarrhythmia.[19]

ATRIAL FLUTTER AND CARDIOMYOPATHIES

The prevalence of AFl in the various cardiomyopathies is difficult to ascertain, due to the common

Table 1		
Atrial flutter in special populations—epidemiology and clinical management		
Patient Population	**Epidemiology**	**Hints for Optimal Clinical Management**
Heart failure	• Prevalence of AFl in unselected patients with heart failure is unknown • Prevalence of heart failure in patients with AFl is 8%–56%	• Use of class I or class III antiarrhythmic drugs (except amiodarone) is contraindicated in patients with heart failure and a reduced ejection fraction • For typical AFl, catheter ablation is a first-line therapeutic option, especially if tachycardia-induced cardiomyopathy is suspected
Arrhythmogenic right ventricular cardiomyopathy	• Prevalence of AFl is 4%–30% • Patients with right atrial enlargement and/or moderate/severe tricuspid regurgitation have increased risk of AFl	• In case of typical AFl, cavotricuspid isthmus catheter ablation has similar effectiveness as in the general population and may prevent inappropriate defibrillator shocks
Hypertrophic cardiomyopathy	• 40% prevalence of supraventricular tachycardia (all subtypes) in studies on Holter monitoring • 10% prevalence of AFl inducibility by electrophysiology study	• High risk of thromboembolism irrespective of CHA_2DS_2-VASc; anticoagulation is always warranted • Catheter ablation of the cavotricuspid isthmus is highly effective for typical AFl
Dilated cardiomyopathy	• Prevalence of AFl in unselected patients with dilated cardiomyopathy in unknown • The highest risk of AFl is seen with lamin A/C cardiomyopathy, which constitutes 4%–6% of all dilated cardiomyopathies; in this subset, AFl has a prevalence of 21% and may be the first disease manifestation	• In case of typical AFl, cavotricuspid isthmus catheter ablation may be of help to rule out tachycardia-induced cardiomyopathy and to improve symptoms • In case of atypical AFl or when catheter ablation is contraindicated or refused by the patient, "ablate and pace" with biventricular defibrillator implantation may be an option
Cardiac amyloidosis	• AFl and AF have been collectively reported in 60% of patients with ATTR amyloidosis and 30% of AL amyloidosis • AFl commonly leads to clinical deterioration • Rate control drugs are commonly not tolerated, and rhythm control is the initial therapeutic approach in most of the cases seen at early-mid stages of disease	• Before cardioversion, transesophageal echocardiography should be performed even in anticoagulated patients, due to the high risk of intracardiac thrombosis • Cavotricuspid isthmus ablation is the first-line option in case of typical AFl • "Ablate and pace" with biventricular or dual chamber pacemakers is an important option for atypical AFl with poorly controlled ventricular rate
Neuromuscular disorders	• Myotonic dystrophy type 1 (prevalence, 2–14/100,000) has the highest reported prevalence of AFl (8%–9%)	• Use of antiarrhythmics often exposes to an inacceptable risk of bradiarrhythmias in the

(continued on next page)

Table 1
(continued)

Patient Population	Epidemiology	Hints for Optimal Clinical Management
	• Atrial arrhythmias (including AFl) are independent predictors of sudden and nonsudden death in patients with myotonic dystrophy type 1	absence of a pacemaker/defibrillator • Anticoagulation should be prescribed according to the CHA$_2$DS$_2$-VASc score • The decision to perform catheter ablation should consider the patient's respiratory and muscular involvement and the inherent risk of procedural complications
Heart transplantation	• AFl has a prevalence of 9%–13% after heart transplantation • AFl is the most common arrhythmia after the first 3 wk • Higher risk of AFl is observed with the now mostly abandoned biatrial technique	• Catheter ablation is very effective and may involve ablation of the cavotricuspid isthmus, atypical sites (ie, mitral isthmus), or receiver-to-donor atrial connections • Multiple arrhythmias are usually ablated in each patient • Repeat procedures are needed 29% of times • Anticoagulation should always be prescribed • Apixaban or rivaroxaban has lower risk of interactions with cyclosporin than warfarin or dabigatran
Chronic obstructive pulmonary disease	• Chronic obstructive pulmonary disease increases the incidence of AFl by 1.9 times	• Beta-1 selective β-blockers are first-line rate-control drugs unless the patient has bronchospasm; β-blockers may also lower risk of chronic obstructive pulmonary disease exacerbation • Theophylline and short-acting beta agonists may precipitate AFl and AF, and prevent adequate rate control • Amiodarone may be used for rhythm control
Pulmonary arterial hypertension	• AFl is equally common as AF, with a 10% incidence over 5 y of follow-up • AFl may contribute to hemodynamic worsening	• A rhythm control strategy is preferable to revert the adverse hemodynamics brought by the loss of the atrial contribution to ventricular filling and by the high ventricular rate seen with AFl • Catheter ablation should be performed early on for typical AFl
COVID-19	• Prevalence of AFl is 4%–10% among hospitalized patients, with higher risk in critically ill patients	• Catheter ablation should be deferred after resolution of the viral infection

(continued on next page)

Table 1 (continued)		
Patient Population	**Epidemiology**	**Hints for Optimal Clinical Management**
		• Electrical cardioversion is indicated in the presence of hemodynamic instability • Digoxin may be a good option to control ventricular rate in critically ill patients under vasopressor support
Athletes	• 10% of athletes with AF also have AFl • Risk of AFl is high among endurance athletes, especially in aging athletes • AFl carries the risk of 1:1 atrioventricular conduction with hemodynamic impairment during exercise	• Cavotricuspid isthmus ablation is the first-line therapy for typical AFl • Return to leisure-time sports is allowed 1 wk after catheter ablation in patients without structural heart disease and without symptoms of hemodynamic intolerance during exercise before catheter ablation • Return to competitive sports may be allowed after 1 mo in asymptomatic patients without structural heart disease and without symptoms of hemodynamic intolerance during exercise before catheter ablation • Anticoagulated patients should not participate in contact sports
Ventricular preexcitation	• The epidemiology of AFl in patients with ventricular preexcitation is unknown, and its ascertainment is complicated by the difficulties in the electrocardiographic diagnosis	• Catheter ablation of the accessory pathway is clearly indicated in patients with preexcited AFl with 1:1 atrioventricular conduction

mixed reporting of AFl together with AF. Theoretically, cardiomyopathies involving the right chambers may have the highest risk of typical AFl, as more widespread right atrial substrate abnormalities could facilitate slow conduction in the cavotricuspid isthmus; noteworthy, cardiomyopathies with left ventricular involvement may also be associated with AFl, either typical or atypical.

Atrial fibrofatty replacement may occur in *arrhythmogenic right ventricular cardiomyopathy* (ARVC) and increase vulnerability to various supraventricular arrhythmias, including AFl.[20,21] The reported prevalence of AFl ranges between 4% and 30%,[22–24] with higher figures (of AFl and AF) in case of atrial enlargement[22] and moderate/severe tricuspid regurgitation.[24] Of note, AFl (and also AF) is associated with high risk of inappropriate shocks in patients with ARVC, in whom implantable cardioverter defibrillators (ICDs) are commonly used.[22] Furthermore, many investigators pointed out that AFl (and AF) may have a negative prognostic impact in patients with ARVC, being associated with increased risk of death and HF, although it is currently unclear whether AFl (and AF) may serve as an independent adverse prognostic predictor or as a marker of disease severity.[22,25] With regard to treatment, antiarrhythmic drugs are commonly used to treat and prevent ventricular and atrial arrhythmias in patients with ARVC.[21] Based on the results of a recent observational multicenter study, catheter ablation may be offered to patients with AFl and ARVC, given that the procedural success of cavotricuspid isthmus ablation is comparable to that of the general population and may help prevent inappropriate shocks.[26,27]

Hypertrophic cardiomyopathy is associated with very high prevalence of supraventricular arrhythmias, which approaches 40% in studies on Holter monitoring.[28] The first reports specifically concerning AFl in hypertrophic cardiomyopathy were published in the 1980s.[29,30] At that time, the focus was on the assessment of clinical significance of arrhythmia inducibility by atrial or ventricular programmed electrical stimulation. Fananapazir and colleagues[30] reported a 10% inducibility rate for reentrant atrial tachycardia, with a mean cycle length of the induced arrhythmia of 275 ± 35 ms; 28% of inducible patients also had evidence of AFl by Holter recordings. In the authors' experience, patients with more severe forms of disease, especially patients with systolic dysfunction (ie, "end-stage" hypertrophic cardiomyopathy), tend to develop atypical left AFl, whereas typical AFl may occur at earlier stages of disease (**Fig. 1**). According to recent observational evidence, catheter ablation of non-AF supraventricular arrhythmias (including AFl) is associated with optimal survival free from recurrences in hypertrophic cardiomyopathy.[31]

Among the various genetic forms of *dilated cardiomyopathy*, that associated with lamin A/C mutations (which constitutes 4%–6% of all cases of dilated cardiomyopathy) has the highest reported prevalence of AFl.[32] Lamin A and C are key structural components of the nuclear membrane and also play a role in the regulation of gene transcription. The various mutations in the gene coding for these proteins (the LMNA gene) are associated with several disease phenoptypes, in which cardiac involvement is either the main clinical manifestation or a common component of a multisystem syndrome (eg, Emery-Dreifuss muscular dystrophy).[32] In a study involving 122 subjects with lamin A/C mutations, who were followed for a median of 7 years, the prevalence of AFl passed from 3% at first clinical contact to 21% at the end of follow-up.[32] Furthermore, there was a high incidence of thromboembolic complications.[32] Notably, patients with atrial arrhythmias as the first disease manifestation had both a 47% prevalence of concomitant atrioventricular block at baseline and a very high risk of subsequently developing ventricular arrhythmias, atrioventricular block, and HF.[32] Therefore, the presence of AFl (or other arrhythmias) and atrioventricular block in young patients with dilated cardiomyopathy should raise the suspicion for lamin A/C cardiomyopathy and prompt genetic testing.[33,34] Because of the very high risk of sudden cardiac death, a diagnosis of lamin A/C cardiomyopathy is currently recognized as an indication for the implantation of an ICD in patients requiring cardiac pacing.[35] Atrial arrhythmias, atrioventricular block, thromboembolic complications, and ventricular arrhythmias in patients with lamin A/C mutations may represent clinical manifestations of progressive fibrofatty replacement of the atrial myocardium[36] and scarring of the basal interventricular septum (**Fig. 2**).[37]

The treatment of AFl in dilated cardiomyopathy is complicated by the scarce hemodynamic tolerance of rapid atrioventricular conduction and by the contraindication for several antiarrhythmic drugs (especially class I drugs and sotalol) in the presence of left ventricular dysfunction, owing to the increased risk of proarrhythmia and mortality.[33] Typical AFl may be effectively controlled by catheter ablation, although biventricular defibrillator implantation with concurrent ablation of the atrioventricular node (ie, ablate and pace) may be considered an important option in selected cases.[33]

Cardiac amyloidoses represent the most common forms of restrictive cardiomyopathy and are characterized by the extensive extracellular deposition of insoluble amyloid fibrils in the myocardium.[38] Besides being associated with very high risk of bradyarrhythmias and infra-His conduction disturbances,[38] amyloidosis is also linked to high risk of AF and AFl, which have been collectively reported in 60% of patients with transthyretin (ATTR) amyloidosis[39] and 30% of patients with AL amyloidosis.[40] The pathophysiology of atrial arrhythmias is related to both tissue infiltration–related slowing of conduction velocity and atrial dilation due to increased ventricular filling pressures.[38] AF and AFl commonly lead to clinical deterioration in this setting, as the loss of atrial contribution to ventricular filling in the context of diastolic dysfunction, as well as the commonly associated high ventricular response rate (especially in case of AFl) may compromise cardiac output, making rhythm control a desirable therapeutic approach.[41,42] According to a recent report,[42] in 80% of patients with ATTR amyloidosis and AF or AFl, rate-controlling drugs were not tolerated and had to be discontinued; rhythm control was attempted in 64% of the cohort, using cardioversion or ablation.[42] After cardioversion, recurrence of arrhythmias was both common (91%) and early (after a median of 6 months).[42] In the case of typical AFl, however, outcomes after cavotricuspid isthmus ablation were good, with 14% risk of recurrence after a median of 5 years.[42] In another report of patients with AL or ATTR amiloydosis,[31] electrical cardioversion was commonly canceled (in 28% of cases), due to the finding of intracardiac thrombi at transesophageal echocardiography, even in adequately anticoagulated

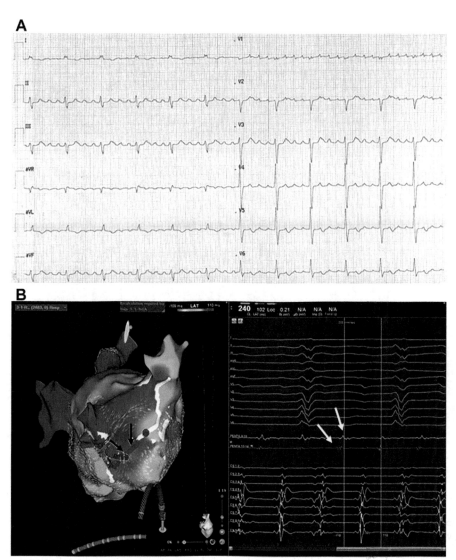

Fig. 1. Atypical atrial flutter in end-stage hypertrophic cardiomyopathy. A 66-year-old male patient with hypertrophic cardiomyopathy is evaluated for worsening dyspnea. The electrocardiogram (ECG) (*A*) reveals atypical atrial flutter, with positive flutter waves in both inferior and precordial leads. The echocardiogram shows severe left ventricular systolic dysfunction. Catheter ablation is performed, and the critical isthmus of the tachycardia is mapped in the left atrium, between the right inferior pulmonary vein and the fossa ovalis. (*B*) The tachycardia activation map in the right anterior oblique view, as reconstructed with the CARTO3 v7 electroanatomical mapping system (Biosense Webster Inc, CA, USA); please note that the multipolar mapping catheter (PentaRay, Biosense Webster Inc, CA, USA) records diastolic and fragmented potentials (*white arrows*) between the right inferior pulmonary vein and the fossa ovalis (*black arrows*). Radiofrequency energy delivery on the critical isthmus leads to arrhythmia termination (not shown); at hospital discharge, ejection fraction is improved to 45%.

patients. The procedure was also associated with high periprocedural risk of complications (14%), mainly ventricular arrhythmias or severe bradycardia.[41] In summary, the management of AFl (and AF) is highly challenging in patients with cardiac amyloidosis, due to the scarce tolerance of rate-controlling drugs and risk of recurrence after cardioversion, but catheter ablation of the cavotricuspid isthmus may be useful in case of typical AFl

(**Fig. 3**).[38,42] Ablate and pace (with biventricular or dual chamber pacemakers) may be an important option among patients with atypical AFl and poorly controlled ventricular rate.[38]

ATRIAL FLUTTER IN NEUROMUSCULAR DISORDERS

Muscular dystrophies encompass a wide spectrum of inherited disorders characterized by

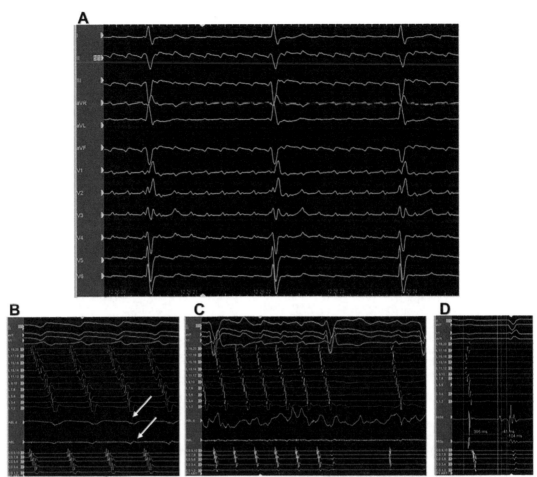

Fig. 2. Typical atrial flutter in lamin cardiomyopathy. A 38-year-old male patient with typical atrial flutter with low ventricular response rate and lamin A/C mutation. (*A*) A 12-lead ECG, showing an 8:1 atrioventricular conduction ratio, complete right bundle branch block, and left anterior fascicular block. (*B*) Intracavitary activation pattern, with proximal-to-distal activation of the coronary sinus (CS, proximal 9,10 to distal 1,2) and counterclockwise propagation around the tricuspid annulus (L, septal 19,20 to lateral 1,2). Please note that the ablation catheter is positioned in the cavotricuspid isthmus and records fragmented, long, and diastolic signals (*arrows*). (*C*) Radiofrequency energy delivery leads to flutter termination. (*D*) In sinus rhythm, after ablation, delayed supra-, intra-, and infra-Hisian conduction were found. Because of the conduction disturbance and a severely reduced left ventricular ejection fraction, the patient underwent cardiac resynchronization therapy-defibrillator implantation and, later on, cardiac transplantation.

progressive involvement of the skeletal muscles, and most of the muscular dystrophies also affect the myocardium.[43,44] Disorders associated with mutations of dystrophin and dystrophin-associated glycoproteins (eg, Duchenne and Becker muscular dystrophies), which connect the myocyte's contractile proteins to the sarcolemma, are associated with progressive loss of myocardiocytes and fibrofatty replacement, leading to dilated cardiomyopathy; arrhythmias (both ventricular and supraventricular) occur late in the disease course.[43] On the other hand, myotonic types 1 and 2, Emery-Dreifuss, limb-girdle type 1B, and facioscapulohumeral dystrophies are characterized by fibrofatty replacement of the basal interventricular septum and of the conduction system, leading to bradyarrhythmias and tachyarrhythmias early in the disease course.[43–45] Of all the muscular dystrophies, myotonic dystrophy type 1 has the highest prevalence of AFl,[46] which may be up to 8% to 9%.[47,48] The propensity for the development of AFl and AF in myotonic type 1 dystrophy is thought to represent a consequence of the extensive right atrial scarring and slowing of conduction seen in the disease, which may be directly proportional to the number of

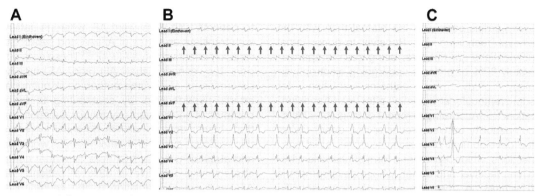

Fig. 3. Atrial flutter in cardiac amyloidosis. A 67-year-old male patient with AL amyloidosis presents with worsening dyspnea. The ECG shows a wide complex tachycardia, with low-voltage QRS complexes in peripheral leads. In (*A*), the tachycardia is regular, with a cycle length of 440 msec; it has an atypical right bundle branch block morphology (monophasic R wave in V1) and extreme axis deviation (monophasic R wave in aVR); both findings raise the suspicion of ventricular tachycardia. The ECG is repeated after some minutes (*B*) and reveals an irregular rhythm with similar QRS morphology. In inferior leads (most notable in DII and aVF), you can appreciate negative flutter waves (*red arrows*), with a cycle length of 440 msec; the R-R interval is «regularly irregular», with 4:3 and 3:2 Wenckebach periodism. A diagnosis of atypical atrial flutter is made and electrical cardioversion performed. The ECG after cardioversion (*C*) shows sinus rhythm, first-degree atrioventricular block (PR interval, 220 ms), right bundle branch block, and extreme axis deviation, together with low limb leads voltages and wide q waves (pseudo-infarct pattern) in inferior leads. Atrial flutter may sometimes mimic ventricular tachycardia in the presence of abnormal intraventricular conduction, as commonly occurs in cardiac amyloidosis.

unstable CTG triplets in the 3′ untranslated region of the 19q13 (DMPK) gene, encoding for the myotonin-protein kinase protein, and affecting the processing of RNA transcripts.[44,49] The presence of AFl (and other atrial arrhythmias) is not only common but also prognostically ominous: atrial arrhythmias were shown to be the only independent predictors of both sudden (by representing a marker of myocardial fibrosis) and nonsudden (by indicating a higher burden of pulmonary involvement with right chamber overload) death in patients with myotonic type 1 dystrophy.[50]

The medical treatment of AFl in patients with neuromuscular disorders should follow general guidelines, anticoagulation being recommended in the presence of conventional risk factor for stroke as per the CHA_2DS_2-VASc score.[46,47] The decision to perform invasive procedures should take into account life expectancy as well as the severity of muscular and respiratory involvement, which may increase the risks of procedural sedation-induced complications.[43] Catheter ablation may be very effective in selected patients with cavotricuspid isthmus–dependent AFl.[46,48]

ATRIAL FLUTTER AFTER HEART TRANSPLANTATION

Over the past decades, the survival of patients after heart transplantation has progressively improved, due to advancements in patient/donor selection, surgical technique, and immunosuppressive treatments.[51] With a median survival after heart transplantation of 12 years,[51] more patients survive to develop arrhythmias during follow-up, and arrhythmias are a major determinant of both quality and quantity of life.[52]

AFl is the most common arrhythmia after the initial postoperative period, with reported prevalences of up to 9% to 13%,[53,54] outnumbering AF after the first 3 weeks.[54] The pathophysiological processes leading to AFl are complex and multiple and may involve rejection (AFl is the most common arrhythmia associated with rejection[54]), progressive atrial remodeling, and receiver-to-donor connections.[52] In regard to this latter mechanism, it is worth pointing out that 2 main surgical techniques may be used for heart transplantation: the original biatrial method, in which portions of the receiver's atria are retained and sutured to the donor's heart, and the now preferred bicaval technique, in which anastomoses are placed at the level of vena cavae, great arteries, and the cuff around the pulmonary veins ostia.[52] The former technique is associated with higher risk of establishment of electrical connections between the receiver's and the donor's heart, allowing conduction of AFl or AF from the receiver's to the donor's atria or reciprocating reentrant tachycardias between receiver and donor atria (in case of multiple electrical connections), potentially explaining the greater risk of atrial tachycardias seen with the biatrial than with the bicaval technique.[52,53] Receiver-to-donor atrial connections are not rare, being seen in approximately 20% of patients undergoing electrophysiology study and catheter ablation for supraventricular arrhythmias after heart transplantation.[55,56] According to recent data, greater histocompatibility between receiver and donor favors the development of receiver-to-donor atrial connections, which represent a form of chimerism between receiver and donor, whose development is facilitated in the absence of donor-specific antibodies.[56]

Other than donor-to-receiver connections–mediated atrial arrhythmias, donor cavotricuspid isthmus–dependent AFl or atypical right or left (especially perimitral) AFl are the main types of macro-reentrant atrial tachycardia encountered in patients after heart transplantation (**Fig. 4**).[55,56]

Catheter ablation is a key therapeutic opportunity, being associated with good arrhythmia-free survival, although repeat procedures are needed in up to 29% of patients.[55,56] The procedural approach depends on the specific type and mechanism of arrhythmia[55,56]; when receiver-to-donor atrial connections are implied, they may be effectively ablated with a limited number of radiofrequency deliveries (usually 1–3).[56]

ATRIAL FLUTTER AND LUNG DISEASE

The association between several acute or chronic lung diseases and AF is well known[57]; less information is available on AFl.

As noted in the introduction, COPD is recognized as an independent risk factor for AFl.[5] Hayashi and colleagues[58] showed that among subjects with COPD undergoing catheter ablation of AF, prevalence of typical AFl was higher than in the control group of patients with AF and no lung disease (68% vs 33%, $P = .06$); furthermore, they demonstrated that conduction velocity in the cavotricuspid isthmus was lower in patients with COPD than in the control group and that prevalence of AFl was related to the severity of COPD itself.[58]

In a prospective study including patients with pulmonary arterial hypertension,[59] Olsson and colleagues[59] showed that AFl could be diagnosed in 10% of the study population (typical AFl, 9%; atypical AFl, 1%) over a follow-up period of 5 years. AFl was equally common as AF, and risk of both arrhythmias was higher in patients with more severe hemodynamic parameters of pulmonary hypertension.[59] Episodes of AFl or AF were associated with clinical deterioration[59]; furthermore, AFl and AF were independent predictors of increased mortality, a finding primary attributable to patients with permanent AF, whereas patients with transient episodes of AFl/AF had similar survival to patients without AFl/AF.[59] These data support the concept that AFl and AF are key determinants of adverse outcomes in pulmonary arterial hypertension, by contributing to further compromising the right ventricular function, and that rhythm control has the potential to reverse this vicious cycle of hemodynamic worsening and atrial arrhythmia.[59] Of note, a rhythm control strategy was effective in 88% of patients with AFl, and catheter ablation of the cavotricuspid isthmus was performed in 67% of cases.[59]

Therefore, we may speculate that conduction velocity in the right atrium may be reduced in case of increased pressure load, further compromising electrical impulse propagation in the cavotricuspid isthmus, thus setting the stage for AFl.[57,60] Atrial fibrosis, hypoxemia, and neurohormonal activation likely play modulatory roles in the process.[57,60]

Similar considerations likely apply for another emerging condition primary involving the lungs, Coronavirus disease 2019 (COVID-19): prevalence of AFl is reported to be 4% to 10% among hospitalized subjects,[61,62] with higher figures in critically ill patients. AFl and other supraventricular arrhythmias have been linked to increased mortality in COVID-19,[62] although their role is more likely that of a risk marker rather than a risk determinant. Catheter ablation should be deferred for patients with active infections, including COVID-19[63,64]; the management of AFl usually involves anticoagulation and rate/rhythm control drugs (paying particular attention to drug–drug interactions and QT interval monitoring), as well as electrical cardioversion in case of hemodynamic instability.[64,65] Evidences to guide medical management are scarce, although digitalis may be particularly suitable to control the ventricular response in critically ill patients with COVID-19 according to some investigators.[66]

ATRIAL FLUTTER IN ATHLETES

Although physical exercise is a key component of a healthy lifestyle, which is associated with reduced risk of cardiovascular events,[67,68] chronic high intensity endurance sports may lead to various bradyarrhythmias or tachyarrhythmias, especially AFl and AF, with potentially serious consequences.[67–69] Chronic endurance exercise induces a series of profound adaptations in the heart's structure and function, which are collectively known as "athlete's heart,"[70,71] a broad term that indicates the combination of symmetric

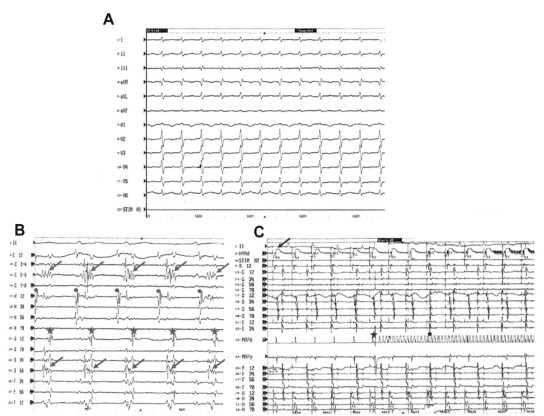

Fig. 4. Atrial flutter after heart transplantation. Five years after heart transplantation with the biatrial technique, a 38-year-old male patient develops incessant atrial tachycardia with cycle length of 375 msec and 1:1 atrioventricular conduction (A) After having excluded acute rejection with endomyocardial biopsy, the patient undergoes electrophysiology study with a multipolar basket catheter (B) which shows 1:1 conduction from the receiver's (*red dot*) to the donor's (*red star*) atrium, with evidence of conduction through receiver-to-donor atrial connections, characterized by long, fragmented, and fused electrograms (*red arrows*). An ablation catheter is positioned over the receiver-to-donor atrial connection, and radiofrequency energy is delivered, with termination of the tachycardia. Further radiofrequency pulses are delivered (C; *blue star*) during pacing from receiver's atrium (*blue arrow*), obtaining block of receiver-to-donor atrial conduction (*blue dot*) after few beats.

eccentric hypertrophy of the cardiac chambers, high vagal tone, bradycardia, and dispersion of repolarization at rest, as well as high adrenergic tone and wall stress during exercise, configurating an ideal milieu for arrhythmogenesis.[71]

There are few reports on the prevalence of AFl among athletes: in a work including 30 athletes with AF, 3 of them also had history of AFl (10% prevalence)[72]; in a study on the very long-term follow-up (38 ± 6 years) of former professional cyclists, there was a 6.5% incidence of AFl, which was higher than in a control group.[73] The mechanisms linking the practice of (especially endurance) sports and AFl have not been completely elucidated; however, we may speculate that the repeated pressure loads imposed by sessions of intense exercise on the thin walled right heart chambers may lead to marked chamber dilation and, consequently, slow conduction at the level of the cavotricuspid isthmus, predisposing to

AFl, and that these phenomena mostly occur in the aging athlete.[74,75]

The management of AFl in athletes is complicated by the fact that the high sympathetic tone during exercise often prevents an adequate rate control, and very high ventricular rates (especially in case of 1:1 atrioventricular conduction) pose the athlete at risk of major injuries. Therefore, catheter ablation of the cavotricuspid isthmus is a first-line therapeutic strategy for leisure-time and competitive athletes and is very effective in preventing AFl recurrences, with more than 90% effectiveness over long-term follow-up.[76] Cavotricuspid isthmus ablation should also be performed in athletes with both AFl and AF (either as a stand-alone procedure or together with pulmonary vein isolation for AF), especially if treatment with class I antiarrhythmic drugs is anticipated, to reduce the risk of 1:1 atrioventricular conduction.[15,77,78] Notwithstanding the effectiveness of cavotricuspid isthmus ablation for AFl, endurance sports have been recognized as a dose-dependent risk factor for AF after AFl ablation, suggesting the opportunity of regular follow-up and periodic reassessment of athletes after cavotricuspid isthmus block.[76]

According to a recent European position statement,[77] return to leisure-time sports is possible 1 week after catheter ablation (as soon as vascular access sites heal) in athletes with AFl, no structural heart disease, and no hemodynamic impact of AFl during exercise before catheter ablation; return to competitive sports may be allowed after a 1-month symptoms-free period, in athletes with no structural heart disease and without hemodynamic impact of AFl during exercise before catheter ablation.[77] Anticoagulation management should follow general guidelines, using conventional risk stratification tools (ie, the CHA_2DS_2-VASc score); participation in contact sports should be avoided in anticoagulated athletes.[77,78]

ATRIAL FLUTTER AND PREEXCITATION: THE BAD COUPLE

Subjects with preexcitation may represent a very high-risk subgroup of AFl: accessory pathways with short effective refractory period (ie, high-risk accessory pathways) have the potential for 1:1 atrioventricular conduction during AFl paroxysms, with a theoretic risk of hemodynamic collapse.[79] The diagnosis of preexcited AFl with 1:1 atrioventricular conduction is not always straightforward, and the arrhythmia is often indistinguishable from ventricular tachycardia, being characterized by a wide complex regular tachycardia with a heart rate greater than 250/min.[79] Initial management involves electrical cardioversion, and although ventricular preexcitation may be suspected based on the QRS morphology with a "precision electrocardiology" approach,[80] the diagnosis of preexcited AFl may only be confirmed with invasive electrophysiological testing.[79] Of note, when considering pharmacologic treatment of a wide complex, regular, and very rapid (ie, with a heart rate of >250 bpm) tachycardia, emergency physicians should be aware of the possibility of preexcited AFl, as drugs impairing conduction over the atrioventricular node (ie, digitalis, β-blockers, nondihydropyridine calcium channel blockers) may be especially dangerous in a patient with the Wolff-Parkinson-White syndrome, by facilitating preferential atrioventricular conduction over the accessory pathway and possibly inducing cardiovascular collapse and/or ventricular fibrillation.[79,81]

Patients with AFl and the Wolff-Parkinson-White syndrome are ideal candidates for catheter ablation of the accessory pathway, which may also reduce AFl/AF episodes: in fact, in subjects with accessory pathways, AF and AFl may occur as a result of degeneration of orthodromic atrioventricular reentrant tachycardia, due to a combination of rapid and eccentric atrial activation pattern, rate-dependent atrial effective refractory period shortening, as well as atrial pressure overload due to atrial systole occurring with closed atrioventricular valves.[82] Nonetheless, risk of AF recurrences during follow-up remains higher than that of the general population, highlighting the presence of an increased atrial vulnerability to AF among subjects with the Wolff-Parkinson-White syndrome, which may persist even after successful catheter ablation of the accessory pathway.[82] No study has examined the effects of cavotricuspid isthmus ablation in addition to accessory pathway ablation in patients with preexcited AFl, but the procedure may be indicated in case of AFl recurrences after accessory pathway ablation.

CONCLUSIONS—ATRIAL FLUTTER: ONE ARRHYTHMIA, MANY CLINICAL SCENARIOS

The science of AFl starts with the electrocardiographic identification of an atrial macro-reentrant arrhythmia. However, it is only through the accurate review of all clinical information, including comorbidities, history of heart surgery/transplant, patients' symptoms, physical examination, as well as a comprehensive approach to the assessment of the other elements provided by the electrocardiographic tracing, that the most appropriate treatment plan can be selected. In many circumstances, catheter ablation may be a key therapeutic opportunity, and its favorable efficacy/safety profile is continuously being improved by the availability of advancing technology.[83–85]

CLINICS CARE POINTS

- Atrial flutter is particularly common in some groups of patients, and may have important implications for patients' management.
- Atrial flutter may be the first manifestation of an underlying cardiomyopathy.
- Catheter ablation of the cavotricuspid isthmus should be offered early in the clinical management of patients with typical atrial flutter.
- After catheter ablation of atrial flutter, athletes may return to play following a brief period of recovery.

DISCLOSURE

A. D. Russo. is a consultant for Abbott. All other authors declared no conflict of interest.

REFERENCES

1. Einthoven W. The telecardiogramme. Arch Int Physiol 1906;4:132–41.
2. Lee KW, Yang Y, Scheinman MM. Atrial flutter: a review of its history, mechanisms, clinical features, and current therapy. Curr Probl Cardiol 2005;30(3):121–67.
3. Capucci A, Compagnucci P. Progressi nel trattamento della fibrillazione atriale [Advances in the treatment of atrial fibrillation]. G Ital Cardiol (Rome) 2021;22(9):689–96.
4. De Martino G, Compagnucci P, Mancusi C, et al. Stepwise endo-/epicardial catheter ablation for atrial fibrillation: the Mediterranea approach. J Cardiovasc Electrophysiol 2021;32(8):2107–15.
5. Granada J, Uribe W, Chyou PH, et al. Incidence and predictors of atrial flutter in the general population. J Am Coll Cardiol 2000;36(7):2242–6.
6. Gula LJ, Redfearn DP, Jenkyn KB, et al. Elevated incidence of atrial fibrillation and stroke in patients with atrial flutter-A population-based study. Can J Cardiol 2018;34(6):774–83.
7. Wijffels MC, Kirchhof CJ, Dorland R, et al. Atrial fibrillation begets atrial fibrillation. A study in awake chronically instrumented goats. Circulation 1995;92(7):1954–68.
8. Goette A, Kalman JM, Aguinaga L, et al. EHRA/HRS/APHRS/SOLAECE expert consensus on atrial cardiomyopathies: definition, characterization, and clinical implication. Europace 2016;18(10):1455–90.
9. Hirsh BJ, Copeland-Halperin RS, Halperin JL. Fibrotic atrial cardiomyopathy, atrial fibrillation, and thromboembolism: mechanistic links and clinical inferences. J Am Coll Cardiol 2015;65(20):2239–51.
10. Guichard JB, Nattel S. Atrial cardiomyopathy: a useful notion in cardiac disease management or a passing fad? J Am Coll Cardiol 2017;70(6):756–65.
11. Olshansky B, Okumura K, Hess PG, et al. Demonstration of an area of slow conduction in human atrial flutter. J Am Coll Cardiol 1990;16(7):1639–48.
12. Waki K, Saito T, Becker AE. Right atrial flutter isthmus revisited: normal anatomy favors nonuniform anisotropic conduction. J Cardiovasc Electrophysiol 2000;11(1):90–4.
13. Guichard JB, Naud P, Xiong F, et al. Comparison of atrial remodeling caused by sustained atrial flutter versus atrial fibrillation. J Am Coll Cardiol 2020;76(4):374–88.
14. Kirchhof P, Camm AJ, Goette A, et al. Early rhythm-control therapy in patients with atrial fibrillation. N Engl J Med 2020;383(14):1305–16.
15. Capucci A, Compagnucci P. Is delayed cardioversion the better approach in recent-onset atrial fibrillation? No. Intern Emerg Med 2020;15(1):5–7.
16. Diamant MJ, Andrade JG, Virani SA, et al. Heart failure and atrial flutter: a systematic review of current knowledge and practices. ESC Heart Fail 2021;8(6):4484–96.
17. Pizzale S, Lemery R, Green MS, et al. Frequency and predictors of tachycardia-induced cardiomyopathy in patients with persistent atrial flutter. Can J Cardiol 2009;25(8):469–72.
18. Oka S, Kai T, Hoshino K, et al. Rate versus rhythm control in tachycardia-induced cardiomyopathy patients with persistent atrial flutter. Int Heart J 2021;62(1):119–26.
19. Crijns HJ, Van Gelder IC, Tieleman RG, et al. Long-term outcome of electrical cardioversion in patients with chronic atrial flutter. Heart 1997;77(1):56–61.
20. Casella M, Bergonti M, Dello Russo A, et al. Endomyocardial biopsy: the forgotten piece in the arrhythmogenic cardiomyopathy puzzle. J Am Heart Assoc 2021;10(19):e021370.
21. Gasperetti A, Cappelletto C, Carrick R, et al. Association of premature ventricular contraction burden on serial holter monitoring with arrhythmic risk in patients with arrhythmogenic right ventricular cardiomyopathy. JAMA Cardiol 2022;7(4):378–85.
22. Camm CF, James CA, Tichnell C, et al. Prevalence of atrial arrhythmias in arrhythmogenic right ventricular dysplasia/cardiomyopathy. Heart Rhythm 2013;10(11):1661–8.
23. Tonet JL, Castro-Miranda R, Iwa T, et al. Frequency of supraventricular tachyarrhythmias in arrhythmogenic right ventricular dysplasia. Am J Cardiol 1991;67(13):1153.
24. Chu AF, Zado E, Marchlinski FE. Atrial arrhythmias in patients with arrhythmogenic right ventricular cardiomyopathy/dysplasia and ventricular tachycardia. Am J Cardiol 2010;106(5):720–2.
25. Saguner AM, Ganahl S, Kraus A, et al. Clinical role of atrial arrhythmias in patients with arrhythmogenic right ventricular dysplasia. Circ J 2014;78(12):2854–61.
26. Gasperetti A, James CA, Chen L, et al. Efficacy of catheter ablation for atrial arrhythmias in patients with arrhythmogenic right ventricular cardiomyopathy-A multicenter study. J Clin Med 2021;10(21):4962.
27. Gasperetti A, Schiavone M, Ziacchi M, et al. Long-term complications in patients implanted with subcutaneous implantable cardioverter-defibrillators: real-world data from the extended ELISIR experience. Heart Rhythm 2021;18(12):2050–8.
28. Adabag AS, Casey SA, Kuskowski MA, et al. Spectrum and prognostic significance of arrhythmias on ambulatory Holter electrocardiogram in hypertrophic cardiomyopathy. J Am Coll Cardiol 2005;45(5):697–704.

29. Schiavone WA, Maloney JD, Lever HM, et al. Electrophysiologic studies of patients with hypertrophic cardiomyopathy presenting with syncope of undetermined etiology. Pacing Clin Electrophysiol 1986; 9(4):476–81.

30. Fananapazir L, Tracy CM, Leon MB, et al. Electrophysiologic abnormalities in patients with hypertrophic cardiomyopathy. A consecutive analysis in 155 patients. Circulation 1989;80(5):1259–68.

31. Zhang HD, Ding L, Weng SX, et al. Characteristics and long-term ablation outcomes of supraventricular arrhythmias in hypertrophic cardiomyopathy: a 10-year, single-center experience. Front Cardiovasc Med 2021;8:766571.

32. Kumar S, Baldinger SH, Gandjbakhch E, et al. Long-term arrhythmic and nonarrhythmic outcomes of lamin A/C mutation carriers. J Am Coll Cardiol 2016;68(21):2299–307.

33. Kumar S, Stevenson WG, John RM. Arrhythmias in dilated cardiomyopathy. Card Electrophysiol Clin 2015;7(2):221–33.

34. Cioffi GM, Gasperetti A, Tersalvi G, et al. Etiology and device therapy in complete atrioventricular block in pediatric and young adult population: contemporary review and new perspectives. J Cardiovasc Electrophysiol 2021;32(11):3082–94.

35. Meune C, Van Berlo JH, Anselme F, et al. Primary prevention of sudden death in patients with lamin A/C gene mutations. N Engl J Med 2006;354(2): 209–10.

36. Fishbein MC, Siegel RJ, Thompson CE, et al. Sudden death of a carrier of X-linked Emery-Dreifuss muscular dystrophy. Ann Intern Med 1993;119(9): 900–5.

37. Kumar S, Androulakis AF, Sellal JM, et al. Multicenter experience with catheter ablation for ventricular tachycardia in lamin A/C cardiomyopathy. Circ Arrhythm Electrophysiol 2016;9(8):e004357.

38. Barbhaiya CR, Kumar S, Baldinger SH, et al. Electrophysiologic assessment of conduction abnormalities and atrial arrhythmias associated with amyloid cardiomyopathy. Heart Rhythm 2016;13(2):383–90.

39. Maurer MS, Hanna M, Grogan M, et al. Genotype and phenotype of transthyretin cardiac amyloidosis: THAOS (transthyretin amyloid outcome survey). J Am Coll Cardiol 2016;68(2):161–72.

40. Sayed RH, Rogers D, Khan F, et al. A study of implanted cardiac rhythm recorders in advanced cardiac AL amyloidosis. Eur Heart J 2015;36(18):1098–105.

41. El-Am EA, Dispenzieri A, Melduni RM, et al. Direct current cardioversion of atrial arrhythmias in adults with cardiac amyloidosis. J Am Coll Cardiol 2019; 73(5):589–97.

42. Dale Z, Chandrashekar P, Al-Rashdan L, et al. Management strategies for atrial fibrillation and flutter in patients with transthyretin cardiac amyloidosis. Am J Cardiol 2021;157:107–14.

43. Groh WJ. Arrhythmias in the muscular dystrophies. Heart Rhythm 2012;9(11):1890–5.

44. Feingold B, Mahle WT, Auerbach S, et al. Management of cardiac involvement associated with neuromuscular diseases: a scientific statement from the american heart association. Circulation 2017; 136(13):e200–31.

45. Pelargonio G, Dello Russo A, Sanna T, et al. Myotonic dystrophy and the heart. Heart 2002;88(6): 665–70.

46. Finsterer J, Stöllberger C. Atrial fibrillation/flutter in myopathies. Int J Cardiol 2008;128(3):304–10.

47. Bhakta D, Shen C, Kron J, et al. Pacemaker and implantable cardioverter-defibrillator use in a US myotonic dystrophy type 1 population. J Cardiovasc Electrophysiol 2011;22(12):1369–75.

48. Wahbi K, Sebag FA, Lellouche N, et al. Atrial flutter in myotonic dystrophy type 1: patient characteristics and clinical outcome. Neuromuscul Disord 2016; 26(3):227–33.

49. Dello Russo A, Pelargonio G, Parisi Q, et al. Widespread electroanatomic alterations of right cardiac chambers in patients with myotonic dystrophy type 1. J Cardiovasc Electrophysiol 2006;17(1):34–40.

50. Groh WJ, Groh MR, Saha C, et al. Electrocardiographic abnormalities and sudden death in myotonic dystrophy type 1. N Engl J Med 2008;358(25): 2688–97.

51. Chambers DC, Yusen RD, Cherikh WS, et al. The registry of the international society for heart and lung transplantation: thirty-fourth adult lung and heart-lung transplantation report-2017; focus theme: allograft ischemic time. J Heart Lung Transplant 2017;36(10):1047–59.

52. Thajudeen A, Stecker EC, Shehata M, et al. Arrhythmias after heart transplantation: mechanisms and management. J Am Heart Assoc 2012;1(2):e001461.

53. Vaseghi M, Boyle NG, Kedia R, et al. Supraventricular tachycardia after orthotopic cardiac transplantation. J Am Coll Cardiol 2008;51(23):2241–9.

54. Cui G, Tung T, Kobashigawa J, et al. Increased incidence of atrial flutter associated with the rejection of heart transplantation. Am J Cardiol 2001;88(3): 280–4.

55. Mouhoub Y, Laredo M, Varnous S, et al. Catheter ablation of organized atrial arrhythmias in orthotopic heart transplantation. J Heart Lung Transpl 2017. https://doi.org/10.1016/j.healun.2017.07.022.

56. Herweg B, Nellaiyappan M, Welter-Frost AM, et al. Immuno-electrophysiological mechanisms of functional electrical connections between recipient and donor heart in patients with orthotopic heart transplantation presenting with atrial arrhythmias. Circ Arrhythm Electrophysiol 2021;14(4):e008751.

57. Simons SO, Elliott A, Sastry M, et al. Chronic obstructive pulmonary disease and atrial fibrillation:

an interdisciplinary perspective. Eur Heart J 2021; 42(5):532–40.

58. Hayashi T, Fukamizu S, Hojo R, et al. Prevalence and electrophysiological characteristics of typical atrial flutter in patients with atrial fibrillation and chronic obstructive pulmonary disease. Europace 2013; 15(12):1777–83.

59. Olsson KM, Nickel NP, Tongers J, et al. Atrial flutter and fibrillation in patients with pulmonary hypertension. Int J Cardiol 2013;167(5):2300–5.

60. Medi C, Kalman JM, Ling LH, et al. Atrial electrical and structural remodeling associated with long-standing pulmonary hypertension and right ventricular hypertrophy in humans. J Cardiovasc Electrophysiol 2012;23(6):614–20.

61. Coromilas EJ, Kochav S, Goldenthal I, et al. Worldwide survey of COVID-19-associated arrhythmias. Circ Arrhythm Electrophysiol 2021; 14(3):e009458.

62. Peltzer B, Manocha KK, Ying X, et al. Outcomes and mortality associated with atrial arrhythmias among patients hospitalized with COVID-19. J Cardiovasc Electrophysiol 2020;31(12):3077–85.

63. Compagnucci P, Volpato G, Pascucci R, et al. Impact of the COVID-19 pandemic on a tertiary-level electrophysiology laboratory in Italy. Circ Arrhythm Electrophysiol 2020;13(9):e008774.

64. Lakkireddy DR, Chung MK, Deering TF, et al. Guidance for rebooting electrophysiology through the COVID-19 pandemic from the heart rhythm society and the American heart association electrocardiography and arrhythmias committee of the council on clinical cardiology: endorsed by the American college of cardiology. Heart Rhythm 2020;17(9):e242–54.

65. Magnocavallo M, Vetta G, Della Rocca D, et al. Prevalence, management, and outcome of atrial fibrillation and other supraventricular arrhythmias in COVID-19 patients. Card Electrophysiol Clin 2022; 14(1):1–9.

66. Siniorakis E, Arvanitakis S, Katsianis A, et al. Atrial fibrillation and flutter in patients hospitalized for COVID-19: the challenging role of digoxin. J Cardiovasc Electrophysiol 2021;32(3):878–9.

67. Volpato G, Falanga U, Cipolletta L, et al. Sports activity and arrhythmic risk in cardiomyopathies and channelopathies: a critical review of European guidelines on sports cardiology in patients with cardiovascular diseases. Medicina (Kaunas) 2021; 57(4):308.

68. Compagnucci P, Volpato G, Falanga U, et al. Myocardial inflammation, sports practice, and sudden cardiac death: 2021 update. Medicina (Kaunas) 2021;57(3):277.

69. Dello Russo A, Compagnucci P, Casella M, et al. Ventricular arrhythmias in athletes: role of a comprehensive diagnostic workup. Heart Rhythm 2022; 19(1):90–9.

70. Fogante M, Agliata G, Basile MC, et al. Cardiac imaging in athlete's heart: the role of the radiologist. Medicina (Kaunas) 2021;57(5):455.

71. Heidbuchel H. The athlete's heart is a proarrhythmic heart, and what that means for clinical decision making. Europace 2018;20(9):1401–11.

72. Hoogsteen J, Schep G, Van Hemel NM, et al. Paroxysmal atrial fibrillation in male endurance athletes. A 9-year follow up. Europace 2004;6(3):222–8.

73. Baldesberger S, Bauersfeld U, Candinas R, et al. Sinus node disease and arrhythmias in the long-term follow-up of former professional cyclists. Eur Heart J 2008;29(1):71–8.

74. D'Ascenzi F, Anselmi F, Focardi M, et al. Atrial enlargement in the athlete's heart: assessment of atrial function may help distinguish adaptive from pathologic remodeling. J Am Soc Echocardiogr 2018;31(2):148–57.

75. Stadiotti I, Lippi M, Maione AS, et al. Cardiac biomarkers and autoantibodies in endurance athletes: potential similarities with arrhythmogenic cardiomyopathy pathogenic mechanisms. Int J Mol Sci 2021;22(12):6500.

76. Heidbüchel H, Anné W, Willems R, et al. Endurance sports is a risk factor for atrial fibrillation after ablation for atrial flutter. Int J Cardiol 2006;107(1):67–72.

77. Heidbuchel H, Adami PE, Antz M, et al. Recommendations for participation in leisure-time physical activity and competitive sports in patients with arrhythmias and potentially arrhythmogenic conditions: Part 1: supraventricular arrhythmias. A position statement of the Section of Sports Cardiology and Exercise from the European Association of Preventive Cardiology (EAPC) and the European Heart Rhythm Association (EHRA), both associations of the European Society of Cardiology. Eur J Prev Cardiol 2021;28(14):1539–51. https://doi.org/10.1177/2047487320925635.

78. Zipes DP, Link MS, Ackerman MJ, et al. Eligibility and disqualification recommendations for competitive athletes with cardiovascular abnormalities: task force 9: arrhythmias and conduction defects: a scientific statement from the American heart association and American college of cardiology. J Am Coll Cardiol 2015;66(21):2412–23.

79. Nelson JG, Zhu DW. Atrial flutter with 1:1 conduction in undiagnosed Wolff-Parkinson-White syndrome. J Emerg Med 2014;46(5):e135–40.

80. Bagliani G, De Ponti R, Notaristefano F, et al. Ventricular preexcitation: an anomalous wave interfering with the ordered ventricular activation. Card Electrophysiol Clin 2020;12(4):447–64.

81. Delise P, Sciarra L. Sudden cardiac death in patients with ventricular preexcitation. Card Electrophysiol Clin 2020;12(4):519–25.

82. Centurión OA, Shimizu A, Isomoto S, et al. Mechanisms for the genesis of paroxysmal atrial fibrillation

in the Wolff Parkinson-White syndrome: intrinsic atrial muscle vulnerability vs. electrophysiological properties of the accessory pathway. Europace 2008;10(3):294–302.

83. Compagnucci P, Volpato G, Falanga U, et al. Recent advances in three-dimensional electroanatomical mapping guidance for the ablation of complex atrial and ventricular arrhythmias. J Interv Card Electrophysiol 2021;61(1):37–43.

84. Bergonti M, Dello Russo A, Sicuso R, et al. Long-term outcomes of near-zero radiation ablation of paroxysmal supraventricular tachycardia: a comparison with fluoroscopy-guided approach. JACC Clin Electrophysiol 2021;7(9):1108–17.

85. Compagnucci P, Dello Russo A, Bergonti M, et al. Ablation index predicts successful ablation of focal atrial tachycardia: results of a multicenter study. J Clin Med 2022;11(7):1802.

Antiarrhythmic Drug Therapy in the Treatment of Acute and Chronic Atrial Flutter

Martina Amadori, MD[a,b], Antonio Rapacciuolo, MD, PhD[c,d], Igor Diemberger, MD, PhD[a,b,d],*

KEYWORDS

- Antiarrhythmic • Rhythm control • Rate control • Cardioversion • Sinus rhythm • Atrial flutter

KEY POINTS

- Atrial flutter and atrial fibrillation are not 2 isolated clinical identities. However, the overlap in terms of substrate, occurrence, and response to specific treatments varies from patient to patient.
- For acute rhythm control of atrial flutter Class III agents are preferable over Class I antiarrhythmic drugs in terms of efficacy and side effects.
- Acute management of atrial flutter needs a comprehensive evaluation to personalize the short and long-term treatment.

INTRODUCTION

Atrial flutter is the most common sustained cardiac arrhythmia after atrial fibrillation. It is classically defined as synchronized supraventricular tachycardia characterized by a regular activation at a rate between 240 and 400/min. The typical atrioventricular (AV) conduction is 2:1, meaning a ventricular rate of 150 beat/min with the usual atrial rate of 300 beats/min. The electrogenic mechanism underlying the development of atrial flutter requires the presence of a macro-circuit of reentry, localized in most cases in the right atrium (typical atrial flutter). However, there are cases in which this circuit has a different localization, such as around scars of a previous surgical intervention or in the left atrium (atypical atrial flutter). These electroanatomic characteristics are relevant for

the pharmacologic treatment as well as for transcatheter ablation.

ATRIAL FLUTTER ELECTROANATOMIC MECHANISMS AND THE RELATIONSHIP WITH ATRIAL FIBRILLATION

Atrial flutter has a macro-reentrant mechanism and in the classic form the reentrant wave front travels up the inter-atrial septum and down the right atrial free wall or vice versa.[1,2] As elegantly discussed by Waldo,[3] the development and maintenance of this reentrant circuit requires 2 elements: the lateral boundaries and an appropriate cycle length. For the typical atrial flutter, we have 2 boundaries: one being fixed (anatomic), the tricuspid valve annulus, and the other almost always being functional, a line of the block between

[a] Department of Experimental, Diagnostic and Specialty Medicine, Institute of Cardiology, University of Bologna, Via Massarenti 9, Bologna 40138, Italy; [b] Cardiology Division, IRCCS AOU di Bologna, Bologna, via Massarenti 9, 40138 Bologna, Italy; [c] Department of Advanced Biomedical Science, University of Naples Federico II, Corso Umberto I 40, 80138 Naples, Italy; [d] Pharmacologic Area of AIAC (Associazione Italiana Aritmologia e Cardiostimolazione), Via Biagio Petrocelli 226, Rome 00173, Italy

* Corresponding author.

E-mail address: igor.diemberger@unibo.it

Card Electrophysiol Clin 14 (2022) 533–545
https://doi.org/10.1016/j.ccep.2022.05.006
1877-9182/22/© 2022 Elsevier Inc. All rights reserved.

the venae cava. This is very important, since as shown in many canine models the easiest way of inducing atrial flutter in the dog is to produce an intercaval incision[4] similarly to what occurs in patients undergoing cardiac surgery. However, there are several models able to provoke atrial flutter in dogs' atria without the need to create any incisional block[5,6] similarly to the larger cohorts of patients with clinical atrial flutter. In these cases the critical site to create the inter-caval block is the crista terminalis.[3] Interestingly, Waldo and colleagues propose that the conversion of atrial fibrillation to flutter that occurs in some patients after the administration of an antiarrhythmic drug is probably due to the development of a functional line of block elicited by their action on the electrophysiological properties of this area. Another interesting observation is that typical atrial flutter infrequently starts after a premature atrial complex such as what occurs in AV node reentrant tachycardia, as in many cases the initial arrhythmia is more similar to atrial fibrillation. The possible explanation is that the fibrillatory conduction creates the inter-caval functional block with the subsequent development of atrial fibrillation. Moreover, another interesting observation regards the importance of the cycle length of the atrial flutter to enable the maintenance of arrhythmia. When the cycle length is too short the final arrhythmia will be atrial fibrillation, while a critical increase in cycle length will lead to the development of atrial flutter. In this regard, it is interesting to analyze the results recently published by Guichard and colleagues[7] on the different impacts of atrial fibrillation and atrial flutter on atrial remodeling. The authors created a canine model of atrial flutter through the production of an intercaval radiofrequency lesion in 24 dogs. All dogs had an atrioventricular node ablation and a ventricular pacemaker implanted and were paced at 80 beats/min, to overcome the bias of different AV conduction. The dogs were divided into 4 groups regarding the rhythm maintained after creating the lesion: atrial flutter, atrial fibrillation (with intercaval lesion), atrial fibrillation (without intercaval lesion), and sinus rhythm (with intercaval lesion). They showed that the effective refractory period (ERP) of the atria was similarly reduced in each of the 3 atrial fibrillation/flutter groups and all showed an enhanced vulnerability to the induction of atrial fibrillation. However, structural remodeling was more pronounced in dogs after atrial fibrillation both in terms of atrial dilatation, fibrosis, and inflammation. While all these considerations underline the strict connection between atrial fibrillation and atrial flutter, not all the patients are similar, leading to a spectrum of subjects ranging from patients with "pure" atrial flutter (usually young patients or subjects with surgical lines of block) to patients with only atrial fibrillation. In the middle, we have a gradient of risk factors increasing the occurrence of both arrhythmias, the expression of different characteristics: CHADSVASC score, inter-atrial conduction delay, associated comorbidities.

CLASSIFICATION OF ANTIARRHYTHMIC DRUGS

The classification of antiarrhythmic drugs still widely used in the clinical setting is that of Vaughan Williams, Singh, and Houswirth, dating back to 1974, with minor changes made later by Harrison and Campbell (**Table 1**). This Classification divides antiarrhythmic drugs according to some electrophysiological effects observed in vitro.

In 1991, the SIC Arrhythmia Study Group revisited this Classification of antiarrhythmic drugs with the introduction of *Sicilian Gambit,* the vulnerable parameter of every single molecule used as an antiarrhythmic. This approach enabled the identification of all the effects of each specific drug, as many drugs have multiple effects that were not considered by the Vaughan Williams classification, explaining the reasons for several clinical findings like the relatively low incidence of torsade de pointes associated with amiodarone despite the prolongation in ventricular repolarization (**Table 2**).

The development of new antiarrhythmic drugs has been progressively reduced over time, due to the finding of low efficacy in the long-term maintenance of the sinus rhythm, the development of ICDs for the control of ventricular arrhythmias, and trans-catheter ablation of foci of atrial or ventricular arrhythmia. Many commercially available antiarrhythmic drugs have been used for the treatment of atrial flutter, although few have been the subject of specific studies.

Later in discussion, we report the characteristics of each individual drug with the main evidence present in the literature, summarizing the main electrophysiological characteristics. We will analyze the current Guidelines in the light of what has already been stated.[9,10]

ANTIARRHYTHMIC DRUGS CHARACTERISTICS AND EFFECTS ON ATRIAL FLUTTER
Class IA Antiarrhythmic Drugs

Quinidine
This drug exerts several electrophysiological effects[11] on Na + channels with the reduction of phase 0 of the action potential, decrease of automatism

Table 1
Antiarrhythmic drugs according to the modified Vaughan Williams classification

	Class I	Class II	Class III	Class IV
	Drugs with direct action on monophasic action potential (Na + channel blockers)	Beta-blockers	Drugs that prolong repolarization	Calcium channel blockers
IA	Phase 0 depression, slowing of conduction, prolongation of repolarization	Acebutolol, atenolol, esmolol, labetalol, metoprolol, nadolol, propranolol, pindolol	Amiodarone, Dronedarone, Sotalol, Ibutilide, Dofetilide	Verapamil, diltiazem
	Quinidine, procainamide, disopyramide			
IB	Reduced effect on phase 0 in the normal tissue; depression in pathologic tissue. Shortening repolarization			
	Lidocaine, mexiletine			
IC	Marked depression of phase 0 and slowing of conduction. Not significant effect on repolarization			
	Propafenone, flecainide			

and slowing down of conduction and I_{kr} enhancing the risk of torsade de pointes. It also blocks I_{TO1} and I_{KUR} at the level of atrial myocytes. The drug also exhibits alpha-blocking and vagolytic effects that can lead to arterial hypotension and compensatory reflex tachycardia.[12] As long as 3 decades ago, quinidine was still one of the most used antiarrhythmic drugs. It was slowly abandoned because of a combination of factors including safety concerns and new, effective, therapeutic alternatives.[13] We lack specific studies on patients with atrial flutter. On the other hand, quinidine has been demonstrated to be a life-saving drug able to control ventricular arrhythmias in patients with channelopathies, in particular the Brugada syndrome, early repolarization syndrome, short QT syndrome and idiopathic ventricular fibrillation.[3] Notably these channelopathies have been associated with atrial fibrillation but unfrequently with atrial flutter.

Procainamide

Procainamide is a medication used to treat several arrhythmias including ventricular tachycardia, atrial flutter/fibrillation, AV nodal reentrant tachycardia, and Wolf–Parkinson–White syndrome.

Procainamide usage has increased in recent years, and it is now seen as a viable option in acute settings. Stambler and colleagues[14] studied the effects of antiarrhythmic drugs in patients with typical atrial flutter. The administration of procainamide provoked an increase in atrial flutter cycle length greater than the increase in monophasic action potential duration. They evidenced that the effect on conduction velocity was more pronounced in the low right atrial isthmus during atrial flutter, which seems the principal effect for conversion to sinus rhythm. From a clinical point of view, procainamide has been used for chemical cardioversion in atrial flutter and atrial fibrillation in patients with emergency department. Stiell and colleagues analyzed the effect of the use of IV procainamide in 341 patients over 5 years. Adverse events were infrequent and included hypotension, bradycardia, atrioventricular block, and ventricular tachycardia. There were no cases of torsades de pointes, cerebrovascular accidents, or death. Most patients (94.4%) were discharged home. IV procainamide had a 52% conversion rate of atrial fibrillation to normal sinus and a 28% conversion rate from atrial flutter to normal sinus.

Table 2
Target of antiarrhythmic drugs according to the Sicilian Gambit Classification

Drug	Fast	Medium	Slow	Ca^{2+}	K$^+$	α	β	M$_2$	P	Na/k ATPasi
		Na$^+$								
Adenosine									++	
Amiodarone	+			+	+++	++	++			
Quinidine		+++			++	+		+		
Diltiazem				+++						
Digoxin								++		+++
Disopyramide		+++			++			+		
Dofetilide					+++					
Dronedarone	+			+	+++	++	+++			
Flecainide			+++		+					
Ibutilide			(+++)a		+					
Lidocaine	+									
Mexiletine	+									
Nadolol							+++			
Procainamide		+++			++					
Propafenone		+++					+			
Propranolol	+						+++			
Sotalol					+++		+++			
Verapamil	+			+++		++				
Vernakalant	+			+	++					

The power of action on specific channels/receptors is expressed as low = +; moderate = ++; high = +++.

ª Ibutilide has a unique mechanism of action for a class III agent as it prolongs repolarization in the atria and ventricle by enhancing the inward depolarizing, slow sodium current.[8]

Disopyramide

Disopyramide exerts a blocking effect of the Na + channels, with a slow recovery from the blockade, and of the I$_{kr}$, I$_{k1}$, and I$_{to}$ channels with consequent depression of the phase 0 of the action potential, slowing the conduction and prolongation of the repolarization and refractory periods. The drug also has important effects of blocking muscarinic receptors and a significant negative inotropic action. Disopyramide can be used in the prevention of recurrence of AF, with a profile similar to that of quinidine; however, the vagolytic effect could cause a compensatory reflex tachycardia for which a combination with rate control drugs is always necessary. In literature, there is no evidence of the use of disopyramide alone to convert atrial flutter, but there are some reports of a hybrid approach combining i.v. disopyramide with atrial pacing, showing some grade of efficacy.[15] After drug infusion, the authors evidenced both a significant increase in cycle length of the arrhythmia and of the ERP. Moreover, the excitable gap of the circuit significantly increased

suggesting that also for disopyramide, the drug exerts its prominent effect by depressing conduction velocity. A wider excitable gap allows easier penetration of the stimulus in the reentry circuit and accounts for the beneficial effects of type IA antiarrhythmic drugs on the termination of atrial flutter by overdrive pacing.

Later in discussion, we summarize the main side effects and drug interactions of class IA antiarrhythmics (**Table 3**).

Class IB Antiarrhythmic Drugs

Class I antiarrhythmic drugs share the ability to reduce the upstroke velocity and the amplitude of the action potential by the block of activated/inactivated sodium channels.[16] They show use-dependent block because this block develops when the channel is used, and it is not removed at the next action potential. For this reason Class I antiarrhythmic drugs would produce only minor effects at normal heart rates, but they inhibit the sodium current to a far greater degree during

Table 3
Side effects and therapeutic interactions of class IA antiarrhythmic drugs

	Adverse Effects	Therapeutic Interactions
Quinidine sulfate Dihydroquinidine	QRS enlargement, asystole, long QT, torsade de pointes, PV, arterial hypotension, cinchonism, acute hemolytic anemia, agranulocytosis, thrombocytopenia, angioedema, asthma, respiratory arrest	Increased plasma concentrations: amiodarone, verapamil, diltiazem, propranolol, digoxin. Increased effect of oral anticoagulants
Procainamide	QRS enlargement, asystole, FV, arterial hypotension, lupoid syndrome, acute hemolytic anemia, neutropenia, agranulocytosis, thrombocytopenia	Increased plasma concentrations: amiodarone and propranolol
Disopyramide	QRS enlargement, long QT, torsade de pointes, arterial hypotension, heart failure	Increased contractile depression: beta-blockers, calcium channel blockers

tachycardia. Notably, class Ib drugs block sodium channels only at the inactivated state, being more effective in tissues with long action potentials (ventricular muscle and Purkinje fibers) than with shorter action potentials (atrial muscle), and they will subsequently be more effective to treat ventricular rather than atrial arrhythmias. Moreover, Classes Ia,c drugs can block the delayed rectifier K (Ik) and the transient outward (Ito) K currents, increasing postrepolarization refractoriness together with decreasing conduction velocity.

Lidocaine
Lidocaine is a local anesthetic that blocks the Na + channels, decreasing the duration of the action potential and refractory period.[17] Former studies on canine models showed a minimal effect on the acute conversion of atrial flutter without any protective effect against recurrences, when compared with class Ia and class III antiarrhythmic drugs.[17,18] The reason advocated by the authors is the action limited to an increase of the cycle length of the arrhythmia, which is less pronounced with respect to class Ia drugs in the absence of any effect on atrial refractory period. From a clinical point of view, this can lead to a relatively high risk of 1:1 AV conduction (both in atrial flutter and atrial fibrillation).

Mexiletine
Mexiletine is an analog of lidocaine with which it shares the spectrum of action but can be used for long-term oral treatment since it does not undergo the hepatic first-pass effect. It has been used in the past for the treatment of postinfarction

ventricular arrhythmias,[19] and there are some reports of its use in patients with recurrent ventricular tachycardia, usually in carriers of implantable defibrillators to interrupt/prevent arrhythmic storms.[20] Similarly to lidocaine, there is no evidence in the literature of the use of mexiletine such as antiarrhythmic agent in atrial flutter and the agents share similar limitations in this setting due to the specific electrophysiologic effect, including the risk of 1:1 AV conduction during atrial flutter due to a decrease in the electrical conduction of the flutter circuit without significant slowing in AV conduction.

Class 1C Antiarrhythmic Drugs

Flecainide
Flecainide exerts its antiarrhythmic effect by blocking Na + channels in the activation phase, characterized by slow constant dissociation and consequent slowing down of the use-dependent and dose-dependent Vmax.[21] A blockade of the ionic current I_{to} in atrial cells and with an unequal distribution between epicardium and endocardium has been observed, leading to dispersion of repolarization between epicardium and endocardium and the appearance of postrepolarization refractoriness at the epicardial level. Flecainide does not exert depressive effects on the automatism or conduction of the sinus node; prolongs the refractory period of the right atrium, right ventricle, and AV node and slows down interatrial conduction. The greatest effect exerted on the His-Purkinje system.[21,22] The principal use of flecainide in current clinical practice, is in the rhythm control strategy of atrial fibrillation[23] either in acute conversion,

by iv or oral administration (ie, pill in the pocket strategy),[24] or for preventing arrhythmia recurrences after sinus rhythm restoration.[25] The use of flecainide in the context of atrial flutter is more debated. There are some positive experiences in animal models after the creation of a fixed anatomic block.[26,27] However, more deluding results were found in clinical settings[28,29] with the exception of some reports in infant, especially fetal, settings.[30,31] The reason for these findings is the specific electroanatomic substrate in adult human atrial flutter versus the canine model and the flutter that occurs in infants. In the first case, the absence of a fixed line of block can enable a more "flexible" variation of the circuit length favoring the stability of the flutter circuit until very prolonged conduction times are reached. Moreover, the dog and infant right atrium has smaller size with respect to the human adult leading to a higher chance that a similar increase in atrial conduction time can reach a critical value leading to instability of the atrial flutter circuit. Notably, the use of flecainide for atrial fibrillation both for acute conversion and prophylaxis is associated with the risk of flutter with 1:1 AV conduction. For this reason, it is recommended the association with calcium channel blockers or beta-blockers which in some cases can also increase the chance of sinus rhythm maintenance in long term.[13]

Propafenone

The most important antiarrhythmic effect of propafenone is the blocking of Na + channels in the activation phase, also there is an action of depression on the channels I_{kr} and I_{kur}. Propafenone also exerts a competitive antagonism action against beta2-adrenergic receptors. High concentrations of propafenone inhibit Ca++ channels on ventricular fibers, with a Verapamil-like effect. From the electrophysiological point of view, the drug reduces the conduction rate of the SA node and increases the atrial, nodal, and ventricular refractory period. Like flecainide, it also has a slowing effect on the conduction of the impulse along the accessory pathways, both in the anterograde and retrograde directions. The clinical uses of propafenone are similar to those of flecainide, in that the drug is effective in preventing recurrences of AF following electrical or pharmacologic cardioversion and can be used as part of the pharmacologic cardioversion of AF. Propafenone as well can be used as a self-administerable home therapy in case of paroxysmal arrhythmic events (*pill in the pocket*). Propafenone is not indicated in the treatment of ventricular arrhythmias. The limitations of the use of propafenone in the context of human atrial flutter are similar to those reported for flecainide (**Table 4**).[29,32]

Class II Antiarrhythmic Drugs

Class II antiarrhythmic drugs are represented by beta-blockers which, through binding to beta-adrenergic receptors, determine a competitive and reversible antagonism action of beta-agonist agents, thus leading to a negative chronotropic, inotropic and lusitropic effect. The rationale for their use in clinical practice as antiarrhythmic drugs lies in the fact that in itself adrenergic stimulation has a pro-arrhythmic effect. They, therefore, have a clinical indication in those conditions in which there is an increased adrenergic tone. Adrenergic stimulation, in fact, represents a pro-arrhythmic factor through various mechanisms: first of all, the increase in heart rate favors the establishment of reentry circuits both in basic conditions and in the presence of ischemic areas of the myocardium, for the establishment of unidirectional conduction blocks in areas of the myocardium with slowed conduction: therefore, one of the mechanisms underlying the antiarrhythmic effect of beta-blockers is the negative chronotropic effect. Other mechanisms of minor importance include the reduction of ventricular refractory dispersion and the reduction of both early and late postdepolarizations (through the inhibition of intracellular Ca++ increase, mediated by adrenergic agonists). Beta-blockers, moreover, together with nondihydropyridine calcium channel blockers and digoxin, represent *rate control* therapy in atrial fibrillation, both in the acute and chronic phases. Similarly to atrial fibrillation, the use of beta-blockers is preferred in subjects with heart failure.[9,23] However, the absence of the concealed conduction that characterizes atrial fibrillation leads to relatively higher ventricular rates during atrial flutter. For these reasons, the use of beta-blockers as a stand-alone strategy for rate-control in patients with atrial flutter is unfrequently successful.

Class III Antiarrhythmics

Such drugs share, as a class effect, the blocking of the K+ channels of cardiomyocytes, resulting in an increase in the duration of action potential and refractoriness.

Amiodarone

Amiodarone is characterized by a very wide spectrum of action, in fact, despite being classified according to Vaughan Williams as a class III drug, it has an effect on multiple targets (see above). Amiodarone is indicated as a first-choice antiarrhythmic drug only in the management of patients with severe heart disease, due to the absence of negative inotropic effects and the very low

Table 4
Adverse effects and drug interaction of class IC antiarrhythmic drugs

	Adverse Events	Therapeutic Interactions
Flecainide	Ventricular and supraventricular arrhythmias, heart failure, tremors, diplopia, headache	Increased plasma concentrations of amiodarone. Increased contractile depression: beta-blockers calcium channel blockers
Propafenone	Ventricular and supraventricular arrhythmias, asthma, constipation, headache, tremors	Increased plasma concentrations: digoxin, metoprolol, propranolol

tendency to proarrhythmic effects[9,23] The use of amiodarone is severely limited by the numerous extracardiac side effects, being reserved to elderly patients or patients with structural heart disease (eg, with left ventricular dysfunction and/or cardiomyopathies). The use for atrial fibrillation includes the prophylaxis of recurrences and pharmacologic conversion to sinus rhythm. However, the time to conversion is relatively long with respect to other antiarrhythmic drugs. With regard to atrial flutter, the use of amiodarone is reserved, in acute, to patients not responsive to first and second-line therapies, having little effect in acute as an antiarrhythmic drug, resulting instead more effective in rate control therapy. During chronic therapy, serious side effects may occur as a result of tissue accumulation of the drug, especially at the level of the cornea, lungs, thyroid, and skin. Maintenance of sinus rhythm with amiodarone was compared with ablation in a randomized study on elderly patients by Da Costa A and colleagues.[33] They enrolled 103 patients (age ≥70) with a first symptomatic episode of ECG-documented atrial flutter with right-isthmus involvement, confirmed by electrophysiology study. No subject had previously received AAD therapy, 61% had structural heart disease, 68% had hypertension, and 24% had histories of atrial fibrillation. Both strategies obtained sinus rhythm restoration (in many cases with the additional use of cardioversion in the amiodarone group). During a mean follow-up of 13 months, recurrence of atrial flutter was significantly less common in the ablation group than in the amiodarone group (4% vs 30%), and the groups had similar rates of recurrent atrial fibrillation (25% and 18%, respectively).

Dronedarone

Dronedarone is an analog of amiodarone, with which it shares pharmacodynamic characteristics, but has a better tolerability profile. As this drug was developed to overcome most of the side effects associated with amiodarone in the chronic

treatment of atrial fibrillation the available studies were focused on this use. However, the efficacy of dronedarone in the maintenance of sinus rhythm is lower with respect to amiodarone and more similar to that of flecainide with a different spectrum of side effects.[34–36] Despite current indication to prevent recurrences of atrial fibrillation or flutter as a whole cohort of subjects, we have no specific data or post hoc analysis on the efficacy of dronedarone for patients with atrial flutter. It is conceivable that dronedarone may share similar efficacy to other class III drugs but data are warranted in this specific field.

Sotalol

Sotalol is a racemic mixture of 2 isomers, d-sotalol, and l-sotalol. Both isomers are blockers of the rapid component (I_{kr}) of the late repolarization current, without the involvement of the slow component (I_{ks}) of that current. Being a blocker only of the rapid component of the late repolarization current, which prevails at low frequencies, sotalol exerts at these frequencies a greater antiarrhythmic effect, which is progressively lost at high frequencies, when late repolarization dominates the slow component of the late repolarization current. Sotalol is inferior in comparison to amiodarone in the atrial fibrillation setting, especially to prevent arrhythmia recurrences after sinus rhythm restoration.[37] The use of sotalol in patients with atrial flutter is supported by several animal studies[38,39] with Y-shaped atrial lesion, showing a selective prolongation of atrial refractoriness with little effect on conduction velocity or flutter cycle length. However, 2 randomized human studies showed limited efficacy to restore sinus rhythm in patients with atrial flutter.[40,41] The use of sotalol for prophylaxis is more supported,[9,42] albeit the proarrhythmic risk should be carefully weighted in these cases. Of particular importance is to avoid combination with other drugs that lengthen the QT interval and QTc should be monitored and in case of a QTc greater than 500 ms the drug should be discontinued. One last comment regards the use in the pediatric population, as there are some promising reports[43] but additional more structured studies are warranted in these settings.

Ibutilide

Ibutilide is a "pure" class III antiarrhythmic drug. At a cellular level, it exerts 2 main actions: induction of a persistent Na + current sensitive to dihydropyridine Ca2+ channel blockers and potent inhibition of the cardiac rapid delayed rectifier K+ current, by binding within the channel pore cavity on channel gating.[44] This combined activity could be the basis of the greater efficacy of this drug in the pharmacologic cardioversion of atrial flutter, compared with conventional antiarrhythmics, which have a very modest efficacy for this purpose. It is also a drug without the negative inotropic effect, which makes it useful in patients with left ventricular dysfunction. Due to the possibility of torsades de pointes, continuous monitoring of the ECG, in a hospital setting, for 3 hours after administration is recommended after administration.[9] For these reasons Ibutilide is, therefore, used as second-line therapy in pharmacologic cardioversion of atrial flutter in hemodynamically stable patients.[9] The use of ibutilide to restore sinus rhythm in patients with atrial flutter has good support both from animal and human studies.[17,45–47] In comparison with other treatment ibutilide showed good conversion rates in several studies ranging between 70% and 90% and being superior to propafenone, procainamide, sotalol, and amiodarone.[41,48–50] Moreover, it showed superior conversion rates also with respect to atrial pacing especially when flutter lasted greater than 48h.[51] Ibutilide has also utilized as a pretreatment for electro cardioversion. Pretreatment with ibutilide, sotalol, or dofetilide may help conversion to sinus rhythm in cases of refractory arrhythmias. Notably, magnesium has been shown to enhance the ability of ibutilide to convert atrial flutter or fibrillation to normal sinus rhythm. Magnesium can also help prevent the prolongation of the QT interval, and it sees frequent use in the treatment of torsades de pointes in hemodynamically stable patients.[52,53]

Dofetilide

Dofetilide has a prominent effect on the blockade of the rapid component of the IKr. It also increases the late sodium current activity at lower concentration; therefore, it prolongs action potential duration in atrial, ventricular, and Purkinje cells. It also increases the atrial ERP more than the ventricular ERP.[54] According to 4 studies on the use of iv dofetilide for the conversion of atrial fibrillation or flutter,

despite the limited number of patients, the drug proved to be more effective than placebo with a conversion rate significantly higher in patients with atrial flutter versus fibrillation (about 55%–65% vs 15%–25%).[55–57] Similar to ibutilide, it can be used as second-line therapy in pharmacologic cardioversion of atrial flutter in hemodynamically stable patients, in view of the potential risk of torsade de pointes.[9] Dofetilide can also be administered as an oral treatment to prevent atrial fibrillation/flutter recurrences in highly symptomatic patients. Available data suggest superiority of dofetilide in patient with atrial flutter versus fibrillation.[58,59]

Class IV Antiarrhythmics

The calcium channel blockers used as antiarrhythmics are verapamil and diltiazem which, unlike dihydropyridine calcium channel blockers, block calcium channels even at the cardiac level. This results in a reduction in heart rate and atrioventricular conduction rate. Their use as antiarrhythmic drugs consists in the prophylaxis and treatment of supraventricular tachyarrhythmias, including reentry arrhythmias for which the atrioventricular node is involved. They are used to reduce the frequency of ventricular response in atrial fibrillation and flutter. In particular, in atrial flutter verapamil and diltiazem are indicated as rate control therapy especially in chronic, as in acute the effectiveness of these drugs, even when combined with other bradycardic agents, is relatively low.[9]

Vernakalant

Vernakalant is an inhibitor of several ion channels, in particular, it exerts a blocking action on the K+, Na+, and Ca++ channels at the atrial level, whereby it prolongs the refractoriness time. It is effective in the pharmacologic cardioversion of short-term atrial fibrillation, while it is ineffective in flutter and persistent atrial fibrillation. Vernakalant is well tolerated, but does not restore sinus rhythm in patients with atrial flutter. In a phase 2/3 randomized, double-blind, placebo-controlled trial only one over 39 patients converted to sinus rhythm after vernakalant administration. The explanation for its lack of effect in converting atrial flutter to sinus rhythm is unclear. It is possible that a more selective and potent blockade of the rapidly activated delayed rectifier potassium current (I_{Kr}), as seen with ibutilide or dofetilide, is required for effective conversion of atrial flutter to normal sinus rhythm. Vernakalant modestly slows atrial flutter and ventricular response.[60]

Adenosine

Adenosine is a nucleoside that exerts its action by binding to the A1 receptor, which physiologically activates a current of K+ sensitive to acetylcholine at the atrial level, of the atrial sinus node, and of the ventricular atrium node. Adenosine also reduces the Current of Ca++ through an antiadrenergic action. It, therefore, involves a hyperpolarization of the cardiac conduction tissue, the suppression of the calcium-dependent action potential, and the increase in the refractoriness of the atrioventricular node. It is used in iv bolus as a drug of first choice in the interruption of paroxysmal supraventricular tachycardia. It has a very short half-life (about 10s) and among the side effects are emphasized: constrictive angor, dyspnea, and transient asystole of a few seconds. Adenosine, by slowing down atrioventricular conduction, reduces the frequency of ventricular response in the flutter, allowing for better appreciation of the F waves in the ECG-graph trace: it, therefore, has a role of diagnostic support and reduction of the heart rate, but does not allow the restoration

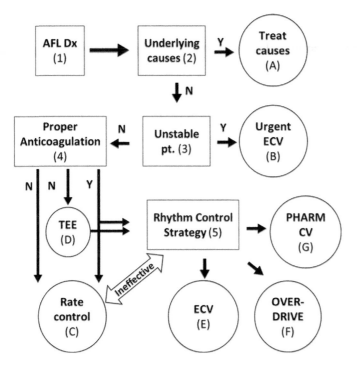

Fig. 1. Proposed algorithm for the acute management of atrial flutter. (1) The first step is the correct diagnosis. Since different supraventricular tachyarrhythmias have different acute/chronic treatments of choice according to the specific substrate it would be appropriate to obtain a definition of the clinical arrhythmia before attempting sinus rhythm restoration (with the exception of hemodynamic instability). Consider the collection of prolong ECGs, record of the effect of vagal maneuvers, and use of adenosine, with the described cautions. (2) Exclude that rapid rate secondary to medical causes (eg, sepsis, bleeding, pulmonary embolism, heart failure, coronary syndromes, and so forth) and in case treat them (A) since both cardioversion and aggressive rate control can be harmful. Clinical characteristics more frequently associated with secondary atrial flutter are: no sudden onsent, absence of palpitation, history or previous documentation of atrial flutter/fibrillation, heart rate less than 150bpm, fever, dyspnea, and pain. (3) Patients can be considered unstable in case of systolic blood pressure less than 90 mm Hg, or signs of shock; ongoing cardiac ischemia; Pulmonary edema: significant dyspnea, crackles, and hypoxia. Notably unstable patients with atrial flutter are really infrequent. In case urgent cardioversion is mandatory (B). (4) Finally proper anticoagulation according to AF guidelines should be followed before restoring sinus rhythm.[23] In subjects not properly anticoagulated rate-control (C) should be preferred or a TEE must be performed to exclude atrial thrombi (D). Notably, rate-control frequently requires multiple drugs in atrial flutter. Some considerations should be made on AV response to atrial flutter. In the absence of drugs that slow AV nodal conduction, a higher degree of AV block (eg, 3:1 or 4:1) suggests AV nodal disease; in these settings, the ventricular rates would be roughly 100 and 75 beats/min, respectively. Even input/output ratios (eg, 2:1 or 4:1 conduction) are more common than odd ratios (eg, 3:1 or 5:1). Odd ratios probably reflect bilevel block in the AV node. Sometimes, variable conduction may occur with alternating or seemingly random patterns of 2:1, 3:1, 4:1, or other conduction patterns, again due to varying levels of block in the AV node. On the other hand, a 1:1 response with typical atrial flutter usually suggests possible hyperthyroidism, catecholamine excess, parasympathetic withdrawal, existence of an accessory bypass tract or drug interference. (5) Rhythm control strategy is generally the preferred approach by all the guidelines, especially the use of direct current electrical cardioversion as low energies are able to restore sinus rhythm in atrial flutter (E). However, in some situation, electrical cardioversion may not be the best solution (eg, sedation issues) for this reason overdrive pacing (F) or pharmacologic cardioversion (G) can be both considered. Ibutilide is probably the best candidate for acute sinus rhythm restoration followed by dofetilide, procainamide, and sotalol. Notably, the addition of magnesium can enhance the effect of ibutilide, while in case of failure overdrive pacing is potentiated by the treatment with ibutilide. The role of amiodarone in the acute setting is more connected to rate control in patients with heart failure and only for selected patients (especially with heart failure). Class Ic and Ib drugs should be avoided. AFL, atrial flutter; ECV, electrical cardioversion; PHARM CV, pharmacologic cardioversion; pt., patients; TEE, trans-esophageal echocardiography.

of the sinus rhythm. Notably, adenosine challenge can be used immediately after cavo-tricuspid isthmus ablation with bidirectional block, or after the abolition of dormant conduction with further ablation to predict spontaneous reconnection.[61]

Digoxin

Digoxin is a digitalis glucoside with a positive inotropic effect and for this reason, it is used as an antiarrhythmic especially in patients with heart failure. It is an agonist of the muscarinic receptor M2 whose activation determines a reduction of the Ca++ current at the level of the atrioventricular node, causing the increase in the refractoriness of the node itself. At the atrial level, digoxin also induces the shortening of the action potential and hyperpolarization through the activation of the K+ channel. Digoxin seems to be superior compared with placebo in reducing the heart rate, but inferior compared with beta-blockers in atrial fibrillation and atrial flutter.

Acute Therapy in Atrial Flutter

Acute treatment of atrial flutter is frequently performed in the emergency department. For this reason, we propose the following treatment algorithm based on ACC, ESC, and CAEP guidelines[9,10,62] (**Fig. 1**).

Chronic Therapy in Atrial Flutter

Patients with recurrent symptomatic atrial flutter should undergo electrophysiology study and substrate ablation as the results are usually good with few recurrence and complications, especially for typical atrial flutter. Some specific considerations should be reserved for postsurgery and/or postablation occurrence of atrial flutter. These conditions tend to evolve within 90 days so antiarrhythmic drugs for sinus rhythm maintenance or rate control should be preferred over a new ablation procedure (during this period). In patients who refuse or fail ablation, the use of oral dofetilide/sotalol/amiodarone can be considered for prophylaxis of arrhythmia recurrence. However, this unfrequently adopted as it is associated with poor outcomes. A final remark regards the efficacy of the hybrid approach with class Ic antiarrhythmic drugs to prevent atrial fibrillation recurrences coupled with isthmus ablation in patients developing the drug-induced flutter.[63] The efficacy reported for such an approach clearly pinpoint the strong relationship between atrial fibrillation and flutter as previously depicted and the importance of a personalized approach to treating patients with atrial flutter.

CLINICS CARE POINTS

- Atrial fibrillation and atrial flutter are a continuum and most patients present both arrhythmias spontaneously or after specific treatments, either ablation or use of antiarrhythmic agents

- Antiarrhythmic drugs are a good choice in selected patients with acute atrial flutter. In particular, ibutilide seems to provide better efficacy/risk profile followed by dofetilide.

- For long-term maintenance of sinus rhythm substrate ablation is the treatment of choice but antiarrhythmic drugs can be used in case of failure or in a hybrid therapy for selected patients with atrial fibrillation combined with isthmus ablation.

DISCLOSURE

The authors have nothing to disclose.

REFERENCES

1. Waldo A. Atrial flutter. In: Podrid P, Kowey P, editors. Cardiac arrhythmia: mechanisms, diagnosis and management. Baltimore: Williams and Wilkens; 2001. p. 501–16.
2. Saoudi N, Cosio F, Waldo A, et al. Classification of atrial flutter and regular atrial tachycardia according to electrophysiologic mechanism and anatomic bases: a statement from a joint expert group from the Working Group of Arrhythmias of the European Society of Cardiology and the North American Society of Pacing and Electrophysiology. J Cardiovasc Electrophysiol 2001;12:852–66.
3. Waldo AL. Mechanisms of atrial flutter and atrial fibrillation: distinct entities or two sides of a coin? Cardiovasc Res 2002;54:217–29.
4. Tomita Y, Matsuo K, Sahadevan J, et al. Role of functional block extension in lesion-related atrial flutter. Circulation 2001;103:1025–30.
5. Page PL, Plumb VJ, Okumura K, et al. A new animal model of atrial flutter. J Am Coll Cardiol 1986;8:872–9.
6. Cox JL, Canavan TE, Schuessler RB, et al. The surgical treatment of atrial fibrillation. II. Intraoperative electrophysiologic mapping and description of the electrophysiologic basis of atrial flutter and atrial fibrillation. J Thorac Cardiovasc Surg 1991;101:406–26.
7. Guichard JB, Naud P, Xiong F, et al. Comparison of atrial remodeling caused by sustained atrial flutter

versus atrial fibrillation. J Am Coll Cardiol 2020;76: 374–88.

8. Naccarelli GV, Lee KS, Gibson JK, et al. Electrophysiology and pharmacology of ibutilide. Am J Cardiol 1996;78:12–6.

9. Brugada J, Katritsis DG, Arbelo E, et al. 2019 ESC Guidelines for the management of patients with supraventricular tachycardiaThe Task Force for the management of patients with supraventricular tachycardia of the European Society of Cardiology (ESC). Eur Heart J 2020;41:655–720.

10. Page RL, Joglar JA, Caldwell MA, et al. 2015 ACC/AHA/HRS guideline for the management of adult patients with supraventricular tachycardia: executive summary: a report of the american college of cardiology/american heart association task force on clinical practice guidelines and the heart rhythm society. J Am Coll Cardiol 2016;67:1575–623.

11. Priori SG, Barhanin J, Hauer RN, et al. Genetic and molecular basis of cardiac arrhythmias; impact on clinical management. Study group on molecular basis of arrhythmias of the working group on arrhythmias of the european society of cardiology. Eur Heart J 1999;20:174–95.

12. Vitali Serdoz L, Rittger H, Furlanello F, et al. Quinidine-A legacy within the modern era of antiarrhythmic therapy. Pharmacol Res 2019;144:257–63.

13. Capucci A, Aschieri D, Villani GQ. Clinical pharmacology of antiarrhythmic drugs. Drugs Aging 1998; 13:51–70.

14. Stambler BS, Wood MA, Ellenbogen KA. Pharmacologic alterations in human type I atrial flutter cycle length and monophasic action potential duration. Evidence of a fully excitable gap in the reentrant circuit. J Am Coll Cardiol 1996;27:453–61.

15. Camm J, Ward D, Spurrell R. Response of atrial flutter to overdrive atrial pacing and intravenous disopyramide phosphate, singly and in combination. Br Heart J 1980;44:240–7.

16. Harrison DC. Antiarrhythmic drug classification: new science and practical applications. Am J Cardiol 1985;56:185–7.

17. Buchanan LV, Kabell G, Gibson JK. Acute intravenous conversion of canine atrial flutter: comparison of antiarrhythmic agents. J Cardiovasc Pharmacol 1995;25:539–44.

18. Feld GK, Venkatesh N, Singh BN. Pharmacologic conversion and suppression of experimental canine atrial flutter: differing effects of d-sotalol, quinidine, and lidocaine and significance of changes in refractoriness and conduction. Circulation 1986;74: 197–204.

19. Mugnai G, Paolini C, Cavedon S, et al. Mexiletine for ventricular arrhythmias in patients with chronic coronary syndrome: a cohort study. Acta Cardiol 2021;1–7. https://doi.org/10.1080/00015385.2021. 1926628.

20. Sobiech M, Lewandowski M, Zajac D, et al. Efficacy and tolerability of mexiletine treatment in patients with recurrent ventricular tachyarrhythmias and implantable cardioverter-defibrillator shocks. Kardiol Pol 2017;75:1027–32.

21. Boriani G, Capucci A, Strocchi E, et al. Flecainide acetate: concentration-response relationships for antiarrhythmic and electrocardiographic effects. Int J Clin Pharmacol Res 1993;13:211–9.

22. Follmer CH, Cullinan CA, Colatsky TJ. Differential block of cardiac delayed rectifier current by class Ic antiarrhythmic drugs: evidence for open channel block and unblock. Cardiovasc Res 1992;26: 1121–30.

23. Hindricks G, Potpara T, Dagres N, et al. 2020 ESC Guidelines for the diagnosis and management of atrial fibrillation developed in collaboration with the European Association for Cardio-Thoracic Surgery (EACTS): the Task Force for the diagnosis and management of atrial fibrillation of the European Society of Cardiology (ESC) Developed with the special contribution of the European Heart Rhythm Association (EHRA) of the ESC. Eur Heart J 2021;42: 373–498.

24. Alboni P, Botto GL, Baldi N, et al. Outpatient treatment of recent-onset atrial fibrillation with the "pill-in-the-pocket" approach. N Engl J Med 2004;351: 2384–91.

25. Boriani G, Diemberger I, Biffi M, et al. Pharmacological cardioversion of atrial fibrillation: current management and treatment options. Drugs 2004;64: 2741–62.

26. Inoue H, Yamashita T, Usui M, et al. Antiarrhythmic drugs preferentially produce conduction block at the area of slow conduction in the re-entrant circuit of canine atrial flutter: comparative study of disopyramide, flecainide, and E-4031. Cardiovasc Res 1991;25:223–9.

27. Inoue H, Yamashita T, Nozaki A, et al. Effects of antiarrhythmic drugs on canine atrial flutter due to reentry: role of prolongation of refractory period and depression of conduction to excitable gap. J Am Coll Cardiol 1991;18:1098–104.

28. Crijns HJ, Van Gelder IC, Kingma JH, et al. Atrial flutter can be terminated by a class III antiarrhythmic drug but not by a class IC drug. Eur Heart J 1994; 15:1403–8.

29. Suttorp MJ, Kingma JH, Jessurun ER, et al. The value of class IC antiarrhythmic drugs for acute conversion of paroxysmal atrial fibrillation or flutter to sinus rhythm. J Am Coll Cardiol 1990;16:1722–7.

30. Aljohani OA, Perry JC, Williams MR. Intravenous sotalol for conversion of atrial flutter in infants. Heart Rhythm Case Rep 2018;4:117–20.

31. Tunca Sahin G, Beattie RB, Uzun O. Favourable outcome for hydrops or cardiac failure associated with fetal tachyarrhythmia: a 20-year review.

Cardiol Young 2021;1–8. https://doi.org/10.1017/S104795112100367X.

32. Levy S, Ricard P. Using the right drug: a treatment algorithm for regular supraventricular tachycardias. Eur Heart J 1997;18(Suppl C):C27–32.

33. Da Costa A, Thevenin J, Roche F, et al. Results from the Loire-Ardeche-Drome-Isere-Puy-de-Dome (LA-DIP) trial on atrial flutter, a multicentric prospective randomized study comparing amiodarone and radiofrequency ablation after the first episode of symptomatic atrial flutter. Circulation 2006;114:1676–81.

34. Diemberger I, Massaro G, Reggiani MLB, et al. Outcomes with dronedarone in atrial fibrillation: what differences between Real-world practice and trials? A meta-analysis and meta-Regression analysis. Curr Pharm Des 2017;23:944–51.

35. Le Heuzey JY, De Ferrari GM, Radzik D, et al. A short-term, randomized, double-blind, parallel-group study to evaluate the efficacy and safety of dronedarone versus amiodarone in patients with persistent atrial fibrillation: the DIONYSOS study. J Cardiovasc Electrophysiol 2010;21:597–605.

36. Wilson H, Patton D, Moore Z, et al. Comparison of dronedarone vs. flecainide in the maintenance of sinus rhythm, following electrocardioversion in adults with persistent atrial fibrillation: a systematic review and meta-analysis. Eur Heart J Cardiovasc Pharmacother 2021;7:363–72.

37. Singh BN, Singh SN, Reda DJ, et al. Amiodarone versus sotalol for atrial fibrillation. N Engl J Med 2005;352:1861–72.

38. Spinelli W, Hoffman BF. Mechanisms of termination of reentrant atrial arrhythmias by class I and class III antiarrhythmic agents. Circ Res 1989;65:1565–79.

39. Boyden PA, Graziano JN. Activation mapping of reentry around an anatomical barrier in the canine atrium: observations during the action of the class III agent, d-sotalol. J Cardiovasc Electrophysiol 1993;4:266–79.

40. Sung RJ, Tan HL, Karagounis L, et al. Intravenous sotalol for the termination of supraventricular tachycardia and atrial fibrillation and flutter: a multicenter, randomized, double-blind, placebo-controlled study. Sotalol Multicenter Study Group. Am Heart J 1995;129:739–48.

41. Vos MA, Golitsyn SR, Stangl K, et al. Superiority of ibutilide (a new class III agent) over DL-sotalol in converting atrial flutter and atrial fibrillation. The Ibutilide/Sotalol Comparator Study Group. Heart 1998;79:568–75.

42. Benditt DG, Williams JH, Jin J, et al. Maintenance of sinus rhythm with oral d,l-sotalol therapy in patients with symptomatic atrial fibrillation and/or atrial flutter. d,l-Sotalol Atrial Fibrillation/Flutter Study Group. Am J Cardiol 1999;84:270–7.

43. Chandler SF, Chu E, Whitehill RD, et al. Adverse event rate during inpatient sotalol initiation for the management of supraventricular and ventricular tachycardia in the pediatric and young adult population. Heart Rhythm 2020;17:984–90.

44. Doggrell SA, Hancox JC. Ibutilide–recent molecular insights and accumulating evidence for use in atrial flutter and fibrillation. Expert Opin Investig Drugs 2005;14:655–69.

45. Buchanan LV, LeMay RJ, Walters RR, et al. Antiarrhythmic and electrophysiologic effects of intravenous ibutilide and sotalol in the canine sterile pericarditis model. J Cardiovasc Electrophysiol 1996;7:113–9.

46. Buchanan LV, Turcotte UM, Kabell GG, et al. Antiarrhythmic and electrophysiologic effects of ibutilide in a chronic canine model of atrial flutter. J Cardiovasc Pharmacol 1993;22:10–4.

47. Ellenbogen KA, Stambler BS, Wood MA, et al. Efficacy of intravenous ibutilide for rapid termination of atrial fibrillation and atrial flutter: a dose-response study. J Am Coll Cardiol 1996;28:130–6.

48. Kafkas NV, Patsilinakos SP, Mertzanos GA, et al. Conversion efficacy of intravenous ibutilide compared with intravenous amiodarone in patients with recent-onset atrial fibrillation and atrial flutter. Int J Cardiol 2007;118:321–5.

49. Sun JL, Guo JH, Zhang N, et al. Clinical comparison of ibutilide and propafenone for converting atrial flutter. Cardiovasc Drugs Ther 2005;19:57–64.

50. Stambler BS, Wood MA, Ellenbogen KA. Antiarrhythmic actions of intravenous ibutilide compared with procainamide during human atrial flutter and fibrillation: electrophysiological determinants of enhanced conversion efficacy. Circulation 1997;96:4298–306.

51. Mazza A, Fera MS, Bisceglia I, et al. Efficacy and safety of ibutilide vs. transoesophageal atrial pacing for the termination of type I atrial flutter. Europace 2004;6:301–6.

52. Caron MF, Kluger J, Tsikouris JP, et al. Effects of intravenous magnesium sulfate on the QT interval in patients receiving ibutilide. Pharmacotherapy 2003;23:296–300.

53. Patsilinakos S, Christou A, Kafkas N, et al. Effect of high doses of magnesium on converting ibutilide to a safe and more effective agent. Am J Cardiol 2010;106:673–6.

54. Shenasa F, Shenasa M. Dofetilide: electrophysiologic effect, efficacy, and safety in patients with cardiac arrhythmias. Card Electrophysiol Clin 2016;8:423–36.

55. Falk RH, Pollak A, Singh SN, et al. Intravenous dofetilide, a class III antiarrhythmic agent, for the termination of sustained atrial fibrillation or flutter. Intravenous Dofetilide Investigators. J Am Coll Cardiol 1997;29:385–90.

56. Norgaard BL, Wachtell K, Christensen PD, et al. Efficacy and safety of intravenously administered dofetilide in acute termination of atrial fibrillation and flutter: a multicenter, randomized, double-blind, placebo-controlled trial. Danish Dofetilide in Atrial Fibrillation and Flutter Study Group. Am Heart J 1999; 137:1062–9.

57. Suttorp MJ, Polak PE, van 't Hof A, et al. Efficacy and safety of a new selective class III antiarrhythmic agent dofetilide in paroxysmal atrial fibrillation or atrial flutter. Am J Cardiol 1992;69:417–9.

58. Banchs JE, Wolbrette DL, Samii SM, et al. Efficacy and safety of dofetilide in patients with atrial fibrillation and atrial flutter. J Interv Card Electrophysiol 2008;23:111–5.

59. Ibrahim MA, Kerndt CC, Tivakaran VS. Dofetilide. Treasure Island (FL): StatPearls; 2022.

60. Camm AJ, Toft E, Torp-Pedersen C, et al. Efficacy and safety of vernakalant in patients with atrial flutter: a randomized, double-blind, placebo-controlled trial. Europace 2012;14:804–9.

61. Morales G, Darrat YH, Lellouche N, et al. Use of adenosine to shorten the post ablation waiting period for cavotricuspid isthmus-dependent atrial flutter. J Cardiovasc Electrophysiol 2017;28:876–81.

62. Stiell IG, de Wit K, Scheuermeyer FX, et al. 2021 CAEP acute atrial fibrillation/flutter best practices checklist. CJEM 2021;23:604–10.

63. Riad FS, Waldo AL. Revisiting an underrecognized strategy for rhythm management: hybrid therapy for patients who convert from atrial fibrillation to flutter on antiarrhythmic drugs. J Innov Card Rhythm Manag 2019;10:3842–7.

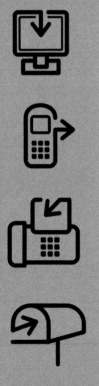